IT CAN BREAK YOUR HEART

WHAT YOU AND YOUR DOCTOR SHOULD KNOW ABOUT SOLVING YOUR WEIGHT PROBLEM

by

J. PERVIS MILNOR, III, M.D., &
GREGORY L. LITTLE, ED.D.
WITH KENNETH D. ROBINSON, ED.D.

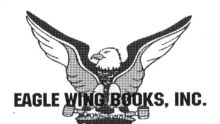

EAGLE WING BOOKS, INC.

It Can Break Your Heart:
What You And Your Doctor Should Know
About Solving Your Weight Problem

Printed in the United States of America.

Published by
Eagle Wing Books, Inc.
P. O. Box 9972
Memphis, TN 38190

email: ewibooks@aol.com
FAX: 901-785-7592
web site: eaglewingbooks.com

Visit the SmartLoss website: smartloss.net

ISBN: 0-940829-31-2

U. S. retail price: $29.95

Dedication

This book is dedicated to the Pima Indian Tribe who have bravely helped uncover the strong genetic link to obesity. The Pimas have allowed us a significant insight into how "thrifty genes" can contribute to obesity and diabetes in the modern world of abundance. All obese and overweight people owe this ancient group of people an enduring debt of gratitude.

Acknowledgments

The authors express a special thanks and acknowledgment to Dr. Tom Hughes of the Department of Endocrinology of the University of Tennessee Medical School for providing superb lectures and information on insulin resistance, metabolic syndrome, and stress defeat syndrome. Dr. Hughes' information was invaluable and played a key role in pointing us in the right directions.

Thanks is also expressed to Alice Ansfield, Founder and Editor of *Radiance Magazine* for permitting us to reprint several covers. *Radiance* stands in stark contrast to the many women's magazines which promote unrealistic thinness and undue social pressure on women and men.

In addition, we wish to express our appreciation to *Environmental Nutrition* for allowing us to reprint their critique of weight loss programs as an appendix.

The authors would like to acknowledge the National Institutes of Health and the Calorie Control Council for making so much quality information readily available. A wealth of information can be accessed on their web sites and in their numerous publications. In addition, credit is due to the Minnesota Attorney General's Office for compiling and making available nutritional data on fast foods. Much of our information regarding fast food content was derived from this excellent source.

Also acknowledged is Jamie Pettit of Eagle Wing Books, Inc., who tirelessly obtained and entered a variety of data groupings. A very special acknowledgment is due to Dr. Lora Little. Her criticisms, suggestions, proofing, and careful indexing of this book resulted in a significantly enhanced text.

Finally, we would like to sincerely thank our families for their support, encouragement, and endurance while this project was being completed. For many months, Vonda Milnor stoically and admirably held the family together (all six children) while Pervis was absorbed in the details of this book. Although Vonda may not have realized it at the time, her efforts were deeply appreciated by everyone involved. Without all of our families, none of this would be meaningful.

About The Authors

Dr. J. Pervis Milnor, III

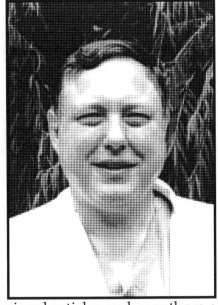

Dr. Pervis Milnor received his M.D. from the University of Tennessee Medical School and is Board Certified in anesthesiology. He has always had an abiding interest in physiology and pharmacology and has battled obesity most of his life: "My mother's earliest remembrance of her grandfather was standing under his stomach to get out of the noon sun. My father, a heart specialist, always told me to eat less and exercise."

Treating obesity has become Dr. Milnor's calling in life. He has coauthored several professional articles and coauthors a monthly column on obesity treatment in Memphis Health & Fitness Sports Magazine. He is a member of the American College of Sports Medicine and the North American Association for the Study of Obesity. *It Can Break Your Heart* is Dr. Milnor's first book.

Dr. Gregory L. Little

Dr. Greg Little received a masters degree in psychology and doctorate in counseling from Memphis State University. Dr. Little is a Licensed Professional Counselor who specializes in counselor training for addictive behaviors treatment. He is the author of 4 books, including the textbook, *Psychopharmacology* (1997), and is

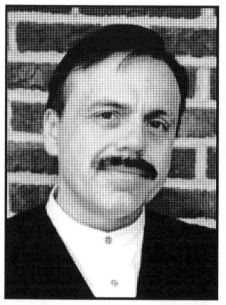

coauthor of 20 other books and workbooks. Dr. Little has published over 200 articles on addictions, drugs, and various other issues. He is the codeveloper of Moral Reconation Therapy (MRT®), a cognitive-behavioral treatment system. Dr. Little's has been a classic weight-cycler throughout the past 30 years. He is a member of the North American Association for the Study of Obesity and the American Counseling Association.

Dr. Kenneth D. Robinson

Dr. Ken Robinson received a masters degree in psychology and a doctorate in educational psychology from Memphis State University. He is President of Correctional Counseling, Inc. and widely speaks on treatment and addictive behaviors. He is the codeveloper of all the MRT® materials and conducts workshops and training in the method. MRT® is in wide spread use in nearly 40 states with nearly 200,000 individuals participating in the program. Dr. Robinson has coauthored 19 books and workbooks and has published and presented hundreds of professional articles. He is a member of the American Counseling Association.

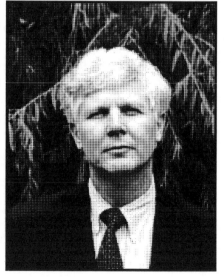

How To Use This Book

This book was begun as an effort to provide a brief overview of the factors related to obesity along with effective weight management strategies for people struggling with weight problems. It also was our initial intention to provide readers with a general understanding of the many causes of the problem. As information and research were compiled for the various chapters, it became more and more apparent to us that a brief overview was insufficient. In order to do justice to the incredible mass of research in the obesity field, it was necessary for us to provide an understandable summary of almost everything known in the field. What gradually emerged was a much more comprehensive (and more important) text than we had originally intended. However, we know of no other book on "weight" or "diets" ever written for the masses that provides so much useful information. We placed a special emphasis on diabetes because it is one of the most frequently seen diseases accompanying obesity. Some of our conclusions could, by "main-streamers," be seen as controversial. For example, the influence of insulin resistance on obesity is debated by some nutritionists and some physicians. But it isn't debated much by obesity specialists. The explanation for the differences in opinion between obesity specialists and others is not obvious.

An important problem in some medical research stems from inadequate technology. There are a lot of bodily processes we can't measure and don't fully understand. In addition, our inability to precisely track the eventual influence of some known bodily responses (i.e., insulin response) is so limited that *proving* almost any speculations on insulin resistance is impossible. There is, however, so much research data available that it is "intuitively obvious" that insulin resistance is especially important. A parallel situation in scientific research once existed. For decades, science couldn't *prove* that cigarette smoking caused cancer. In fact, cigarette smoking was sometimes advertised as healthy and lots of medical professionals took the position that cigarette smoking wasn't harmful. It was "intuitively obvious" back then to just about everyone familiar with the research that cigarette smoking was harmful.

It is intuitively obvious to almost all obesity researchers that insulin response and insulin resistance represent key issues.

We have made every effort to make each chapter understandable for everyone. Some of the information is, by necessity, technical. However, we have made every attempt to provide easy-to-understand examples and definitions. Our apologies are offered to the medical community if we have oversimplified some issues.

We have divided the book into chapters based on how we believe the problem of obesity can be best comprehended. Each chapter is organized so that readers can easily locate specific issues of interest. In addition, an index is provided at the back of the book. A glossary, containing definitions of all technical terms, can also be found in the back of the book.

Each chapter has a summary at its beginning that provides an overview of the material covered. Readers may wish to simply read the summary of some chapters and focus on issues of interest. The book begins by exploring the plight of the obese in America along with a historical review. The medical definitions and methods of diagnosis of obesity follows along with a review of the many associated health risks. We then present chapters detailing the five components of obesity: biological & genetic factors, psychological issues, environmental and life-style, exercise, and diet. Effective coping strategies for each of these components are presented. Finally, we outline a comprehensive approach to management of weight problems which we term SmartLoss. A "special issues" appendix covers a wide range of issues: children, surgical techniques, smoking, and commercial programs to name a few.

We believe that every person who has suffered because of weight has much to gain from this book. Misinformation and contradictory suggestions are the norm in diet books, and we hope to provide readers with a truly balanced perspective. Most obese people worry about their condition and can be confused about their options. Putting worry to rest and making informed decisions is our primary goal.

TABLE OF CONTENTS

Chapter 1
THE TANGLED PUZZLE
OF OBESITY

I'm fat, but I'm thin inside. Has it ever struck you that
there's a thin man inside every fat man?
— George Orwell, *Coming Up For Air*

Chapter Summary — Obesity is one of the most misunderstood and difficult to treat health problems in existence. It is a physical condition — a disease — that has many deep-seated causes. Very few people comprehend the nearly impossible circumstances with which obese people have to contend every day of their lives. Unfortunately, few doctors and even fewer other health professionals have a true understanding of obesity. Inevitably, the obese person receives the entire blame for the problem. Social, psychological, and behavioral issues have become so entwined with obesity that the nature of the problem — and its solutions — have become obscured.

Obesity has its deepest roots in genetics. Some people are born with "thrifty" genes. Their genetic makeup has predetermined a fairly high body weight to ensure that they can survive in times of famine. When these people try to lose weight, their body responds by lowering their energy needs. The more they starve themselves in an effort to lose weight, the lower their bodies set their energy needs. Thus, as obese people lose weight, their bodies respond by making it more and more difficult to lose. When such a person "slips" — as most of us inevitably do — the body responds by rapidly replacing its fat stores. In addition, the body is often programmed to add even more weight to prepare for the next period of "voluntary starvation." The situation is like being in a river and having to swim upstream. Going against the current is difficult, but the problem worsens because the further upstream the person swims, the swifter the downstream current becomes.

Medical and supportive interventions do hold some promise for the obese and overweight. Becoming educated about the problem and making informed decisions are also critical. However, the obese person must, in the final analysis, take one of two paths. One path is to accept being fat with its many physical complications and coping with the resulting problems as they arise. The other path is to directly attack the problem by using the best methods medicine and science have to offer. This is then combined with making life-long, behavioral and life-style changes that alter eating habits, activity levels, and recreation. In truth, obesity is not an issue of character, but character is an issue in escaping its trap.

• • •

Pretend that you find yourself dreaming comfortably. The dream isn't scary, but it has an important message for you.

Imagine yourself floating effortlessly in a small river. You don't know how you got there, but you are trapped in it. The two sides of the river have steep, vertical rock walls. You have no choice but to stay in the river until you can get to a point where you can *try* to get out. The problem is that the only "better place" to get out of the river is somewhere *upstream*. You think you know where this better place is and it seems like a long distance.

As you float in the river, you realize that the current is gradually carrying you further and further downstream. You recognize that the situation gets even worse downstream and that there might even be real danger there. Now you suddenly become aware that you've got to begin to swim upstream and you've got to start swimming *now* — before it's too late.

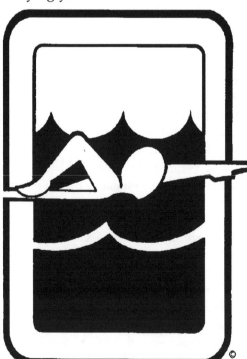

The water is flowing downstream steadily as you begin swimming against the current. At first, the swimming is easy and steady, and you seem to be progressing against the current fairly well. But the constant kicking and arm movements become tiring and boring. So you decide to rest for a few moments. Resting feels good at first, but you realize that once you stop swimming the current sweeps you back downstream. You repeat this cycle again and again, each time progressing against the current for some distance — but each rest period results in the current sweeping you back downstream. You also notice that occasionally you get bored, stressed, or distracted while swimming, and each time it happens, you slow down or stop swimming. This also results in the current pushing you back.

Now you become firmly resolved to make a successful, consistent swim to the "better place." Every distraction, every rest period must be controlled or avoided. It takes enormous effort, discipline, and constant vigilance, but you keep at it. Slowly, gradually, you begin to see the better place where you can escape the river. But the current going against you at this point becomes swifter and swifter. All it seems you can do is barely maintain the place where you are by continuing to swim against the current as hard as you can.

There have been people watching you throughout your swim. Some of them encourage you and yell support. They tell you that you can do this if you really want to. They tell you that you don't try hard enough. They don't seem to realize that *you are swimming against an increasingly strong current* — but they mean well. Others may laugh at you and ridicule you — and tell you it's all your fault. But you really do want out, and you have tried and tried.

The next thing you realize is that you seem to have stopped swimming without even wanting to — at least for the moment. This just seemed to happen to you suddenly. You begin to feel "guilty and weak" as the now-swifter current rushes you all the way back downstream.

Suddenly, you understand that this is a recurring dream. You find yourself floating in a small river gradually being carried downstream. You don't know how you got there, but you are trapped in it and it is very familiar — much to your dismay. The two sides of the river have steep, vertical rock walls, so you have no choice but to stay in the river and try to get to a point where you can get out. The problem is that the only "better place" to get out of the river is even further upstream than last time. "Here I go again," you think, as you start to swim once more.

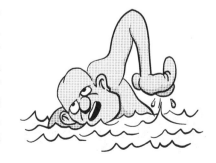

Obesity Is A Genetic, Physical, Metabolic Disease With Behavioral, Psychological, & Social Factors

Hopefully, you have already figured out the meaning of the river "dream" image presented above. It can be very helpful in understanding the dilemmas involved in obesity, being overweight, and weight loss. You might not fully understand all of the specific symbols in the river image, but each one of them represents an important part of the obesity puzzle. This chapter will introduce the pieces of the obesity puzzle. Later chapters will examine various medical, behavioral, psychological, and social pieces in depth. But for now, let's briefly review them in relationship to the river image.

Being Stuck In The River Is Simply Nature (Genetics)

Nature has bestowed upon all of us specific physical characteristics. Body size, shape, complexion, hair color and texture, race, and almost all of our physical attributes are bestowed upon us by genetics.[1] Why nature picked Cindy Crawford for her body and Oprah Winfrey or Roseanne for theirs is not the issue right now. Understanding that nature predetermines many basics about our physical bodies (a predisposition — a blueprint — laying out how our bodies will develop over our lifespan) is the important issue. In the river image, you *neither chose* to be in the river nor did you *have any control over the natural current* of the river. In addition, the river's steep sides kept you from getting out. You simply found yourself in this uncontrollable situation. This is similar to what genetics has done to all of us. We didn't choose our eye color, shoulder width, height, hip width, bone structure — it simply was bestowed upon us. Body mass, fat stores, and basic body shapes are recognized by science as being strongly genetic.[1, 2]

Going Downstream Is Gaining Weight

Going downstream, of course, represents putting on weight. It was easy for you to go downstream. (It's probably easy for you to put on weight, too.) All you had to do was nothing at all. Just by floating in the river's unavoidable current you will move downstream. In this case, it is the result of nature. Genetic predispositions create the river's current. The speed of the current is determined by your body's rate of burning energy (metabolic rate) and how "thrifty" your genes are in storing energy (fat) for possible future use. Both metabolic rate and fat storage rates are genetic.[2]

Your Body's Ability To Conserve Energy Is Genetic

Think for a moment about the many generations of relatives who preceded you on earth over literally tens of thousands of years. Many of them probably worked long and hard to simply feed themselves and their families. Having a genetically regulated metabolism (based on the amount of work done and food available) kept them alive. "Thrifty genes" were once an excellent survival mechanism. During times of famine, the body would survive on its stored energy (fat) and even slow down its rate of burning energy to conserve. When food was available, the body retained the lower metabolic rate forcing it to rapidly store more fat for the next famine. Each cycle of "feast or famine" caused the body to add more energy stores. Of course, in the past, periods of starvation occurred routinely and people had to be much more physically active to survive. As a result, they seldom got to the point of obesity. Today, however, people who have "thrifty genes" often go through a similar "feast or famine" cycle. Yo-yo dieters will rigidly diet & exercise for a time and lose weight. The weight loss is followed by relapses where all of the weight is regained — and then some. If you have been overweight all of your life and others in your immediate family are overweight, you probably have inherited these once life-saving thrifty genes.

Some People Are Born With A Slow Metabolism That Can Become Even Slower To Conserve Energy — Some People Are Born With A Metabolism That Will Increase To Burn Excess Energy
There is another important point to understand in the river current symbol. The downstream current's flow speed (that is, the *strength* of the tendency to add weight) *is different for different people. Some people may have a very slow, drifting current that is easily resisted.* In fact, some people have no current at all. It's almost as if these people are

in a long pond with no upstream or downstream movement. They stay right where they are by doing nothing at all. *In such people, it matters little what they eat or do — their weight stays the same.* While such people are fairly rare, it is their genetic makeup that has created this tendency. It also appears that some of these people have an underlying ability to burn off excess energy intake (eating too much) by nervous fidgeting and increased movement. This is also a consequence of genetics.

The Body Of An Obese Person Tends To
Resist Weight Loss And Easily Gains Weight

Most people tend to have a slow but steady downstream current. There is a slight tendency in almost everyone to add weight as time passes. This is sometimes referred to as **creeping obesity.** If we become less active as we age, weight will increase unless food intake is decreased. Many people do become less active and sedentary as they age. But again, the current, the ability of the body to slow down metabolic rate in times of starvation, is different in different people. The bodies of obese people tend to resist losing weight and will try to regain lost weight quickly. Again, this comes as a result of the inherited genetic blueprint.

In the river, you realized that *it was up to you* to try to swim to a "better place." That place, of course, is represented by what you see as an ideal body size for yourself. (This ideal is greatly influenced by society and the media.)

As you got closer and closer to this "better place," you realized that the current working against you was stronger. You may not have understood what was happening, but you did recognize that it was more and more difficult to just stay where you were. Any small lapse in

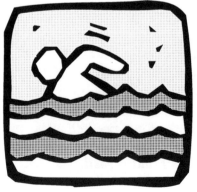

behavior resulted in you rushing back downstream (regaining weight). *The current working against you symbolizes the way your genetic makeup compensates* for the great expenditure of energy you were making. As you got farther and farther upstream (lost more and more weight) the force working against you got stronger. What this represents is *your body metabolism actually slowing down* as your

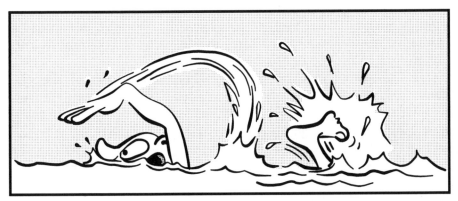

"thrifty genes" make an attempt to conserve energy in light of obviously depleting supplies.

Every time you stopped to rest, every time you lost your resolve, every distraction or bored or stressed moment that caused a momentary letdown in the swimming led to a rush back downstream. So too it goes with dieting. Sometimes it seems like months of rigorous dieting and exercise can be lost in a few weeks of lapse. These downstream rushes become quicker and quicker the further you make it upstream, since the force working against you increases. Your body resists weight loss when you reach a certain point. *With dieting and weight loss, the body's thrifty genes will usually try to add even more weight than before to prepare for your next attempt at forced starvation.* In short, genetics bestows certain physical limitations and characteristics upon everyone which greatly complicate weight loss and gain — especially in obese people.

Small Lapses In Behavior Can Result In Quick Weight Gain Leading To Self-Blame — Psychological & Social Issues Become Entangled In The Puzzle

It was obvious to you that your behavior in the river determined whether you would float downstream or swim upstream. Some people who find themselves in that situation for the first time might give up — especially if important people in their lives encourage it. Others might panic and swim to the point of exhaustion. Then, of course, they'd float back down the river. A few might manage to swim very steadily at a fast pace. However, it's very difficult to maintain such consistency and concentration for long periods. In addition, it is extremely frustrating when a small slip or lapse in behavior leads to a sudden weight gain (quickly moving downstream). This repeating cycle of trying to swim upstream only to be swept back leads to self-doubt, self-blame, low self-esteem, and a host of other problems.

These problems can begin in childhood with the earliest ridicule, blame, put-downs, or derisive comments directed at overweight children. Complicating the problem even more are the ingrained, obesity-producing eating and exercise habits instilled in children by parents who have good intentions, but who don't have appropriate knowledge or resources. All of these psychological and behavioral issues become so entangled in the problem that a seemingly impossible puzzle has been formed. Gradually, the psychological and behavioral problems become the most noticeable part of the puzzle. Thus, most people, including doctors, simply say, "eating less and exercising more" is the solution.

Few People Truly Understand The Plight Of The Obese

It's obvious that there are other people involved in the obesity puzzle who create a "social" influence. Their ridicule, encouragement, and frustration all have effects on you. Because they aren't in the same river, they can't understand what is happening. And even when you are struggling in the river, it's difficult for them to understand. Other's suggestions and coping tricks can often seem to help, but it's always only temporary. In such a situation, it's easy to give up. It's also easy to blame yourself.

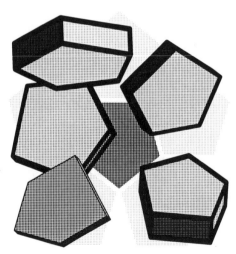

Losing weight is a lot like being in the "dream" river. It's true that your behavior has a lot to do with your movement up or down the stream. But it's also true that the true nature of the

The puzzle obesity presents is huge and can occasionally seem to be contradictory. It is not what it appears to be. Most people focus on only one or two pieces of the puzzle in their attempts to control weight. "Eat less and exercise more" is an example of this. You have to attend to all of the pieces of the puzzle to solve it.

situation you are in is difficult to understand — especially for those people who don't experience it. To make matters worse, many of the so-called experts (this may include your family physician) also aren't aware of how the process of the river's current works.

Although Obesity Is Not A Character Issue, Ironically, Only Great Strength Of Character Can Permanently Change The Situation

Obesity is not a character issue. But the escape from obesity does involve developing great will power, desire, vigilance, and self-control. You do have to swim against the stream constantly. You have to resist the constant temptation to stop swimming. You have to be careful to not do too much at once. (Lots of people want to lose lots of weight *now* — quickly. But such efforts are usually doomed from the start.) You have to be careful to establish new habits and routines that support weight loss *and* maintenance. These new behaviors have to become a part of your day-to-day life and become so ingrained (as a habit) that they happen automatically. Certain medications can make the process easier, but the medicines won't do the job alone. **So, while obesity is not the result of character, the escape from it is.**

Before You Rush To Make Changes, Gather Information And Make A Realistic Plan Of Action

People's motivation about weight control and management of health risks tends to wax and wane. Losing weight is usually viewed as a task to be completed as quickly as possible. Diets are viewed as temporary. When the weight is lost, the task seems to be completed and motivation declines. As a result, many people rapidly slip back into their old habits. The current then quickly rushes them back down the stream. Why do so many of us do this? Why do we have this repeating cycle of weight loss and gain? The answer, in large part, is lack of understanding about the nature of obesity and acceptance of certain realities. You have to see the entire puzzle in order to understand it. Seeing and understanding the obesity puzzle is the first step in making a good decision about how to cope with it.

The Obesity Puzzle Is Enormous

You probably have put together a jig-saw puzzle or two during your lifetime. All of them had at least one common element: there was some sort of picture that you knew — in advance — the pieces formed. With obesity you might stand in front of a mirror and think you see the picture. You might then wonder, "what were the pieces that formed me?" That may be a starting point, but it obscures the genuine puzzle. The size of the obesity puzzle can be understood by a visual image that has been employed to explain other complex mysteries.[3] The visual image depicts obesity as a puzzle that extends for miles and miles in every direction. Wherever you stand on the puzzle, you can't see it in its entirety. A few pieces of the puzzle seem to stand out the most: "eat less and exercise more." However, only using these two pieces results in the same outcome: failure. You have to understand that these are not the only pieces.

This book presents all of the pieces of the obesity puzzle as they are known today. The scientific community doesn't have a full understanding of all of them yet, but enough is understood to make a difference in people's lives. Fortunately, you don't need to understand all of them to the same extent as a scientist. But you do need to be aware of them and know how to cope with the unique problems each piece presents. The vast majority of people struggling with excess weight or obesity will overcome the problem only by confronting each and every puzzle piece. We hope to supply you with knowledge in this book and teach you how to apply it so that you can confront the pieces of your own puzzle.

Obesity must be viewed as a life-long problem with biological, environmental, social, emotional, behavioral, and psychological components. The more of these components you understand, the better prepared you can be to cope with them. You can learn to manage the problem of weight and obesity by gathering information and making a realistic plan of action. One way of looking at it is that you are on a life-long, life changing mission. This book serves as a primary tool for this task. Remember the example of swimming against the current which we presented earlier. Remember that you have to swim steadily and not stop. Using this visual example, keep in mind that the swimming never ends. Going against the current can be done successfully as many people have shown. And it doesn't have to be unpleasant. There are many things you can do that help in fighting the current. But before these are presented, you have to understand what is now known about obesity, weight, and the various contributing physical factors.

Some People Need
To Know A Lot, Some Don't

Readers who have fought weight and fat problems for a large portion of their lives and who also have serious health risks may wish to fully understand all of the information in this book. Those who hope to influence their children (who are developing the multi-generational problem of obesity) may also wish to deeply understand the issues. People who are simply overweight and wishing to shed a few pounds or more might find the information too detailed. If you find it necessary to skip some technical material, don't fret. Each chapter begins with an overview summarizing what you need to know. Some chapters may be more relevant and interesting to you. Explore them. Other chapters may not seem as relevant or interesting to you. Read the chapter summary and skip the rest of it.

We have attempted to present what is known scientifically about the biology of obesity and overweight in an understandable way. We have also attempted to detail the psychological, social, and behavioral aspects of the problem. But some of the information is, by its nature, technical. Some people may find it difficult to absorb or understand all of the information. With this in mind, we have tried to provide you with the overall picture presented in the obesity puzzle and, by the end of the book, enough tools to use in your efforts to make changes. If you can truly comprehend the "swimming in the river" example given at the start of this chapter, you probably know all you really need to know to begin.

Weight problems and concerns have plagued the first two authors of this book throughout their lives, and we want you to know that it has been an ongoing struggle for us. There are a lot of people in the "river of obesity" with you. That may not help you lose weight, but it should help you to understand that your character or strength of will is not the primary cause of the problem. This insight may provide you some comfort. We hope it will also encourage you to take control of the problem and do what you can.

Chapter References & Notes

[1] M. R. Cummings (1997) *Human heredity*. Belmont, CA: Wadsworth.

[2] Treating The Obese Patient by Drew A. Anderson, & Thomas A. Wadden. (1999) *Archives of Family Medicine*, 8, 156-167; A brief review of obesity and genetics.

[3] *Grand Illusions* by Gregory L. Little. (1994) Memphis: White Buffalo Books.

Chapter 2
BEING OVERWEIGHT
CAN BE HEARTBREAKING

More die in the United States of too much food than of too little.

John Kenneth Galbraith — *The Affluent Society*

Chapter Summary—America is a society obsessed with fat. We idolize thin people, yet we are more overweight than at any other time in history. Many people are so obsessed with thinness that they are constantly on drastic diets ignoring the negative health consequences. Fat obsession causes worry and is related to binge eating in a cycle of eating, guilt, and worry followed by more binge eating. Yet fat is necessary for health. Health problems come from having too much fat — medicine calls this condition obesity. Obesity is a disease that is related to many other diseases and several emotional problems. Worrying about obesity is very common, yet the worry serves no useful purpose. In fact, constant worry about weight can actually cause overeating. *Worrying about the problem is not the same thing as actually doing something about it.* We suggest that you become informed about your condition and then make one of two choices. First, you can choose to accept your condition and stop worrying about it. You are a person of worth regardless of your body size. Some people believe that trying to be thin goes against nature and leads to suffering and grief. If you make the choice to accept your body as it is, you should focus your efforts on being fit rather than thin. Second, you can choose to take charge of your condition and make reasonable changes after you form an appropriate course of action. Either decision requires that you first become informed about your condition.

One of the biggest problems people have in becoming informed and knowledgeable about obesity and fitness is the mass of "information" available about it. The thousands of books on diets, fitness, exercise, and health sometimes give conflicting advice. This is because most of them are based on a narrow point of view and have an underlying bias. For example, few diet/exercise proponents take genetics into account and even fewer try to explain the influence of genetics on weight loss. Most books are clearly against the use of medication, yet some medicines can certainly help some overweight people. Many books also are unrealistic about how daily responsibilities can keep people from rigidly following diet and exercise routines. Furthermore, diets don't really work in the long run, yet countless people are manipulated by the hype of each new "miracle" diet. Finally, the deep emotional, psychological, and social consequences of obesity are often denied or not addressed by weight and diet books. This book has been written to provide a comprehensive overview of the facts about being overweight in order to help people make good decisions.

● ● ●

America is drowning in fat. Our children are fatter now than at any time in recorded history[1] and more adults are overweight today[2] than ever before. We're a fat-obsessed society wallowing in our fat-generated misery. We talk incessantly about eating a fat-reduced diet, losing fat, sucking fat, jiggling fat, pinching fat, and hiding fat. Television programs that hawk weight-reducing exercise equipment, miracle diets, herbal diet aids, and fitness routines bombard us constantly. Advertisements "guaranteeing" we will "lose 30 pounds in 30 days" seem to be posted everywhere. Health food stores carry so many "fat burners" and "weight control" supplements it's mind boggling. Yet we're still fat — and we are getting fatter. Our obsession with fat increases more and more as the American populace grows heavier and heavier.

In America we have become so fat that we idolize people with little — or no — fat despite knowing that being too thin can be more unhealthy than being fat. American girls are given the nearly impossible role model for desired thinness early in their lives — the Barbie Doll. If Barbie was life-sized, she'd measure 38-18-34 and have less than 8% body fat.[3] Some people, most of them women, become so fearful of becoming "fat" that they literally starve themselves to death in a misguided effort to be "attractive" and thin. Other people are so obsessed with fat that they worry about it constantly with the end result frequently being a repeating pattern of binge eating, guilt, and more worry. At the same time the availability of food is more prevalent than ever. We are tempted with larger portions and attractive food preparations at easy access buffets and fast food outlets. "Super size it" for a few cents more has become part of our vocabulary. Everything encourages us to eat more yet we're punished brutally if we don't stay thin.

Something is very, very wrong in our society. Everywhere we look we are exposed to our societal obsession with losing weight. Fad diets come and go and come back again. Many people lose weight only to find that they quickly regain it all back — and then some. And then they repeat the cycle again, and again, and again. It should be obvious that obsessive worrying about fat doesn't make it go away. In one way or another, our worry about fat leads to even more worry about our health — and we get larger.

But there is a simple truth about fat. Some fat is **necessary** for your health and well-being. Your brain cells are made from fat. Every part of your body needs some fat for healthy cell growth. Health problems come from carrying around *too much* fat.

The medical term for having too much fat is *obesity*. You may not be overweight enough to have the term applied to you, but many reading this book are probably well on their way toward meeting its definition. So, what *is* obesity?

Most of us define obesity as a person who is fatter than we are! We've all heard people say things like, "Well, at least I'm not *that* fat," as they compared themselves to someone else. But those comparisons aren't useful. In fact, they can keep people from honestly confronting their own condition. *Obesity is a disease* associated with early death and a host of physical and emotional problems.

Worrying about weight accomplishes nothing useful. As you may know, worry can even cause you to overeat. It's possible that worrying about being fat has actually kept many people from truly understanding *why* they are fat, and even more importantly, kept them from learning how to cope with it.

In his many writings on spirituality, Father Bill Stelling discusses how worry and fear get in the way of taking responsibility and action.[4] Father Stelling explains that we worry about all kinds of things. He once wrote that, "worry is the one thing I do really well and people are telling me all the time to quit doing it." He said he worried about that, too. Father Stelling wrote about alcoholics and drug addicts and how they often worried about their behavior and feared the consequences. He playfully asks, "why *do* we worry and fear so much?" Then he answers his own question. We worry, he says, "because it gives us the illusion that we are actually doing something." But these illusions, unfortunately, can cause a lot of grief.

If it seems that all you can "successfully" do about being fat is worry, we'd suggest that the worry may be more unhealthy than the fat. Worrying is an endless game of doing nothing constructive. Often, worriers "medicate" the unpleasant feelings caused by worry by scarfing down a bag of chips or a slice of cheesecake.

Being worried and concerned about fat isn't the same thing as actually doing something about it. It's true that having obvious health problems can help motivate a person to act in more healthy ways. *But worrying serves no useful purpose beyond making us aware of a difficulty.* You can use the awareness from your worries to help yourself make decisions; however, at some point you've got to let go of the worrying and make one of two decisions:

1) *You can accept the condition in which you find yourself and embrace it. Understand that being this way is your choice and that you are still a person of worth.* This idea has caught on in recent years. Some people believe that the obsession with being thin "goes against nature" and causes suffering and grief. They propose that overweight people should not be concerned about losing weight unless it is for obvious health reasons. There are several groups today that support this idea and we'll discuss them in later chapters.

2) *You can become better informed about the condition you find yourself in, make choices about the best course of action, and then take charge of making the changes you have selected.* One of the problems with this choice is the diversity of information and viewpoints available to us regarding how to go about making changes. Bookstores have hundreds — some have thousands — of different books on weight loss, diets, and exercise. Some of this information is valid — some isn't. It is very difficult for people to distinguish fact from hype in the consumer-oriented world of the diet industry. For example, some diet books will tell you to eat no carbohydrates while others tell you to eat almost no fat. These are two vastly different recommendations that cause the typical dieter lots of grief and confusion. You have to know the facts to make good choices. We wish you could simply ask your family doctor about it, but unfortunately, few doctors know enough about obesity to make good recommendations to their patients. And the family doctor really doesn't have enough time to spend with patients to explain all of this. *You* have

to become knowledgeable so you can make your own choices. Understanding what has caused you to be overweight can help you make good decisions. Having the **facts about fat** will help you to be better prepared to make choices.

We can't tell you which of the two decisions we proposed earlier in this chapter is right for you. We can tell you that you'll probably be better off mentally to **make one of these two choices** and **stop** worrying. Most overweight people experience some misery, unhappiness, and worry about their physical condition and chances are that you have too. The constant mental stress of worry exposes the body to harmful physical processes. The biochemical changes caused by worry can, by themselves, lead to a host of physical problems — including heart-related diseases. Of course, one of the main risks of obesity is heart disease. *In short, worrying about excess weight is unhealthy — and so is the excess weight.* Something has to give — or *it can break your heart.*

Making an active choice — taking responsibility for yourself — will alleviate some of the worry. (Chances are that you won't stop worrying until you choose.) Susan Powter's wonderful book, titled *Stop The Insanity*, demonstrates what we mean. "Insane" means a person doesn't know the difference between right and wrong. In the realm of dieting and exercise information, with contradictory advice coming from assorted "authorities," how can anyone know what's right and what's wrong? It *is* insane — but worrying doesn't make it less insane.

Our Mission

We decided to write this book for a number of reasons. One crucial purpose is to help you become a better consumer and a better decision-maker. We want to present the choices and options about weight as well as what scientific research actually shows about them. Being *informed* and *knowledgeable* is a fundamental starting point in making good decisions.

There are literally thousands of diet books, nutrition books, exercise books, health books, and web sites devoted to weight and health, with countless magazines, newsletters, and support groups adding to the information overload. Most of these materials and resources are accurate — but only to a point. That is, they tend to take a narrow point of view and fail to look at the totality of the problem. All of them have a bias. For example, most books fail to recognize the genetic component in obesity. And those books that do mention genetics fail to really explain it. Other books don't consider that the basic responsibilities of day-to-day living in our society can cause genuine, uncontrollable situations for dieters. Oprah can lose weight and usually keep it off, but most people don't have a personal gourmet chef, their own trainer, or several hours available each and every day for exercise. The diet and exercise routines of the "stars" often work for them, but for mothers balancing homemaking responsibilities with jobs, well, it is just unrealistic to expect to do what the "stars" do.

Diets don't work, yet countless people continue to accept the hype and promises of each new "miracle breakthrough" diet book. Few information sources confront the underlying personality issues involved in obesity and most have an obvious bias against medical intervention. Medical research *has* made a number of important discoveries, and people concerned about weight issues need to know them. In this book we will rationally present the facts about obesity and health as they are understood today. We will attempt to show each of the pieces of the obesity puzzle and make them understandable. More importantly, we want to show how each piece can best be handled.

This book will also help you to understand how you got to this point in your life. **Obesity is an extremely complex, multi-factorial problem involving** *genetics, childhood upbringing, environment, personality, diet, and behavior.* This is a fact that many "naturally thin" people don't seem to understand — nor do many obese people seem to get it, either. Drastic dieting doesn't really solve the problem of obesity. In fact, as many of you already know, drastic diets tend to result in even more weight gain. You need to understand why this happens and what reasonable courses of action are available. We also want to show you how obesity effects *every area* of your life.

Almost everybody is aware of health problems caused by too much fat. Medicine defines obesity by the risk of developing health problems. *Obesity is the level of fatness that significantly increases your risk of developing other diseases.* These diseases include heart disease, adult-onset diabetes, high blood pressure, arthritis, certain cancers, and certain sleep disorders among many others. Knowledge of these conditions can help you make an informed decision about your own weight.

Obesity renders a heavy psychological and social price that is too often denied or ignored by some groups. Many overweight people are embarrassed by the way they look. They are embarrassed by the real or imagined stares from others as they sweat at inopportune times or just walk into a crowded room. Social contacts, close relationships, and job opportunities are all affected by obesity. The toll obesity inflicts on a person's self-esteem and mental health is staggering. This, too, is a complex problem that will be addressed. It is certainly true that one's self-esteem and self-worth are determined, in part, by appearance. And whether we like it or not, whether it's fair or not, a lot of judgements about people are made based solely on looks. Obesity can cause heart-breaking social and interpersonal problems.

Ironically, body fat once served a useful purpose for humanity. In the not-too-distant past, body fat kept people alive during times of famine, illness, and social unrest. Being overweight was actually a sign of prosperity and success. Extra weight was nature's way of ensuring survival. And with the primitive medical assistance available then, few people survived long enough to develop the health problems that go along with long-term obesity. But now, in a society with all-you-can-eat buffets on every city street corner and in every small town, with super-markets offering a constant over-abundance of every imaginable food, with fast-food outlets everywhere, famine is something we read about in other cultures, history books, and novels. With medical advances such as vaccines, antibiotics, and pharmaceuticals as well as surgery for almost every ailment, we are living longer and longer. As a result, those of us with nature's survival mechanism built in too strongly face the long-term negative consequences of extra fat.

Almost all overweight and obese people know and acknowledge that their weight impedes their quality of life. Perhaps this is the most important concern for many people who will read this book. We don't know anyone who enjoys being fat. We don't know anyone who wants to be fat. For many people who are chronically overweight, the problem always seems to occupy the center of their attention. For others, being overweight seems to be the only issue in their lives that they just can't seem to handle. Weight affects our quality of life, our purpose in living, our self-worth and self-esteem, and our influence on others. We suspect that you are probably aware of many of these issues already and that, in all likelihood, something in this chapter "hit home."

Your reasons for reading this book are probably found somewhere within the prior pages. Our hope is that this book will help you to become better informed about your condition and that it will motivate you to choose to take responsibility for it. *You can choose to accept your condition and become content with it or you can choose to take meaningful steps to exert some real control over it.* The choice is completely yours, but consciously choosing will, in itself, improve your self-worth and quality of life. We know that life has an underlying significance that is missed when people constantly struggle in a war with themselves. By becoming knowledgeable and truly understanding the struggle, you can make peace with yourself and end the inner war. And in so doing, you can put worrying to rest and discover the higher meanings and purposes in life.

Chapter References & Notes

[1]*Morbidity and Mortality Weekly Report* (June 14, 1996; U.S. Public Health Service) reported that, the prevalence of overweight among youth (age 6-17 years) more than doubled in the past 30 years with most of the increase occurring since the late 1970s. This the highest level ever. It is estimated that 11% of youths in this age range are seriously overweight (obese).

[2]*Socioeconomic Status and Health Chartbook, Health, United States — 1998* (published by the National Center for Health Statistics) reported that, from 1980 to 1994, the percentage of overweight adults in the U.S. increased by about 35%. In 1994, 36% of adult men and 39% of adult women were overweight — the highest level ever.

[3]Schneider, K. S. (1996) Mission impossible. *People Magazine*, June 3, 71.

[4]Father Bill Stelling began writing about worry and fear in the newspapers *Recovery Times* and *Common Sense* in 1990. His books *Simply Spiritual* (1992) and *Spiritual Reflections on Everyday Living* (1998) expanded on the idea that worry and fear keep us from finding our true selves, our purpose, and developing a deep spiritual life. These books were published by Eagle Wing Books, Inc., PO Box 9972, Memphis, TN 38190.

Chapter 3
OBESITY IN HISTORY & THE DEVELOPMENT OF MYTHS

Let me have men about me that are fat ...
Cassius has a lean and hungry look.
He thinks too much. Such men are dangerous.
— Shakespeare

Chapter Summary — Solid archaeological evidence proves that, for at least 27,000 years prior to modern times, obesity in women was seen as a sign of health and fertility. Until recent times, large women were worshipped as goddesses as numerous archaeological finds have proven. The "ideal" woman had lots of extra body fat because large women were much better able to survive childbirth and the periodic starvation cycles common in primitive cultures. Obesity was associated with health, high social status, and material success until the 1800s. Even today, some cultures view obesity as a sign of importance and success. Especially in American women, obesity became stigmatized as society began prizing self-control and virtue. Unrestrained sexuality and lack of self-discipline were linked to over-eating at the same time that goddess figures were demonized. By the mid-1700s, being overweight was judged as a character flaw and the temperance movement in America stressed both controlling alcohol and food intake. Thinness was viewed as being spiritual and Godly.

The idealized woman in America became thin as women increased their involvement in sports and physical activity beginning in the early 1900s. As the developing women's magazine market increased, clothing styles changed allowing women to display their figures. Advertisers used slim women as models and depicted health, success, and slimness as related. Fad diets became vogue just after World War I, and the quest for thinness was on.

During the great depression, attitudes about food and body size switched between social classes. The poor were proud of being able to provide food for the family and waste became a sin. The rich saw eating and overweight as signs of poor health, low social standing, and character flaws. Psychological theories of the 1930s supported the view that obesity was a defect in character. But obesity has now been recognized to have a strong genetic component with complicated biochemical processes unrelated to character. Nevertheless, society and the majority of the medical profession continue to believe that obesity is solely a character problem. Many myths about obesity and overweight persist.

• • •

So many myths about obesity and weight exist that it is difficult to find an appropriate starting point in presenting them. The genesis of myths comes from humanity's history, biases, and observations. Shakespeare's quote at the beginning of this chapter was written in the early 1600s and clearly shows the belief that fat people are more docile, content, agreeable, and less ambitious than thin people. Was that really true then or now? Probably not, but understanding where the belief comes from is useful.

An understanding of obesity myths is closely intertwined with understanding history and the context of the era. This fact may not be apparent on first glance. But think about Shakespeare's time — the 1600s. The average life span then was under 40 years.[1] People who lived longer than 40 years were considered unusual and they often had special abilities attributed to them. People who were overweight in the 1600s had abundant food sources available and were, more often than not, found in wealthy families successful in business, politics, or professions. Food was expensive since food supplies were inconsistent depending upon weather and other growing conditions, and what food was available was usually bland, poorly prepared, and ill-tasting. People who were overweight in those times had to be able to afford food supplies, thus, they were usually well-to-do. In addition, these people were usually older

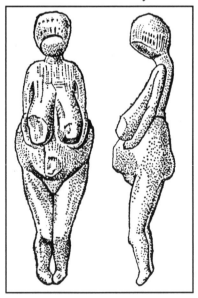

This 27,000 year-old "Venus" figure, about 2 inches tall and carved from mammoth bone, was found in the Ukraine. It is in the Museum de l'Homme in Paris.

than average and had already achieved success in life[2] as Shakespeare observed.

Obesity & Fertility

Being overweight was not always seen as a negative quality. Most people are aware that, at one time, the "ideal woman" was not viewed as thin, but rather was quite large and shaped much like a pear. In the remote past, obesity in women was also asso-

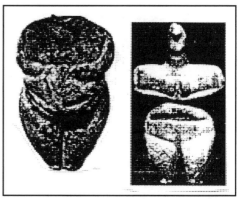

8,000 year-old figures above are typical neolithic-era depictions of fertile females. Left figure is carved from green limestone and was found in Turkey. Right figurine was found in Greece and is made from white stone.

ciated with fertility. Archaeologists have uncovered many small figurines of women in Russia, France, and Italy that have been dated to 27,000 B.C. The figures are formed from carved mammoth ivory, stone, or fire-hardened clay. They are all similar. The women are depicted as very large with huge hips, protruding stomachs, and large breasts. Cave drawings in France and Germany dated to even earlier times show the same large female figures. Archaeologists assume that they depict pregnant women — a sort of idealized "mother" goddess who is sometimes referred to as the "earth mother."[3] Neolithic humans (about 6,000 B.C.) produced thousands of obese "earth goddess" fertility figures. These have been found in vast areas of Europe, Asia, and Africa. Ancient Jericho has yielded similar artifacts.

An understanding of why the idealized mother was obese is fairly simple. Pregnancy puts obvious stress on a women's body. Women who were best suited to survive the 9-month strain of child-bearing had the ability to rely upon supplies of stored energy to carry them through times of famine. Nature ensured human survival by genetically encoding some women with the ability to easily store energy (fat) during times of plenty so that when food was scarce these child-bearing women could survive. Early man quickly came to the understanding that large women were the most valuable to the survival and perpetuation of the family. Obese females were seen as the most desirable mates and they were literally worshiped.

Weight and Social Status

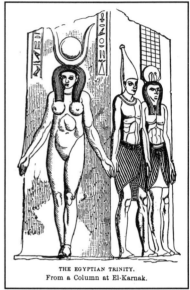

THE EGYPTIAN TRINITY.
From a Column at El-Karnak.

Isis is figure on left. From Ridpath's *History of the World* (1911)

Throughout history, being overweight has often been viewed as synonymous with being successful. "Rarely, if ever, has an entire people had more than enough to eat for any prolonged period of time. As a result, throughout history, as in many underdeveloped areas today, obesity has been restricted to the privileged classes. In many cultures, it was even a status symbol..."[4] Obesity remains a sign of success, high status, and prestige in some societies.[5]

Massive obesity has been identified for at least 27,000 years as evidenced by the earliest revered artifacts. However, the way that obesity is viewed by societies has varied greatly. The mores and religious values held by a given society have determined how obesity is judged. In addition, obesity in men and women have usually been judged differently. You probably are very aware of this fact and have perhaps noticed how girls will adore Barbie but boys certainly don't adore Ken.

In ancient Egypt, the Goddess Isis was often depicted as being large and fertile and even as being physically larger than her mate Osiris. Enhotep, believed to be the architect of the pyramids, was shown in most statues as being overweight by today's

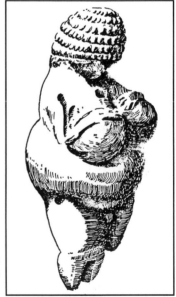

Right —
Female goddess carved in limestone from ancient South Africa. Most ancient African cultures and their descendants revered large females.

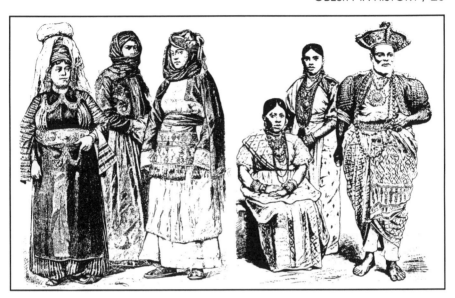

Above —
Right: Sri Lanka, 1880. Left: Turkey, 1880.
Below —
Prince, 1650. From Dover's
Historic Costumes in Pictures (1975)

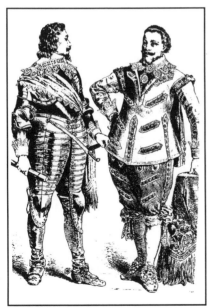

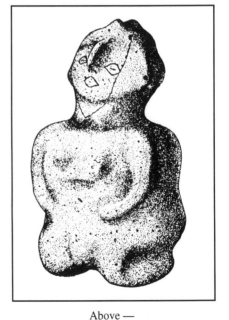

Above —
Even Native American artifacts over 1,000 years
old depicted large females as goddesses. This
effigy was uncovered from a mound in Tennessee.

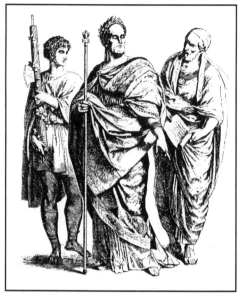

Left —
Roman emperor (center), is the largest figure, nobleman (right) is the next largest, common standard bearer (left) is thin. From Dover's *Historic Costumes in Pictures* (1975)

standards. History tells us that the leader of the 1800s' Shiite Muslims, the Aga Khan, was weighed each year. An annual increase of weight was viewed with pride and optimism. In India, weight and obesity increased as status and class standing in society increased.

Dover Publications (1975) book, *Historic Costumes in Pictures*, shows 1,450 illustrations of people in various classes covering the time period of about 2,000 B.C. to the late 1800s. Nobles, members of ruling classes, and middle-class businessmen and their families are consistently shown as overweight. Commoners and people from lower classes are consistently depicted as thin.

The Idealized Female Loses Weight: Obesity Becomes A Moral Issue

The shift of the idealized female from obese to slim was gradual and has taken place over the past 3,000 years. As humanity progressed in knowledge and food-cultivating efficiency, people began living longer and longer. Developing religious beliefs progressively associated obesity (especially in the young) with excess and lack of self-discipline. Fertility symbols still portrayed the idealized mother as overweight, but in the young, being overweight was slowly stigmatized in everyone but the older, wealthy, and ruling classes.

In ancient Turkey (*ca* 1300 B.C.), the cult of Cybele celebrated the obese Earth Mother — the Goddess of fertility — and her obese male consort Attis. Greek and Roman mythology assimilated the beliefs associated with Cybele. Dionysus, the 13th god of the Greeks, retains a distinctive similarity to Attis. Dionysus celebrates excess - excess in wine, food, sex, and "letting go" of vain attempts to moderate human urges. Paintings, inscriptions, and pottery depicting Cybele, Attis, Dionysus, and their festivals and celebrations all show obese men and women happily embracing their "excesses,"[6] and, as a result, overeating and being overweight — especially in women — were gradually seen as an immorality.

Hippocrates (*ca* 460-377 B.C.), acknowledged as the "father of medicine," was perhaps the first person to record his observations of the problems associated with obesity: "Sudden death is more common in those who are naturally fat than in the lean." Hippocrates' prescription for treating obesity had a distinctive moral tone to it:

> "Obese persons with laxity of muscle and red complexion ... need dry food during the greatest part of the year. Obese people and those desiring to lose weight should perform hard work before food. Meals should be taken after exertion and while still panting from fatigue ... meals should be prepared with sesame or seasoning ... and be of a fatty nature as people get thus satiated with little food. They should, moreover, eat only once a day and take no baths and sleep on a hard bed and walk naked as long as possible."

Hippocrates' observation was not wrong, per se. Obese people are *not* normal physically and very likely have to adhere to a markedly changed, restrained life style. (We do not, however, recommend the walking naked part.)

> "I'll never forget going to the Ramses II exhibitions in Memphis in 1989. Each visitor was provided with a tape player with earphones to guide us through the exhibit. The recorded message explained each artifact and took us step-by-step through this phase of ancient Egypt. Among the wonderful artifacts on display was a small statue of Enhotep, the architect of the pyramids. The message simply said, 'Note that the statue of Enhotep portrays him as portly.' That is because fatness was associated with wealth and success in ancient Egypt. Even recent history shows the same: in some Pacific Island cultures obesity was a badge of high social rank. Even Hawaiian kings and queens are pictured as morbidly obese — and they were proud of it." — *P. Milnor*

The Greeks and Romans embraced conscious efforts to resist excess and, by 100 B.C., prized self-restraint and moderation. In some places celebrations of the cults of Dionysus and Cybele were outlawed or severely restricted by age and marital status.[6] Obesity was gradually associated with negative personal traits such as lack of self-discipline and unrestrained sexuality. Obesity was the product of out-of-control behavior that could be cured only by severely limiting life-style.

The Roman physician Galen (ca 129-199 A.D.) was the first to divide obese people into types. One type, *moderate obesity*, Galen saw as a natural consequence of life and aging. With age, occupational success, marriage, and child rearing, moderate obesity was acceptable and bestowed an aura of success. Immoderate obesity, though, Galen viewed as a character flaw: "The hygienic art promises to maintain a good health to those who obey it; but to those who are disobedient, it is just as if it did not exist at all." Overindulgence in the "lustful" parts of the soul led to an imbalance that severely affected health. Galen believed that people who consciously chose to overindulge were difficult or impossible to treat and were in open defiance of nature itself. Galen's own struggles with overindulgence are described in his work *On Passions*.

As Christianity developed in its early years, fertility images were literally demonized and seen as devil-worship. Fasting, self-denial, moderation, and simplicity were prized and obesity was sometimes seen as an outward sign of sin — especially for women. By the middle ages, a "lady of chivalry" was supposed to show an "anti-sexual ideal" in her body size. She was described as "slender, narrow-waisted, with small breasts and low hips, and above all, she is deathly white in colour ... 'whiter than snow on ice, whiter than snow in sunshine.' "[7] In short, thinness was associated with a lack of sexuality and a refinement of tastes and interests desired in chaste, young women. Obesity came with marriage, sex, and child-bearing. "Whiteness" — lack of skin color or a tan — became associated with purity, chastity, and refinement. Obviously, women who worked outside developed tans and wore clothing that was functional rather than designed to narrow their waist. Upper classes believed that lower-class "commoners" were to be exploited and used. Almost all illustrations of working class people from the middle ages depict thin, muscular people wearing baggy clothing. Thus, body size and clothing were a visible way of determining a person's status in society and quick judgements about people based on their looks — discrimination — became the norm.

Langdon-Davies[7] has described the gradual transition of the roles of the ideal woman as a form of systematic degradation of women. He believes it represents a form of enslavement and subservience to men. Many people today similarly believe that young women's obsession with being thin is a form of enslavement. Some modern fitness "gurus" like Susan Powter express their anger at this form of female degradation, yet go on to encourage women to lose weight and get fit to take their revenge on the men who have degraded them.

Obesity In The Recent Past

By the 1700s, most people viewed obesity as a character disorder. Obesity was a sin and overweight people should be ashamed of themselves. Physicians in the 18th century believed that all diseases and conditions came from the air, the type and quantity of food consumed, what a person drank, their bowel habits, their ability to balance rest and labor, and their emotional state. While this set of beliefs represented a great advance from prior times, it was far from adequate or accurate. Unfortunately, until recent times, medicine, psychology, and the public all have held those beliefs. The prevailing view in society remains that overweight people are completely responsible for their condition: they eat too much, exercise too little, and have no self-control; they willingly engage in one of the deadly sins — gluttony — and are lazy. Physicians came to believe that they had to *cure* obesity by first educating and then controlling the patient's behavior.[8]

In America, the nature of eating and obesity drastically changed in harmony with social movements. Americans were known for eating quickly, eating a lot, and for having poor food quality and taste. Europeans often were repelled at American eating habits and the poor quality of the food itself. The temperance movement that began in earnest in the 1830's not only attempted to restrict alcohol consumption in Americans, but also to change basic patterns of food intake. Eating more vegetables and less meat was a hallmark of the temperance movement. Eating less was seen as godly and spiritual. Those who continued to overeat — or eat the wrong foods — were seen as defective and in need of outside control.

Eating too much was a character issue just as drinking was a character issue.[2]

The reversal of body shape ideals was complete in America by the 1940s, but the social factors that led to it actually began with changes in female roles. In the early 1900s, women began rebelling against the idea that they were weak and frail. Women began actively participating in sports. Fitness became a focal point in the many emerging fashion magazines of the time. Being thin and fit, being an active, modern women in the Roaring 20s, was the new ideal. Advertisers moved in and quickly promoted new fashions that showed off the female physique. How a woman looked became more important than what she did or who she was. Women were told they had to be thin to be attractive. Fad dieting began in earnest just after World War I with the banana/skimmed milk diet proposed by Johns Hopkins professor George Harrop and the 18-Day Hollywood diet centering on grapefruit. In 1926, physicians first described women who purged themselves by vomiting after eating in the quest to eat and be thin.[9] Understanding the causes of obesity then became important to scientists, and all fingers of responsibility pointed to the character and morality of the individual.

In the 1930s, the theories of Sigmund Freud dominated psychology. Freud's psychoanalytic theory pointed to early life character development flaws as the source of overeating. Psychiatry has long held an interest in treating obesity and overweight patients, and Freud's ideas about the "oral" stage (in the first year of life) somehow going haywire was an ideal explanation of obesity. Obesity and overeating became the perfect model to "prove" Freud's theory correct. To Freudians, overeating was the logical result of obsessive orality. Defective parenting resulted in defective children who ate until they became fat. Something, they speculated, was wrong with the personality of the obese and their family. Physicians, psychologists, and the public quickly embraced the connection between being overweight and having a personality flaw — a psychological abnormality. "An apparently irrefutable formula became popular: ... **Psychopathology causes obesity**."[8]

The influence of Freudian ideas on society's opinions about obesity is hard to overestimate. Even today, many well-educated people see an "oral fixation" as the source of overeating. Overeating is still viewed as a character flaw, and being thin somehow shows others that the thin person isn't flawed. The character of the overweight person is still the focus of society and many weight-reducing specialists. Even modern behaviorism focuses on identifying and then modifying the *behaviors* that lead to overeating and obesity. Thus, behavioral treatments see controlling the individual's behavior and character as the main issue.

And Today?

Physicians who specialize in obesity now tell us that the once irrefutable formulation that obesity is a psychopathology of eating too much, "has been turned on its head."[8] Medical research has uncovered a multitude of factors underlying obesity that were unheard of — and unimagined — only 40 years ago. *Obesity has a complicated genetic basis not yet completely understood.* Obese patients who restrict their food intake have a genetic mechanism that quickly adjusts to the lower energy by reducing the fat-burning metabolic rate of their body. If obese people "successfully" starve their bodies into losing weight, their metabolic rate is set artificially low so the body can easily regain the weight. If they go back to their "normal" eating habits, the low metabolism rapidly forces the body to regain all of the lost weight — and more — to prepare itself for the next period of "intentional" starvation.

Insulin, a variety of hormones, fat cell secretions, and other physical processes have been identified as underlying components of obesity. We know more about nutrition today than ever. Researchers are chasing each of these processes in the hopes of finding a magic bullet to cure the disease. Complicating factors are childhood upbringing, learning, habits, and numerous psychological issues — all of which remain elusive but are becoming increasingly understood.

With all of these new understandings, where is the compassion today for the overweight person? Society still views obesity as a cosmetic problem brought on by the weak character of the obese. The obese person is weak and lazy — an overeater. Many physicians and the people who hawk diets and exercise plans view obesity the same way. The blame for our fundamental lack of compassion and understanding for overweight people is a collective responsibility for all of society. But the fundamental problem in attitude lies with the physician, not the patient.

Physicians want to win and are trained to fight diseases with all of their resources. Physicians tend to be systematic and active in diagnosing and treating disorders, in order to do something — to prescribe a drug, perform a surgical procedure and see positive results. But obesity, in many ways like alcoholism and drug addiction, has long resisted treatment efforts. Through the process of elimination, by trying one failed treatment after another, **medicine has gradually adapted the attitude that obesity is the fault of the patient.** Like Hippocrates did in 400 B.C., most physicians today have labelled obesity as a character flaw. Although most physicians are not really conscious of this attitude, it is nevertheless present.

In truth, little has changed over the past 2,400 years in the treatment of obesity by the general physician. Doctors don't like patients they can't cure. Drug addicts and alcoholics have been scorned by most of medicine since treatments that can cure the problem don't exist. So, too, have the obese been scorned by physicians as they tell patients to "eat less and exercise more." Thoughts of gluttony and sloth enter many physician's minds as they attend to obese patients. The famous line, "close your mouth and push away from the table," shows how difficult it is for many people to relate to the pain of obesity.

Obesity remains stigmatized as a disorder of character. People who want to lose weight for "cosmetic" reasons are often ridiculed by those who spend hours putting on makeup and styling their hair. The overweight person is still thought of as weak-willed and lazy. Arguments about whether obesity is a disease or not continue to rage. Every time a new diet drug is proposed, many physicians protest its approval because of potential side-effects. Debate continues to rage in medicine and state licensing boards over whether physicians should even be involved in treating obesity. Physicians who treat obesity are scorned by their peers as well as by the very people they treat.

Despite the current state of obesity treatment and societal perceptions of the problem, it is important to keep two issues in mind. First, while many people still view obesity and overweight as character issues, a strong counterforce has emerged. We know for certain that obesity has a fundamental genetic basis and a substantial amount of scientific research is rapidly piecing together the complex jig-saw puzzle that underlies it. **Modern medicine does have some tools and some knowledge that can truly help the overweight person.** But like all tools, they only do the job as well as the person who handles them.

Second, there is a complex interplay of psychological factors related to obesity. People struggling with weight deserve the same compassion as those who struggle with other diseases. Telling an overweight person to "eat less and exercise more" is like telling a person who is depressed to "cheer up." Neither statement works. Depression involves more than needing to "cheer up," and obesity involves more than "eating less and exercising more."

Common Obesity Myths

Myth: Overweight people are generally happy, content, and unambitious.

Fact: Overweight people are basically no different from others in happiness, contentment, and ambition.

Myth: Being overweight has always been seen as a sign of weakness and failure.

Fact: Only in recent times and in societies where food is abundant has obesity been viewed as a negative trait. Obesity was previously associated with success and having important stature in society.

Myth: The ideal woman has always been depicted by men as being thin.

Fact: Idealized women were depicted as being obese or certainly overweight until recent times. Overweight women were generally more fertile and healthier than thin women. Today, thinness in women is admired although primarily in Western culture. In some parts of the world today thinness in women is still viewed with disdain.

Myth: Thin people are healthier than overweight people.

Fact: There are few, if any, differences in the health of moderately thin and overweight people. The obese — severely overweight persons — do have significant health problems. By the same token, extremely thin, underweight persons also tend to have a myriad of health problems.

Myth: Obesity is simply caused by eating too much.

Fact: Obesity results when the body stores excess energy in fat. The body is programmed through genetics to store fat for times of emergency and famine. Some people and specific cultural groups have extremely "thrifty genes." This means that their bodies are efficient in regulating metabolism up and down depending upon the availability of food. The "thrifty" aspect of the genes means that the gene is stingy in that it hordes too much fat.

Myth: It is always better for the overweight person to lose weight.

Fact: Some people experience severe problems, both physical and psychological, when they lose weight to the levels often shown in "idealized" weight tables.

Myth: Fat is fat, no matter where on the body it is found.

Fact: Fat around the abdomen, stomach, and upper body is a much greater health risk than fat in the lower part of the body (hips, thighs).

Myth: Most diets will lead to long-term weight loss.

Fact: Almost everyone who loses weight on a diet will gain all of the weight back within a year. It is estimated that less than one half of 1% of dieters permanently lose weight through dieting.

Myth: Fat people tend to have greater psychological problems than those who aren't fat.

Fact: Fat people do not have greater levels of psychopathology. They do experience discrimination and ridicule and often have self-image and self-esteem problems. They also have higher than average levels of anxiety and depression.

Myth: Obesity is caused by psychological and behavioral problems.

Fact: Obesity is caused by underlying genetics interacting with the individual's environment, personality, and habits. Some psychological problems are caused by obesity.

Myth: There are no safe medications that assist in weight loss.

Fact: *There are no completely safe medications.* All medicines have side effects and risks. But several medicines with minimal risks exist today that assist in weight loss when used in conjunction with other strategies.

Myth: "Natural" weight loss supplements and over-the-counter diet aids are completely safe.

Fact: No natural supplements or over-the-counter diet aids are completely safe. In fact, many of these carry higher risks than prescribed medicines because the actual quantity and quality of these supplement formulations can vary greatly. In addition, some of them have serious side effects.

Myth: Most people try to lose weight for health reasons.

Fact: Most people try to lose weight to look and feel better.

Myth: If you exert total control over your diet and exercise enough, you can reach your desired weight and shape.

Fact: Your basic body shape and overall size is primarily determined by genetics. You can lose weight and become fit with appropriate diet and exercise, but your desired weight and shape may be unattainable. In addition, if you are successful in losing weight below your genetic set point, maintaining the low weight may be nearly impossible.

Chapter References & Notes

[1] *Grollier's Encyclopedia* (1992).

[2] W. J. Rorabaugh (1979) *The Alcoholic Republic: An American Tradition.* New York: Oxford University Press. Rorabaugh's major concern in this book is alcohol consumption in the United States during its early years. He describes how food consumption and alcohol were related and how poor food quality increased American's drinking. Early American's tended to eat quickly and consumed everything that was set before them. The food was poorly prepared and basically tasteless. Religious convictions played a large role in how and why food was consumed.

[3] *The Dawn of Civilization* (1961) London: Thames & Hudson. This massive book depicts the earliest figures ever found by archaeologists and shows how carvings and statues of very large, overweight women were essentially worshipped. The "earth mother" is sometimes also referred to by the name "Venus." Fertile women were revered in ancient society and the women who were most fertile were obese (by today's standards).

[4] Albert J. Stunkard, M.D. Obesity, Pp 1648-1655. In: A. M. Freedman (Ed.) *Comprehensive Textbook of Psychiatry - II.* (1975) Baltimore: Williams & Wilkins.

[5] Sobal, J. & Stunkard, A. J. (1989) Socioeconomic status and obesity: A review of the literature. *Psychological Bulletin*, 105, 260-275.

[6] Richard Cavendish (Ed.) (1970) *Man, Myth & Magic* Encyclopedia. New York: BCP Publishing. Numerous illustrations of these early cults celebrating the earth mother and later manifestations all show obese people obviously enjoying themselves. It is interesting to note that it was the Greeks who began to focus on personal discipline and moderation in all things. It was about this time that a stigmatization of obesity began. Obesity gradually became associated with drunkenness, lack of discipline, uncleanliness, and weakness. Overweight women, however, were still revered as fertile.

[7] Cited in John Langdon-Davies (1927) *A Short History of Women*. New York: Viking Press.

[8] Albert J. Stunkard. Obesity. In: R. Hales & Frances, A. J. (Eds.) (1985) *American Psychiatric Association Annual Review — Vol 4*. APA: Washington, D.C.

[9] Fraser, L. (1998) *Losing It*. New York: Penguin.

Chapter 4
AM I FAT, OVERWEIGHT, OR OBESE?

Fat is an efficient storage form for energy, because each gram of fat holds more than twice the energy content of either carbohydrate or protein. Excess fat in the diet is stored in fat cells (called adipose tissue) located under the skin and around internal organs.
Total Fitness — 1996

Chapter Summary — Most people "eyeball" themselves and others to determine fatness and body desirability. However, America's idealized body standards are usually based on actors, actresses, and models who are paid vast sums of money to stay thin and fit. We often forget that these people represent a very small percentage of the population and that they have a great deal of motivation to rigidly diet and exercise. Medicine uses the terms overweight, overfat, and obesity to describe weight-related problems. Overweight usually means that, based on a height/weight chart established by averaging large groups of people, a particular person's weight exceeds the established, average "desired" weight. Overfat is a much better term and means that a person's percentage of body fat exceeds the normal limits for his/her sex. For women, the "ideal" body fat percentage (the amount of fat that shows the least health problems) is 24% to 26%. For men, the ideal body fat percentage is 15% to 17%. Obesity is a medical diagnosis that is defined as the level of fatness where the risk of developing a number of diseases significantly increases.

In 1998, two National Institutes of Health agencies issued unified standards on definitions of obesity based on body mass index (BMI). BMI is an estimate of fatness based on height and weight. This chapter contains a BMI chart for reference, but it must be kept in mind that it is an estimate only. The "ideal" BMI is defined as being 19 to 24.9. BMIs above 30 are defined as obesity. BMIs above 30 indicate increased risk for developing a host of diseases.

Overall body shape can also be used to assess potential health risks. Apple shapes, also called android obesity, are often seen in men. People who take on rounded, apple shapes with fat accumulating on the hips, mid-section, and upper body have the most health risks. Pear shapes, also called gynecoid obesity, are most often seen in women. Pear-shaped people accumulate fat in the lower body including the hips, thighs, and legs. Pear shapes have less health risks than apple shapes. Waist circumference is the simplest measure of basic body shape. Women with waist sizes 35 inches and above and men with waists 40 inches and above are at the greatest risk.

Body fat percentage measurements are the most important to weight-management specialists. The simplest measures of body fat percentage are the most utilized (because of their low cost), but are also the most inaccurate. These include the use of skin fold calipers and BMI. Cheap, fairly accurate bioelectrical impedance devices have recently become available to measure fat percentage. However, the correct use of these devices relies on a number of requirements often ignored. The most precise measurement tools for body fat are the most cumbersome and expensive. Underwater weighing is extremely accurate, but it presents cumbersome problems. The Bod Pod® also gives accurate measurements but is very costly. Other precise medical methods that measure body fat are the DEXA®, MRI, and CAT scans. All of these are costly.

Precise measures of body fat percentage are important because the best way to accurately assess health risks is in actual body fat percentage. Many patients don't understand why their "weight" problem necessitates a measurement of fat. The health risks that accompany obesity aren't weight problems, they are fat problems.

•   •   •

Whether a person is "fat" or not can be evaluated from several perspectives. The most frequently used method is the "eyeball" test: "If a person looks fat, he or she probably is fat." The eyeball test, of course, depends upon a comparison to a desired (or undesired) body shape. The idealized body shape norm in America is established by often abnormally thin super-models posing in ads for clothing, cosmetics, perfumes, jewelry, or even food. Not only does advertising bombard us with examples of "perfection," but we are subjected to these same exacting standards by actors and actresses in movies, television, and glamour magazines. How many obese people are seen in ads for jeans, perfumes, shoes, cigarettes (yes, even here), cars, and candy? How many fat people have leading roles in movies or plays? Contrarily, how often are fat actors and actresses portrayed as negative or foolish foils to the "beautiful people" starring in movies? In the past, obese actors were usually stereotyped as fairly happy simpletons. But that depiction has subtly changed. *Star Wars, Seinfeld, The Spy Who Shagged Me,* and even *Jurassic Park* portray obese people as villains. Being overweight is gradually being associated with having sinister motives. And you know when everything ends: "When the fat lady sings!" But modern standards of thinness are warped. Based on today's standards, even Marilyn Monroe would be considered on the pudgy side.

Most of us, whether we're 10 or 60 years old, compare our appearance and body to a very small, carefully selected subset of the population. We forget that these people represent less than 2% of the total population. We don't keep in mind that part of their job is staying thin and fit. They make millions of dollars from their looks, thus, they are highly motivated to rigidly diet and exercise. It is probably true that many overweight people could lose substantial amounts of weight and keep fit if they were paid millions of dollars to do it. The "beautiful people" to whom we compare ourselves don't represent the real world, yet they strongly influence our personal images by establishing societal standards. **The truth is that these standards are almost an impossible-to-achieve goal for people living in the normal world.**

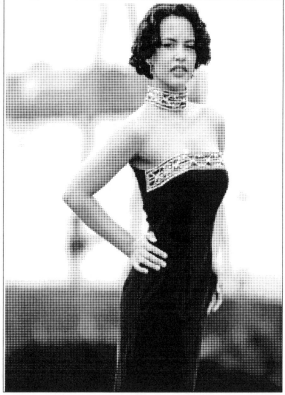

Another way of looking at fatness is the "volume" test. Sit in a coach class seat of an airliner or try to get yourself into the rear seat of a Honda Civic and you will quickly find out if you have a "volume" problem.

Volume tests are usually passed only if you are under 5'10" tall and weigh 175 pounds or less. Bar stools and restaurant booths also provide a volume measurement that cause many an embarrassing moment as we wiggle and squeeze ourselves into places not designed for us. But these are not measurements of obesity. In reality, they are an indication of the average size of people.

Obviously, the eyeball and volume methods don't take into account the unique physical characteristics of individuals. Nor do they account for differences in diverse groups such as Asians, Europeans, Africans, or Americans. Simply put, our ideal body images don't reflect the real world. So, how do we *really* know who is overweight or obese? The answer lies in ongoing medical research determining what amount of fat is healthy or unhealthy. This perspective can help us differentiate between "normal" and "healthy" — regardless of size. For example, we know that being a little overfat is associated with living longer, but being too skinny isn't. Being a little fat is therefore healthy and normal. The question is how much fat is normal.

Definitions of Overweight, Overfat, and Obesity

Overweight, overfat, and *obese* are confusing terms. These terms are often defined differently by patients and doctors. Doctors sometimes define them differently among themselves. But in order to diagnose a problem, we have to accurately describe it. In this chapter we have attempted to explain why the terms are confusing and give a simple definition for each.

Overweight

Overweight is the broadest term. Overweight usually means that, based on a particular height, a person should weigh no more than a given weight. Height/weight standards are somewhat arbitrary although efforts have been made in medical science to make them more uniform. One problem is that anyone who exceeds the given weight for their height is considered to be overweight — regardless of where the weight comes from. Based on the typical height/weight charts, Arnold

Schwartzenegger is overweight. So was the comedian John Candy. The "eyeball" test shows obvious differences between the two men. Schwartzenegger isn't fat, but John Candy certainly was. Height/weight standards **are** rather arbitrary — a fact that will be apparent from their history.

In 1901, American insurance companies first published idealized "weight tables" detailing what men and women of various heights should weigh to remain "healthy." Health was conveniently defined, at that time, as remaining *alive* until age 55. Of course, **staying alive** was the most important measure of "health" for life insurance companies (as it still is). These early charts were based on average weights of "healthy" men — all of them older and white. Women were later added to the charts. In 1959, The Metropolitan Life Insurance Company produced a new height/weight chart listing the "desirable" weight for various heights. Desirable weight was determined by longevity (what weight showed the lowest mortality). Life insurance tables remained the most utilized method to define "overweight" until public health agencies began to more carefully devise tables based on better data. According to these new weight charts, overweight was defined rather simply: you were overweight if you exceeded the "optimum" weight for your height.[3]

Most physicians, insurance companies, and lay people still rely on height/weight charts as an easy way to assess overweight. It takes minimal equipment to assess a person with a weight chart. All you need are a ruler and scales. If you exceed the listed weight, physicians usually then apply the "eyeball test." Sometimes they remark, "You don't look that fat! Maybe you're just big boned."

It is recognized that height/weight charts are far from perfect. The charts do not distinguish between muscle, fat, bone, or water weight and will often unfairly and inaccurately categorize some people as overweight. Bluntly put, it's absurd to assume that all men of a certain height should weigh the same or that all women of a particular height should weigh the same. It's also absurd to assume that any excess weight is harmful. Yet many insurance companies and pre-employment physical evaluations still use nothing but standard weight charts to predict future health risks.

Simple definition of *overweight*: **If your weight exceeds the "optimum" weight for your height listed on a height/weight chart, you are overweight.**

Overfat

The term **overfat** is more restrictive than overweight. It also is more accurate in estimating potential health risks. Overfat (having too much fat) does not rely on a measure of weight. Fat is often thought of as being somewhat "fluffy" — light in weight but expansive in size. Fluffy is a *volume* term. Therefore, overfat is defined by body volume, not weight. Overfat is defined as an unhealthy, high percentage of fat in relation to the remainder of the body (e.g. water, bones, muscle, other tissues). If we measured the body volume of a group of healthy, normal adults and determined their fat percentages, we could come up with an average and a range of body fat percentages that we'd label "normal." Anyone with a body fat percentage higher than "normal" would be overfat. This, of course, has been done. For men, the ideal percentage of body fat is about 15%-17% while for women it is 24%-26%. Making exact measurements of fat percentages can be difficult and requires specialized equipment. Later in this chapter we'll review the methods used to measure fat percentage.

Simple definition of *overfat*: **If your percentage of body fat exceeds the normal limits for your sex, you are overfat.**

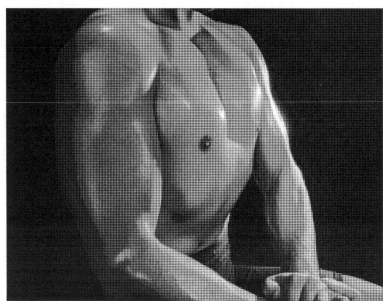

This weightlifter is overweight but not overfat.

Obesity

All people who are obese are overfat, but not all overfat people are obese. **Obesity** is being overfat to the extent that it can lead to significant increases in a number of related diseases. Research on the health conditions of groups of people at varying percentages of body fat has found an imperfect dividing point where being overfat becomes obesity. Women with a body fat percentage of 36% and higher and men with a fat percentage of 26% and higher are considered to be obese. At these fat percentages a dramatic increase in heart disease, high blood pressure, diabetes, arthritis, and a number of other diseases occurs. Later chapters will address these conditions.

> If your weight exceeds the "optimum" weight for your height listed on a height/weight chart, you are **overweight**.
>
> If your percentage of body fat exceeds the normal limits for your sex, you are **overfat**.
>
> When your body fat percentage reaches the level where related diseases show dramatic increases, you are **obese**.

Simple definition of *obesity*: **When your body fat percentage reaches the level where related diseases show dramatic increases, you are obese.**

Mild, Moderate, & Severe Obesity

Physicians have long used differing definitions in describing and diagnosing levels of overweight, overfat, and obesity. Overweight has long been defined in medicine as *an excess of body weight* in comparison to the standard weight in typical height/weight tables. Most people that are categorized as overweight are *not* obese. These people simply have more weight than the "standard" recommends, but they typically have the same relative health risks as those within the acceptable weight guidelines.

Modern medical definitions of overfat and obesity don't use weight as a measurement. You should quickly realize that a person could have a "normal" weight but still be overfat and perhaps even obese if their fat percentage reached a high level. And the reverse is also true. Some people can be very overweight according to the charts but not obese or overfat. A glance at some professional football players, basketball players, female aerobics participants, and even some wrestlers (i.e. *American Gladiators*) will indicate that many of them have very low levels of body fat but high weight.

Obesity is usually divided into three categories of increasing health risk severity. The older definitions of obesity (based on height/weight charts) are still used by some practitioners and utilized in books and articles you may encounter. It is for that reason we are listing them. It is important to remember that the following three definitions have been replaced by more precise standards that use body fat percentage rather than actual weight. At the same time, some practitioners will apply these terms.

Older Definitions Of Obesity. **Mild obesity** is diagnosed when an individual is 20% to 40% overweight. **Moderate obesity** is diagnosed at 41% to 100% overweight. **Severe obesity** is diagnosed when a person is more than 100% overweight (double their standard ideal weight). Some specialists employ the term **malignant obesity** for people at least 60% above desirable weight who are also 100 pounds overweight. Severe obesity is also called **morbid obesity.** Morbid obesity is defined by being twice one's ideal weight or at least 100 pounds overweight.[5,6]

Body Mass Index & Obesity
1998 Federal Guidelines

Until 1998, there were no recognized accepted national standards using height and weight tables. Many governmental agencies had published height/weight guidelines, but these were inconsistent and needed to be standardized. In June 1998, two National Institutes of Health agencies, the National Heart, Lung and Blood Institute and the National Institute of Diabetes and Digestive and Kidney Diseases, issued the first federal obesity standards based on the health risks that increase as weight increases. A panel of 24 experts combined with 8 other members and a consultant reviewed the results of 394 published studies to arrive at its results. Based on the new standards, an astonishing *97 million Americans are considered to be overweight* (overfat or obese). This figure represents **55%** of the adult population.[4]

The new national federal obesity standards were created based on research relating excess body fat to an increase in health problems. The most **frequently used** measurement of overweight and overfat is called **body mass index (BMI)**.[7] BMI is based on height/weight charts, so it represents an estimate rather than a precise measure. BMI is a fairly simple mathematical formula that can appear complicated.[8] BMI is calculated by dividing body weight (in kilograms) by height (in meters) squared.

$$BMI = Weight\ (kg)/Height^2\ (meters)$$

BMI is an easy, fast way to screen patients or large populations, but it can be grossly inaccurate on an individual basis. BMI does not distinguish among muscle, fat, bones, or water, but it is based on averages of large samples of people. Thus, BMI can be used as a screening tool since it compares individuals to the overall average. For example, chances are that a 200 pound person who is 5 feet 2 inches tall has a fairly large amount of excess fat. But what if that person had engaged in serious weight lifting and had huge muscles? BMI doesn't take individual characteristics into account — it is based on the averages of large numbers of people.

BMI Definition of Obesity

Life insurance and health studies show that the **least** health problems are seen in people who have a BMI of between 20-25. The 1998 Federal standards consider BMIs between 19 and 24.9 as "healthy" with BMIs *above and below* that range showing increased health risks. This book doesn't address the severe health risks associated with being underweight. But it should be noted that people who are underweight have similar mortality and overall health problems as those who are overweight and, in some cases, higher mortality levels.

Body Mass Index Chart (from federal guidelines)

Find your height on the top row. Go straight down until you find your weight.
Then go the far left column for estimated body Mass Index (BMI).

BODY MASS INDEX	HEIGHT IN INCHES																		
	58	59	60	61	62	63	64	65	66	67	68	69	70	71	72	73	74	75	76
19	91	94	97	100	104	107	110	114	118	121	125	128	132	136	140	144	148	152	156
20	96	99	102	106	109	113	116	120	124	127	131	135	139	143	147	151	155	160	164
21	100	104	107	111	115	118	122	126	130	134	138	142	146	150	154	159	163	168	172
22	105	109	112	116	120	124	128	132	136	140	144	149	153	157	162	166	171	176	180
23	110	114	118	122	126	130	134	138	142	146	151	155	160	165	169	174	179	184	189
24	115	119	123	127	131	135	140	144	148	153	158	162	167	172	177	182	186	192	197
25	119	124	128	132	136	141	145	150	155	159	164	169	174	179	184	189	194	200	205
26	124	128	133	137	142	146	151	156	161	166	171	176	181	186	191	197	202	208	213
27	129	133	138	143	147	152	157	162	167	172	177	182	188	193	199	204	210	216	221
28	134	138	143	148	153	158	163	168	173	178	184	189	195	200	206	212	218	224	230
29	138	143	148	153	158	163	169	174	179	185	190	196	202	208	213	219	225	232	238
30	143	148	153	158	164	169	174	180	186	191	197	203	209	215	221	227	233	240	246
31	148	153	158	164	169	175	180	186	192	198	203	209	216	222	228	235	241	248	254
32	153	158	163	169	175	180	186	192	198	204	210	216	222	229	235	242	249	256	263
33	158	163	168	174	180	186	192	198	204	211	216	223	229	236	242	250	256	264	271
34	162	168	174	180	186	191	197	204	210	217	223	230	236	243	250	257	264	272	279
35	167	173	179	185	191	197	204	210	216	223	230	236	243	250	258	265	272	279	287
36	172	178	184	190	196	203	209	216	223	230	236	243	250	257	265	272	280	287	295
37	177	183	189	195	202	208	215	222	229	236	243	250	257	265	272	280	287	295	304
38	181	188	194	201	207	214	221	228	235	242	249	257	264	272	279	288	295	303	312
39	186	193	199	206	213	220	227	234	241	249	256	263	271	279	287	295	303	311	320
40	191	198	204	211	218	225	232	240	247	255	262	270	278	286	294	302	311	319	328
41	196	203	209	217	224	231	238	246	253	261	269	277	285	293	302	310	319	327	336
42	201	208	215	222	229	237	244	252	260	268	276	284	292	301	309	318	326	335	344
43	205	212	220	227	235	242	250	258	266	274	282	291	299	308	316	325	334	343	353
44	210	217	225	232	240	248	256	264	272	280	289	297	306	315	324	333	342	351	361
45	215	222	230	238	246	254	262	270	278	287	295	304	313	322	331	340	350	359	369
46	220	227	235	243	251	259	267	276	284	293	302	311	320	329	338	348	358	367	377
47	224	232	240	248	256	265	273	282	291	299	308	318	327	338	346	355	365	375	385
48	229	237	245	254	262	270	279	288	297	306	315	324	334	343	353	363	373	383	394
49	234	242	250	259	267	278	285	294	303	312	322	331	341	351	361	371	381	391	402
50	239	247	255	264	273	282	291	300	309	319	328	338	348	358	368	378	389	399	410
51	244	252	261	269	278	287	296	306	315	325	335	345	355	365	375	386	396	407	418
52	248	257	266	275	284	293	302	312	322	331	341	351	362	372	383	393	404	415	426
53	253	262	271	280	289	299	308	318	328	338	348	358	369	379	390	401	412	423	435
54	258	267	276	285	295	304	314	324	334	344	354	365	376	386	397	408	420	431	443

BMIs above 30 have increased mortality and risk for a host of diseases. A BMI of 30 *roughly* means the person is 30 pounds overweight. The new federal obesity guidelines define **overweight as a BMI of 25 to 29.9. Obesity is defined as a BMI of 30 and above.**[4] BMI can be estimated by the new 1998 height/weight table which we have reproduced on the adjacent page. It is important to remember that weight/height BMI tables cannot tell you whether weight comes from muscle, fat, bone, or water. Nor can they evaluate fitness or fatness! They should only be used for preliminary screenings and estimates. If your BMI places you in a danger zone, a more precise measurement should be made to determine your exact fat percentage.

Body Shape & Obesity As A Risk Assessment

As we are often reminded, obese people seem to be grouped into one of two primary body shapes — **apples** or **pears**. These body shapes can help predict the development of heart disease, strokes, and a host of other conditions. These two shapes are determined by where fat deposits accumulate on a person's body. The pear shape, referred to in medicine as *gynecoid obesity*, shows less health risks and is seen primarily in women. It is also called *female type obesity*. Pear shapes tend to accumulate fat around the lower body on the hips, thighs, and legs.

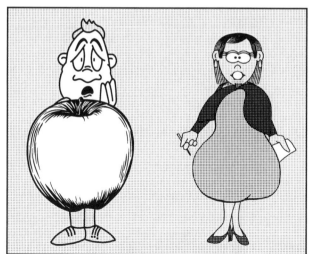

Apples and Pears
Apple shapes (android obesity) are predominantly seen in men. They tend to accumulate body fat in the mid-section and upper part of the body. The apple-shaped person has the greatest health risks because of the high metabolic activity level of fat in the abdominal region. Pear shapes (gynecoid obesity) are predominantly seen in women. Fat accumulates on the hips, thighs, and legs of people with pear shapes.

Those people whose fat accumulates on the hips, mid-section, and upper body tend to take on a "rounded," apple-shaped form. This apple-shape is referred to as *android obesity*. More men than women are apple shaped, so android obesity is sometimes referred to as *male pattern obesity*. The most serious medical problems tend to be seen mainly in the android, or apple-shaped, group.

Central to the problem of android obesity (the apple shape) is abdominal fat. Although a large stomach is obvious, what is not so apparent is that a tremendous amount of fat is located inside the abdomen of apple shaped people. The intestines and the *omentum* (a tissue covering the intestines) are two abdominal areas that accumulate high amounts of fat. This abdominal fat is metabolically very active and poses a major health risk. Intra-abdominal fat is intimately involved with the serious diseases associated with obesity. Later chapters will discuss the reasons for this.

Assessing Abdominal Fat

Because it poses such a risk to health, abdominal fat is evaluated in people who exceed recommended BMI standards. The simplest method used to measure the amount of abdominal fat is **waist circumference**. The inches around a person's waist can be used as a simple, but some-what unreliable, indicator of health risk. The 1998 federal guidelines

The "Humor" Of Obesity

Obese people are a frequent target of attempts at humor. Fat people seem to be the only group of people remaining in America who can be still be discriminated against. "Jokes" about the obese seem to be especially acceptable if they contain put downs of a region of the country. Down south, there is a lasting stereotypical joke still told about men with apple-shaped, android obesity. They are said to have Dunlop's Disease. A man with Dunlop's Disease is simply described as, "his belly done lopped over his belt." A noticeable feature of this problem is that the center of their rear end is usually visible riding high above their underwear which is typically sticking out of old blue jeans at least one size too small. A clever commercial poster depicts this aspect of Dunlop's Disease. It shows the backside of a large man sitting on a ball field bench. Below the man's exposed expanse is printed, "say no to crack." It is also occasionally described in the South as "biscuit and gravy poisoning."

state that women's risk for the development of diseases increases when waist size is 35 inches and up. Men with waist sizes 40 inches or more show increased risks. Health risks are especially high when both BMI and waist size exceed the standard levels.

Waist-To-Hip Ratio

Another easy and fairly reliable measurement for determining risk from abdominal obesity is a **waist-to-hip ratio**. It is the waist circumference measured at the belly button divided by the circumference of the hips at their widest spot.

Waist-To-Hip Ratio = waist in inches/hips in inches

The resulting number (the ratio) indicates the degree of "apple shape" and the presence of abdominal fat. For example, a woman with a 37 inch waist and 47 inch hips has a 0.79 ratio (37/47 = 0.79).

Women with ratios above 0.8 and men above 1.0 are at greatest risk. (The higher the number, the greater the "apple" shape tends to be — indicating higher risks.)

Determining Body Fat Percentage: Some Techniques Are Precise, Some Aren't

Up to this point, we have covered the simplest and most common measurement techniques. They are primarily used as quick screening tools (a simple risk assessment) to determine how a given person compares to others in terms of height, weight, or girth. Newer and far more accurate body fat measurement methods exist, and obesity specialists typically employ at least one of them to precisely determine body fat percentage.

The most important thing to keep in mind about the modern definition of obesity and fatness is that the problem is not one of weight. It is a fat problem. The percentage of body fat is too high. *Thus, knowing the exact percentage of body fat on each individual patient is extremely impor-*

tant to physicians who sincerely seek to treat obesity. The primary goal is to reduce health risks by reducing body fat percentage. Body fat percentage can be calculated in many different ways. Unfortunately, these measurement techniques range from the simple to perform (but yielding somewhat inaccurate and unreliable results) to more cumbersome or expensive measurements that have significantly greater accuracy.

The Most Common Body Fat Measurement Methods: Simplest But Least Accurate

The most frequently used method of calculating body fat percentage is measuring skin fold thickness with calibrated calipers. The second most frequently used method is measuring the circumference of certain body areas (wrist, neck, waist, upper arm, etc.).

After taking a person's measurements, both of these methods adjust for the individual's height. Then, using a mathematical formula to manipulate the numbers, presto-change-o, a body fat percentage emerges.

The primary problem with both methods is in reliability. Measurements differ depending on who is taking them and when they are taken. Even the same person making repeated measurements will often demonstrate inconsistent measurements. Some diet/fitness programs market calipers in their product lines, but they are likely a waste of the typical person's money, time, and effort. Accurate and reliable estimates of body fat percentage with calipers or measuring tape requires some training and skill. Even then, the method can be marginal at best, yielding approximations varying from 90% to 97% in accuracy. Perhaps that seems satisfactory, but it isn't to medical specialists.

Bioelectrical Impedance: A Better Method For Determining Body Fat Percentage

A fairly easy method for determining body fat percentage is through bioelectrical impedance. In this procedure, electrodes are placed on predetermined places on the body or the patient may be asked to stand on two electrodes with bare feet. A mild current is sent through the electrodes and the body's resistance to the current is measured. Body fat is a poor conductor of electricity while fat-free body tissues and bones are good electrical conductors. (Body fluids and electrolytes account for this.) The technique determines the amount of fat free body mass. Body fat percentage is easily calculated by subtracting the fat free mass from total body weight.

At first glance, bioelectrical impedance might appear to be completely accurate — but it, too, has some problems and stipulations. Individuals should have eaten a light meal 2-4 hours prior to being measured by the device. In addition, no exercise is allowed for the previous 24 hours. Body water content and potassium levels (K^+) effect electrical conductivity adding some unreliability to this technique.

Consumers can now buy fairly cheap ($100 or less) home versions of bioelectrical impedance scales. These scales measure weight and give a read out of body fat percentage when you stand on the electrodes with bare feet for a specified period of time. The reliability of these depends upon the quality of the scales as well as one's ability to rigidly follow the stipulations each time a measurement is taken. Used correctly, these impedance scales can accurately reflect fat-reducing progress. Measurements should be taken the same time each day under the same conditions.

Precise Measures of Body Fat Percentage

The "gold standard" for obtaining body fat percentage has long been *underwater weighing* (also called *water displacement*). The technique is cumbersome and has been employed mainly by academic research institutes and some specialized (and expensive) obesity treatment centers. The patient is first accurately weighed (dry). Next, he or she is carefully seated in a tank of water on a special chair. A weight belt is attached. The person expels as much air from the lungs as possible and then completely submerges for almost 10 seconds. (Air in the lungs changes both volume and weight.) The person is then weighed underwater and the amount of water displaced by the body is recorded. This is repeated up to 10 times to get a good average of underwater weight and water displacement. We won't go into the complex calculations employed to come up with body fat percentage, but the key to understanding it is simple — fat floats, the rest of the body sinks.

Underwater weighing is extremely accurate with people whose body fat percentages fall into the range of 4% to 30%. Outside of that range it loses some accuracy. In addition, the technique is too cumbersome, time consuming, and intrusive for patients treated in a routine medical office practice. Finally, young patients, older patients, and those who have difficulty submerging themselves in water (especially after exhaling) further restrict the use of underwater weighing.

Advanced, Accurate Fat Percentage Measuring Methods

A newer tool for measuring body fat percentage is the Bod-Pod®. This expensive piece of equipment is ideally suited to routine office measurements of body fat percentage. The Bod-Pod® uses the same principles of displaced volume employed in underwater weighing. However, the Bod-Pod® displaces air rather than water. A computer controls the device and accurately calculates body fat percentage. It yields accurate and reliable results and can be used in a gym or small office. It requires minimum space and is much easier to use for most patients — especially the elderly, very heavy patients, and those with water anxieties.

All clothing except underwear has to be removed prior to entering the Bod-Pod®. The Bod-Pod® measures volume, so clothing and even hair can give false readings. After a tightly fitting bathing cap is donned, the patient simply sits in the sealed pod for a few moments and exhales when told. The main disadvantage of the Bod-Pod is its high cost.

Another new instrument is the DEXA®. DEXA® is a type of X-ray machine capable of measuring body fat percentage directly. It can also measure bone density — as it was initially designed to do. It is very easy to use and yields accurate and reliable results. The amount of radiation the patient is exposed to is so low that no shielding is required. It is ideally suited to a physician's office, but high cost is a major factor.

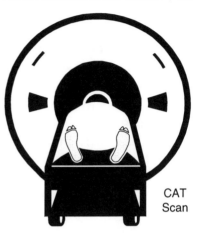

CAT Scan

A few other accurate ways of measuring body fat percentage exist and merit mention. Magnetic Resonance Imaging (MRI) is an excellent procedure that shows body fat in specific tissues and can accurately measure fat percentage. But MRI equipment costs about $1.5 million and requires a large, shielded area for safe operation. Each test can cost over $1,000, which is a major limiting factor to both the physician and the patient.

Computer Axial Tomography (CAT) Scans are almost as accurate as MRI in obtaining body fat percentage. CAT scans are a computer-driven series of x-rays that produces significant levels of radiation limiting repeated measures and requiring shielding. Cost and space factors also limit the use of CAT scans.

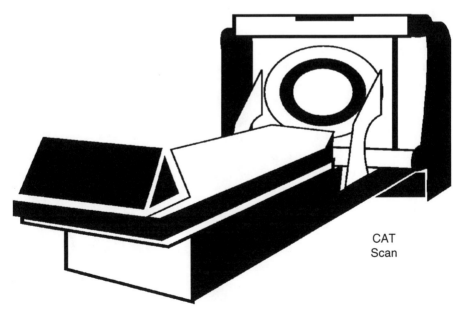

CAT Scan

Precise Body Fat Percentage Measurement Is Important To Assess Health Risks: Summary

There are several reasons why this chapter presented various techniques that estimate or measure body fat. First, keep in mind that obesity isn't really a weight problem. It's a fat problem that is evaluated in two broad ways. The most important way is in measuring exactly how much fat is present — expressed in body fat percentage. Recall that the ideal percentage of body fat for men is about 15%-17% while for women it is 24%-26%. Obesity is present when body fat percentage reaches 36% in women and 26% in men. A person's health risks increase as body fat percentage increases above the "ideal" or normal range. Health risks rapidly escalate when body fat percentage reaches the diagnosis of obesity. Physicians should do more than a quick estimate of BMI or utilize an inaccurate body fat measurement technique. Precise measurement of body fat percentage can give both the patient and physician enough information to yield a realistic and accurate health risk assessment, indicate exactly how much fat should be lost, and provide accurate and consistent feedback on progress (much like cholesterol tests).

Many patients go to physicians for "over-

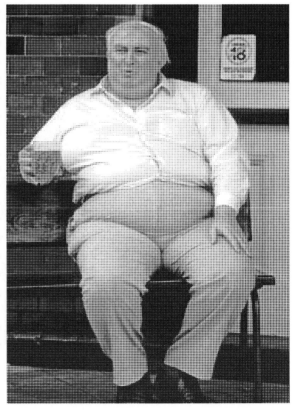

What do your eyeballs
tell you?

weight" problems. They are typically weighed, their BMI is estimated, they are "eyeballed" for overall shape, blood pressure and a brief history are taken. Sometimes blood tests are done. The physician may discuss how much weight should be "lost" by the patient, hand them a brief diet plan, and give them a prescription. Many patients have come to expect this routine and, when it varies, it can cause anxiety. In addition, some patients simply don't really want to know — exactly and precisely — how much fat they carry around. Thus, physicians who use precise measurement techniques for body fat are sometimes avoided. Patients may find the Bod Pod® unusual and water-weighing cumbersome. Even many health professionals who have weight problems don't understand why a precise measure of body fat percentage is desirable. They typically don't know that body fat, not weight, is the important issue. Patients can take an important cue from the information presented in this chapter. Avoid practitioners who tell you that obesity is simply a matter of weight. Look for specialists who use techniques that precisely measure body fat percentage.

Chapter References & Notes

[1] Atkinson, R. (1992) Treatment of obesity. *Nutritional Reviews,* 50, 338-345.

[2] Pamuk, E., Makuc, D., Heck, K. Reuben, C., & Lochner, K. (1998) *Socioeconomic Status and Health Chartbook. Health,* United States — 1998. Hyattsville, MD: National Center for Health Statistics.

[3] Fraser, L. (1997) *Losing It: False Hopes and Fat Profits In The Diet Industry.* New York: Plume.

[4] National Institutes of Health (1998) *Clinical Guidelines on the Identification, Evaluation, and Treatment of Overweight and Obesity in Adults.* Washington, DC.

[5] Stunkard, A. J. (1985) In: R. E. Hales & A. J. Frances (Eds.) *American Psychiatric Association Annual Review.* Washington: APA Press.

[6] Black, et. al. (1992) Prevalence of mental disorder in 88 morbidly obese bariatric clinic patients. *American Journal of Psychiatry,* 149, 227-234.

[7] Body Mass Index is also referred to as the "Quetelet" index.

[8] It helps to use a small calculator to compute BMI. It can be calculated two ways. The first method uses metric measurements that requires changing inches and pounds to meters and kilograms. Here we give an example of calculating the BMI of a 217 pound man who is 5 feet 10 inches tall. BMI is calculated by starting with a person's weight in kilograms (kg). One kilogram is about 2.2 pounds. Our 217 pound man weighs 98.6 kg (217/2.2 = 98.6). Next, the height of the man needs to be calculated in meters (m). One meter is about 39.4 inches. Our man is 70 inches tall (5'10"). His height is 1.78 meters (70/

39.4 = 1.78). Finally, we need to square (multiply by itself) the height in meters. This gives us 3.17 (1.78 X 1.78 = 3.17). The BMI is computed by dividing the kg weight by the height in meters squared (W_{kg}/H_m^2 = BMI). The BMI of the 217 pound, 5'10" tall man is 31.1 (98.6/ 3.17 = 31.1).

The second method for measuring BMI leads to the same results. The weight in pounds (217) is divided by the height in inches squared (70 inches X 70 inches = 4900) with the result multiplied by 704.5: 217/4900 = .0442857 X 704.5 = 31.1.

[9] S. C. Wooley, & O. W. Wooley (1984) Should obesity be treated at all? In: A. J. Stunkard & E. Stellar (Eds.) *Eating and its disorders*. New York: Raven Books.

[10] Consensus Development Conference (1985) Health implications of obesity. *Annals of Internal Medicine*, 103, 1073-1077.

[11] P. Ernsberger, & P. Haskew. (1987) *Rethinking obesity: an alternative view of its health implications*. New York: Human Sciences Press. This book reviews obesity-related health research up until the mid-1980s. It clearly shows how much of the research was flawed and indicates that, at the time, there wasn't a true consensus on the health risks of obesity.

[12] Many statistics books have used smoking and health problems as an excellent example of using correlation to prove causation. Smoking has long been known to be related to health problems, but whether it actually caused them was very difficult to prove. Edward Brecher's (1972) *Licit & Illicit Drugs* (Consumer's Union) reviews the long-term history of smoking problems and the slow march made by science to prove causality.

[13] J. T. Doyle, et. al. (1964) The relationship of cigarette smoking to coronary heart disease. *Journal of the American Medical Association*, 190, 886-890.

[14] For those interested, the internet site maintained by the National Institutes of Health contain the complete report and other related features. The web address to access this information is www.nhlbi.nih.gov/nhlbi/cardio/obes

[15] S. K. Powers, & S. L. Dodd (1996) *Total fitness: exercise, nutrition, and wellness*. Needham Heights, MA: Allyn & Bacon.

[16] D. G. Myers (1992) *Psychology*. New York: Worth Publ.

Chapter 5
DOES BODY FAT CAUSE HEALTH PROBLEMS?

(Fat) ... is really a most harmless, healthful, innocent tissue. ... The fat man tends to remain fat, the thin woman to stay thin — and both in perfect health — in spite of everything they can do.
— Woods Hutchinson, **Cosmopolitan (1894)**

Chapter Summary — Until recently, the question of whether too much fat causes health problems has been argued vigorously. While a fair number of obese people are healthy and lots of thin people are unhealthy, the basic facts are simple. In general, obese people have significantly more health problems as compared to normal weight people. But whether fat in and of itself causes these problems has been debated. Research begun in 1948 — and still in progress — has followed large groups of people over their lifetimes discovering many important health facts. For example, this research found that high blood pressure triggered heart attacks and caused increased risk for strokes. It also uncovered the relationship between cholesterol and heart disease. This same research was the first to prove that exercise and increased activity levels lowered the risk for heart disease and that being overweight increased the risk for heart disease. Obesity has subsequently been classified as a "risk factor" for the development of many other diseases.

While obesity is clearly linked to an increased risk for developing other diseases, it also increases mortality rates. In general, the more severe the level of obesity, the higher the death rate. For example, moderately obese people, those whose weight exceeds their "standard weight" on BMI charts by 30%, show a 35% higher mortality rate than do people whose weight is in the standard range. Morbidly obese people have an astonishing 1000% increase in death rates.

Up to 20% of all deaths in America are related to obesity. Obesity increases the risk of developing at least 26 diseases. Heart disease is the major cause of obesity-related deaths and is very strongly linked to weight. High blood pressure, strokes, high cholesterol levels, and high triglyceride levels are also linked to obesity.

The development of adult onset diabetes (now called type 2 diabetes) is strongly associated with obesity. A set of diabetes-related problems is also linked to obesity. These include impaired tolerance to blood sugar, insulin resistance, hyperinsulinemia, and leptin resistance. Unfortunately, once these problems develop, they set in motion a series of bodily changes that can lead to even more weight gain (e.g., the body stores more and more fat). This increased level of fat, in turn, worsens blood sugar, insulin, and leptin problems resulting in even more fat storage. And on and on this cycle goes.

Obese women tend to suffer from menstrual cycle irregularities and other endocrine problems. PolyCystic Ovary Syndrome is a hormone-related disease that is more often associated with obesity than not.

The risk of developing various cancers escalates as obesity level increases. In men, the development of colorectal and prostate cancer is linked to obesity. In women, the development of breast cancer, uterine cancer, and ovarian cancer is linked to obesity.

Obesity is also implicated in rheumatoid arthritis and osteoarthritis. Gout, a painful inflammation of the joints, is obesity-related as are various other arthritic conditions.

A number of sleep and breathing disorders stem from obesity. These include sleep apnea, shortness of breath, and a substantially lowered lung capacity.

Reflux esophagitis (heartburn) is related to obesity and some of the poor eating habits that often accompany the disease. The obese have increased levels of various skin disorders as well as higher accident risks.

The good news is that weight loss and exercise can lower a person's risk for these diseases as well as alleviate symptoms. Even moderate weight loss lowers the risk of developing all of these diseases and lessens the severity of symptoms in people who have already developed some of them. Greater weight loss tends to result in even more improvement and lowered risk levels. Increasing one's activity level also improves all of these conditions.

Gallbladder disease is strongly related to obesity — especially in women. Almost a third of obese women will develop gallbladder disease by age 60. Gallstones, formed by crystallizing cholesterol in the gallbladder, are often painful and can require surgery. However, rapid weight loss — especially through liquid, very-low-calorie diets and gastric bypass surgery — increases the risk of developing gallstones by 4% to 6%. Anyone attempting to lose weight rapidly should take notice of this. Obese people who have pre-existing gallstones should be extremely cautious and thoroughly discuss weight loss plans with a physician.

In deciding whether to lose weight or not, the risk of developing an obesity-related disease should be evaluated. Most of these diseases "run in families" and have a genetic component. Thus, if your family has a medical history showing these diseases, your risk for them is probably elevated. If you already have obesity-related diseases, you should understand that losing weight tends to result in improvement of all of them with the sole exception of gallstones.

While most people seem to recognize the health benefits of weight loss and regular exercise, few actually take sustained action to make appropriate changes. Why? We believe that people place their health relatively low on their list of priorities. Many will deny this although their behavior and habits demonstrate that lots of other things are more important than health. A pattern of excuses such as, "Tomorrow I'll start my diet and exercise, but today I'm going to rest and indulge myself," seems to develop in the vast majority of people. When tomorrow actually comes around, the same excuse is used. "There's always tomorrow," seems to be the rule. But for some people, tomorrow doesn't come. We truly understand this excuse cycle and the rationalization underlying it because we've used it. We want you to recognize the risks obesity poses in lowering quality of life and shortening lifespan.

Psychological issues and life-long habits are intimately related to both weight problems and our resistance to making changes. These issues must be confronted in genuine attempts to permanently alter life-style. However, in assessing the urgency to lose weight and increase fitness, a number of questions should be considered. These include your age, the chances of future health problems, the presence of obesity-related disease, and the issues of happiness and quality of life.

F • • •

or many years, controversy has swirled around the question of whether being fat, in and of itself, *causes* health problems.[1] As stated by the quote at the beginning of this chapter and in the chapter on the history of obesity, fat has not been considered a health problem until relatively modern times. Increase in life span and improved medical treatment are the main factors in our recent observations linking obesity to health problems. If fat does cause medical problems, at what exact point of "fatness" do these health problems arise? Some professionals question whether medical providers should treat obesity. For example, as recently as 1984, Susan and Orland Wooley wrote that the health risks often cited as related to obesity are probably overstated and that some treatments for obesity are actually harmful. The Wooley's suggested that the best approach to obesity is to do nothing.[2] However, in 1985, the National Institutes of Health termed obesity a "killer disease" encouraging weight loss for people 20% above their standard weight.[3]

As a result, increased attention is being shown to the health problems of obesity and Americans are gradually becoming aware of the risks. If you are overweight, you are among at least 80 million other Americans. At any given time, about 40% of adult women and 25% of adult men are dieting — continually trying to shed unwanted pounds.[4] Until very recently, medical guidelines categorized 39% of adult women and 36% of adult men as overweight.[5]

Literally thousands of studies have investigated the links between weight and health, with some results seeming to be contradictory and conflicting.[6] But it should be recognized that medical research progresses rapidly with controversies being resolved and some research becoming outdated. Lots of *current* diet and fitness books still cite dated research on obesity and the controversy over health problems accompanying obesity. Many of these books fail to acknowledge newer findings. The outdated and obviously biased information presented in many weight and diet books has caused confusion among the multitudes of people worrying about their weight problems. And you should keep in mind throughout this book that worry is essentially useless.

The Health Implications Of Obesity Are Becoming Much Clearer

The links between obesity and health problems *are* certainly complicated. They are also difficult to understand. Some obese people are very healthy and physically fit. Some thin people are unhealthy and physically unfit. **Yet it is true that obese people, in general, have more physical health problems as compared to people whose weight (and body fat percentage) fall into the normal range.** At the same time, we know that many health problems have a strong genetic component. So, does obesity itself actually cause any health problems?

The controversy over obesity and health problems is similar to another historical health controversy — cigarette smoking. Cigarette smoking is responsible for causing a host of health problems. Yet medical science was unable to prove that cigarette smoking actually caused health problems until fairly recently.[7] The research problem is often described by statisticians as *correlation doesn't mean causation.*

When researchers say things like, "health problems are related to obesity or smoking," they are usually citing findings from correlational studies. Correlational studies are used to find meaningful relationships between events and facts, but this type of research can't discover for certain whether one event *actually causes* the other. When studies use terms like "related to," "associated with," or "correlated to," they are almost always citing results from correlational research.

Cigarette smoking was long known to be related to (correlated with) a host of physical diseases, but the correlations didn't adequately prove that smoking caused the problems. In fact, cigarette companies even advertised smoking as a health-promoting activity sometimes stating that some brands were used by physicians. Celebrities such as Lucille Ball and Ricky Ricardo appeared in television ads touting health benefits. The tobacco industry cited research showing that many cigarette smokers didn't develop health problems and occasionally argued that people who developed health problems would have developed them whether they smoked or not. What would normally be required by science to prove that cigarette smoking caused disease would be an unthinkable experiment. A group of healthy nonsmokers would have to be randomly assigned into two groups: one group would not smoke while the other would be forced to smoke at a predetermined level. If cigarette smoking caused health problems, over time, the smokers would develop a lot more health problems than the nonsmokers. Since an experiment of this type couldn't be done, it took decades of clever correlational studies to prove causality.

Obesity research is currently in a position similar to that of smoking research perhaps 30 years ago. If we could take a large group of healthy, average weight people and then randomly assign them into two groups we could easily resolve lots of important issues. If we could force one of the groups to become obese while the other was forced to stay at a "normal" weight — and then look at their health problems over the next 30 years or so — we'd be able to show exactly what problems the extra fat caused. We could also look at the effects of exercise, fitness, diet, and more. But, of course, we can't do this. What has been done is the next best thing. Researchers have followed large groups of people over their lifetimes carefully recording their diets and behavior while measuring health problems.

The Framingham Study

In 1948, a National Institutes of Health group recruited 5,209 residents of Framingham, Massachusetts to participate in a long-term study designed to uncover what had caused a sudden increase in heart disease and stroke in Americans after World War II. Every two years, the residents were interviewed and given a physical examination. In 1971, another 5,124 Framingham residents were entered into the study. Over 1,000 research studies have been published based on the Framingham study. Much of what we know about diet, obesity, and the development of many diseases has been uncovered by this research. In fact, the relationship between cigarette smoking and heart disease was one of the most important early findings from the study[8] and the term "risk factor" was itself coined in 1961 as a result of this study. Some of the relevant findings from Framingham research include:

- **High blood pressure triggers heart attacks and increases stroke risk**
- **High levels of blood cholesterol increase heart attack risk**
- **High-density lipoprotein (HDL) in the blood lowers heart disease risk**
- **Physical exercise lowers the risk of heart disease**
- **Being overweight increases the risk of heart disease**
- **Diabetes is a cause of heart disease**

Framingham Study

In 1948, when very little was known about what caused heart attacks and strokes, the National Heart Institute sent researchers to Framingham, Massachusetts to recruit volunteers for an ambitious research project. The town was chosen because it was considered to be fairly representative of the U.S. population, however, almost no Blacks were included in it. The goal was to discover the causes of heart disease and strokes. A total of 5,209 men and women between the ages of 30-62 were recruited — none of them had suffered heart attacks or strokes. Life-style interviews, lab tests, and physical exams were given to each subject every two years. In 1971, another 5,124 people were added to the study. These were the original subjects' adult children and spouses. Boston University now has primary responsibility for the ongoing study. Over the past 50 years, over 1,000 articles have been published from data gathered at Framingham. Much of what has been proven in medical science (the negative effects of cigarette smoking, secondhand smoke, psychological issues related to heart attack and high blood pressure, cholesterol, and obesity; the beneficial effects of exercise and weight loss) comes from this research.

Current Medical Consensus On Obesity And Health Problems: Obesity Causes Increased Mortality From Many Related Conditions

Recent medical research confirms what most obesity treatment specialists have long proposed: **obesity is intimately related to the development of various health problems.** In addition, the loss of weight by obese people results in a lessening of physical problems. The 1998 National Institutes of Health guidelines contain excellent summaries of obesity-related health problems.[9] Each of these health problems will be briefly reviewed here.

It is important to remember that *obesity causes increased mortality* (early death). The increased mortality rate in obese populations is caused by a host of obesity-related physical problems and diseases. Perhaps just as important, though, is that *weight loss decreases* these problems and decreases the risk of mortality. The significance of these facts to the reader is simple. If you are deciding whether or not you should lose weight, the presence of health problems would be a factor in this decision. Overweight people who already have some of the health problems associated with obesity would probably find that losing weight would result in better health. Losing weight tends to decrease many health problems and increase the lifespan of obese people.

Another factor in making informed decisions about weight loss is family history. Obesity and many of its health problems have a strong genetic component — these conditions tend to run in families. If members of your immediate family have had a history of weight-related health problems (especially diabetes, heart disease, high blood pressure, and stroke) you should consider yourself at a higher than average risk for developing the same problems. Losing weight lessens that risk.

How overfat a person is (as diagnosed by the level of obesity present) is a predictor of future health problems and mortality. Body fat percentage, discussed in the prior chapter, is the most precise way to determine obesity level. The modern idea is that the presence of other health problems in a person who is also obese, significantly increases the need for weight loss.

Obesity & Its Associated
Health Risks, Diseases, and Problems

"Obesity increases the risk for at least twenty-six diseases."[10] The National Institutes of Health (NIH) conclude that somewhere between **15% to 20% of all deaths in America** are caused by obesity-related disease.[3] Health risk assessments performed on obese patients include screening for the presence of a wide range of various diseases, familial background, behaviors related to activity level, and habits. Each disease could be caused or worsened by obesity, increase the health consequences of obesity, and also measure the risk of mortality.

In making statements regarding obesity-related risks, the NIH utilized BMI "standard weight" charts rather than body fat percentage. This is because, as the prior chapter discussed, body fat percentage is generally too difficult to assess for most physicians. But all physicians have a set of scales and a ruler. So, for the sake of simplicity, risk statements are typically given in terms of how much over the standard weight a given person is. For example, men who are at least 20% above their standard weight on BMI charts show a lifetime 20% increase in death rates from any cause. What this means is that obese men have a 20% greater chance of dying in any given time period than do normal weight men. As the level of obesity increases, the mortality risk increases even more rapidly. Later chapters will discuss some of these diseases and disorders in greater detail. Only a brief synopsis of obesity-related problems is presented here.

Coronary Heart Disease

The increased risk for early death in obese persons comes mainly from coronary heart disease. High cholesterol levels and elevated blood pressure are both closely related to blood vessel damage in the heart and sudden deadly heart attacks. Although heart disease, blood vessel disease, and high blood pressure occur in normal weight people, they are all seen to increase in many, if not most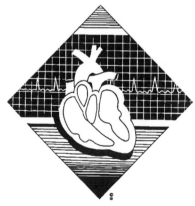

people, as their body fat increases. Individuals whose weight exceeds their standard weight on BMI charts by 30% have a 35% increased risk of death. People whose weights are 50% higher than the standard weight have a 50% increased death rate. The morbidly obese (weights double their standard or 100 pounds over it) show an astonishing 1000% increase in death rates (a rate 10 times greater than "normal" weight people).

High Blood Pressure & Stroke

High blood pressure is related to obesity. The NIH summary panel evaluated 76 studies finding "strong and consistent evidence" that reducing weight can reduce blood pressure. There is some evidence that abdominal fat (apple shapes, android obesity) is also related to high blood pressure. A reduction in fat in the abdomen lowers blood pressure in some people. Regular aerobic exercise also reduces blood pressure. Obese people (20% above standard weight) show a 10% increased risk of deaths from stroke. Obese adults aged 20-45 are six times more likely to have high blood pressure than normal weight adults the same age.

Elevated Cholesterol & Triglycerides

Elevated levels of total cholesterol, LDL (bad cholesterol), and triglycerides are associated with obesity as are low levels of HDL (good cholesterol). The NIH panel evaluated 65 studies researching these factors. Losing weight lowers total cholesterol, LDL, and triglycerides as well as increasing HDL. Regular aerobic exercise also aids in these beneficial changes.

Type 2 Diabetes & Blood Sugar Levels

The NIH panel evaluated 49 research articles investigating diabetes and blood sugar (glucose). Obesity is associated with higher blood sugar levels and the amount of abdominal fat is associated with impaired glucose tolerance. Insulin resistance, hyperinsulinemia (high levels of insulin), and leptin resistance all seem to be coupled to obesity. These conditions, in turn, may cause the body to store even more fat. The increased level of fat worsens the insulin resistance, hyperinsulinemia, and leptin resistance leading to more and more fat accumulation. This self-perpetuating cycle appears to be present in a fairly large percentage of obese patients seeking treatment. (A later chapter will examine impaired glucose tolerance, insulin resistance, and diabetes in more detail.)

Obesity, especially apple-shaped, android obesity, increases the odds of a person developing **non-insulin dependent diabetes mellitus** by a factor of 10. This is now simply referred to as **type 2 diabetes** (also formerly called **adult onset diabetes**). It typically occurs in an overweight person after age 40. Some people do develop the disease at an earlier age, but a genetic component is often present. In Type 2 diabetes, the pancreas does not produce sufficient insulin or the body has become resistant to insulin. In insulin resistance, the pancreas has to produce increasing amounts of insulin to maintain normal blood sugar levels. Insulin facilitates the passage of sugar circulating in the bloodstream into the body's cells (fat and muscle cells). Sugar (glucose) is the primary energy source for muscles and the brain. Thus, when high blood sugars are evident, this is probably a strong sign that a problem with insulin action is present.

Uncontrolled type 2 diabetes can cause blindness and kidney failure. Blood vessel problems can often occur in the extremities and especially the legs, sometimes leading to gangrene requiring amputation. These circulation problems can also cause skin ulcers or bruises that don't heal.

Insulin resistance is lessened by weight loss and exercise. Some people with insulin resistance have normal blood sugar levels, but many don't. Weight loss lowers insulin resistance in both obese people who have type 2 diabetes and obese people who do not have diabetes. Reducing abdominal fat may reduce glucose intolerance and lessen insulin resistance. Exercise combined with weight loss improves glucose tolerance and can aid in type 2 diabetes.

Weight loss, exercise, and control of diet can markedly improve the condition of the diabetic person. Obesity and inactivity are keys to declining health in patients with type 2 diabetes.

Endocrine Abnormalities

Obesity in apple-shaped women causes menstrual cycle irregularity and other menstrual abnormalities. Pregnant women who are obese show numerous increased risks including high blood pressure and blood abnormalities. Obesity in young girls hastens initiation of menstruation (the first menstruation is termed *menarche*).

There is also strong evidence that obesity in women can lead to abnormally high levels of the hormones androstenedione and testosterone. These are male sex hormones that stimulate the ovaries and the pituitary gland to produce other hormones at abnormally high levels. Infertility, amenorrhea, and excess body hair can result. The disease *PolyCystic Ovary Syndrome* (PCOS) is intimately associated with insulin resistance and abnormally high insulin levels (hyperinsulinemia).

Cancer

Cancer risks escalate as a person becomes overweight and obese. Obesity in men is related to the development of colorectal cancer and prostate cancer. In women, obesity is linked to the development of breast cancer, uterine cancer, and ovarian cancer. Upper body fat in menopausal women (the apple-shape) is strongly related to breast cancer. It is not known exactly how obesity relates to increased cancer development, only that it does.[11]

Arthritis And Joint Conditions

Arthritis is a painful inflammation of the body's joints. *Rheumatoid arthritis* is caused by an overproduction of certain antibodies that attack other antibodies in the joints causing inflammation. Obesity is related to the development of rheumatoid arthritis.

Uric acid is often found present in elevated levels in overweight people, and the elevated levels of uric acid crystals cause *gout* — a painful inflammation of joints. Studies show that the risk of developing gout is about double for obese people. In addition, inflammation in weight-bearing joints, like the knee, can be caused by excess weight. *Osteoarthritis* is also associated with obesity. Patients with osteoarthritis have been shown to have increased problems with weight-bearing joints. An unexplained observation is that these 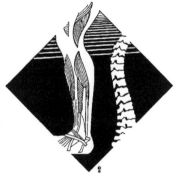 same patients can also have increased problems in nonweight-bearing joints. Many overweight middle age women suffer from osteoarthritis of the knee. Other arthritic conditions occur in obese people in their hips, feet, back, and spine. Weight loss will significantly reduce these symptoms.

Respiratory/Sleep Impairment

Many obese men and some women suffer from *obstructive sleep apnea* (OSA). In sleep apnea breathing can be obstructed during sleep for a minute or more. The lowered oxygen level in the bloodstream is sensed by brain centers that cause the person to briefly awaken and loudly snort

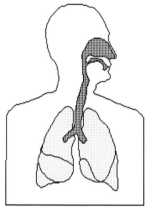

in air. The loud snorting sounds like snoring, but is far more serious. People who suffer from sleep apnea can briefly awaken literally hundreds of times each night, but the awakenings aren't usually remembered. During the day, the sufferer is chronically sleepy and tired but is seldom aware of the cause.[13] Weight loss usually lessens the problem substantially.

Many obese people also suffer from *shortness of breath* and a *lowered lung capacity*.[11] This can markedly impair exercise ability and even simple movement to the point where small physical exertions are extremely difficult. Obesity causes resistance to the lungs' expansion and total lung volume is reduced. In short, breathing becomes increasingly difficult as the level of obesity increases. Weight loss results in substantial improvement in both sleep disturbances and respiratory problems.[11]

Miscellaneous Health Problems

Reflux Esophagitis occurs in increased levels in obese patients. Reflux Esophagitis is also called *heartburn*. It is an unpleasant sensation in the chest caused by stomach acids "leaking" into the esophagus due to an anatomy structure change. A muscle where the esophagus connects to the stomach normally acts like a valve closing off the esophagus from

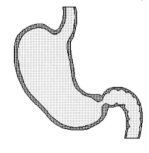

the stomach. When reflux occurs, the muscle isn't properly working and the stomach acids backflow up into the esophagus. The symptoms are similar to a heart attack and are often quite painful. It is a sometimes difficult-to-treat disorder that is worsened by obesity and eating prior to sleep. Weight loss and sensible eating habits greatly lessen the symptoms.

Obesity is also related to an *increase in accidents*. Many obese people are accident-prone resulting in physical injuries.[14] Finally, obesity causes skin folds and stretching, the development of fatty skin tags (especially on the neck and under the arms), and other minor problems.

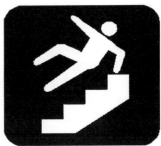

Gallbladder disease

Gallbladder disease is strongly related to obesity. Obese women aged 20-30 show a 600% increased chance of developing gall bladder disease and almost 33% of obese women will develop gall bladder disease by age 60. The gallbladder lies under the liver where it stores bile. Gallstones form when the liver secretes substantial amounts of cholesterol into the gallbladder. The cholesterol forms crystals as it lumps together and various salts harden the stone. In many obese people the liver produces too much cholesterol. The excess cholesterol becomes oversaturated in the gallbladder leading to the stones. From that information, you might conclude that losing weight reduces the risk of developing gallstones. But that's not the case.

People who lose weight rapidly increase the risk for developing gallstones. *"Gallstones are one of the most medically important complications of voluntary weight loss."*[12] Very-low-calorie diets (800 calories or less each day often taken in liquid forms) are especially related to gallstone problems. Research has shown that between 10% to 25% of obese people who lose weight on very-low-calorie diets develop gallstones. About 67% of these were "silent" gallstones — that is, they produced no symptoms. But the remaining third suffered symptoms with many requiring surgery. *"In short, the likelihood of a person developing symptomatic gallstones during or shortly after rapid weight loss is about 4 to 6 percent."*[12]

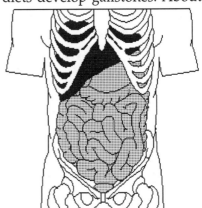

No one knows what effect weight cycling (yo-yo dieting) has on gallstones. In addition, exactly why the risk of gallstones increases with very low calorie diets is not understood. Researchers speculate that restrictive "dieting may cause a shift in the balance of bile salts and cholesterol in the gallbladder.... If the gallbladder does not contract often enough to empty out the bile, gallstones may form."[12] Enough research on the relationship between the nutrient composition of diets and gallstone formation has not been conducted to clarify what causes the increased risk. It is speculated that "some very-low-calorie diets may not contain enough fat to cause the gallbladder to contract enough to empty its bile. A meal or snack containing approximately 10 grams of fat is necessary for the gallbladder to contract normally."[12]

What are the implications of this particular medical problem to the obese? First, becoming obese clearly increases the risk of developing gallbladder disease. However, once a person is obese, if weight loss is rapid, the risk of gallbladder disease increases even more. This finding is not only present in very-low-calorie diets, but also occurs with gastric bypass surgery. Some research shows that more than a third of patients who had gastric bypass surgery develop gallstones — most within a few months post-surgery. The NIDDKD (National Institute of Diabetes and Digestive and Kidney Diseases) asserts that the other health risks of obesity are so serious that the increased risk of gallstones is frequently worth taking. Obese patients with pre-existing gallstones should be cautious and always check with their physician before embarking on diets. Finally, it is strongly suspected that more gradual weight loss methods won't produce the same gallbladder disease risk as rapid weight loss. Thus, restrictive diets producing rapid weight loss should perhaps be avoided by many, if not most, obese patients.

Do You Need To Decrease Fatness? What Are Your Risks?

Health risks can increase a person's motivation to lose weight and become fit. If you have already developed obesity-related health problems, we'd ask you, "How much more motivation do you need? How much worse does your condition need to be?" But too many people wait until they actually develop serious physical problems before they make genuine efforts to manage their weight and fitness level. We have discussed this observation among ourselves many times, and believe that a couple of important factors account for it. First, physical health is not the number 1 priority in most obese people's lives. Many people will say that it is, but their behavior contradicts their words. We have reasons without number for failure to be physically active. There are countless reasons for eating the wrong foods and overeating. Many of us struggling with weight make endless promises to ourselves: "Tomorrow I'm going to start my diet; tomorrow I'll exercise." Health is important, but not as important as work, home, family, television, cheesecake, chips, and candy. Sometimes the cost of treatment seems too high. People will balk at spending $40 a month for necessary medicines, but they won't hesitate to spend that much on cigarettes, cable TV, or sodas. One of the things you must do is truly assess your priorities in life. Work and family are important — perhaps they are the most important things in your life. But where does your physical health fit into your priorities? If you suddenly have a heart attack or a stroke, won't your priorities change just as suddenly?

If the health problems described in this chapter are present in your close relatives (such as parents, siblings, grandparents) then you probably have an increased risk of developing them too. Losing weight and becoming fit lessen almost all of these risks. But if your behavior shows that the possible future health risks are outweighed by the desire — or the habit — to simply stay the way you are, chances are that you won't change even if these health problems develop.

Why Isn't Health A Higher Priority?

Part of the difficulty people have in making health a higher priority is that health problems from obesity seem to be remote possibilities somewhere in an ill-defined future. They aren't in the here-and-now. Putting things off one more day doesn't seem to be all that bad. Besides, you've put it off before and here you are. "There's always tomorrow."

You've probably never heard anyone say, "I was wrong, there wasn't a tomorrow." Perhaps you've already guessed why. They were dead. Dead people aren't generally known for coming back and telling others how that "last time" was *really* their "last time." Unfortunately, that's how it is with many severely obese people. They put off exercise, reasonable dieting, and confronting health problems. Each day they wake up fully aware of their plight, but because they've awakened every day in their life, they expect to awaken tomorrow. "Tomorrow I'll walk and start my diet," they say to themselves as they continue to watch television and eat themselves to death. It's all rationalization, flimsy excuses to maintain eating and habits of inactivity. We recall times in our lives where we knew we were young and health problems seemed only a possibility in an ill-defined future. It was easy for us to make empty promises to change tomorrow — or maybe the next day. We've been there too, and we still struggle with life-long excuses and rationalizations. It may well be a fundamental human trait to put off making changes that drastically effect behaviors like eating and leisure. But if severe, life-limiting health problems — or early death — are probable outcomes of staying the same, making changes seems the smartest and most sensible course.

Confronting The Underlying Psychology And Behavior

Another essential problem in making beneficial changes is that obese people often have deeply ingrained habits that go in the exact opposite direction of those required for health. Inactivity, eating the wrong foods, eating too much, avoiding confrontation with eating-

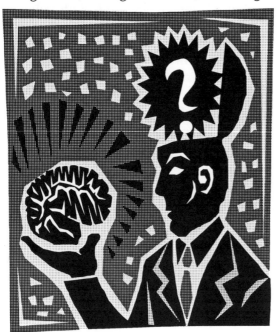

related stress and emotions, and delaying healthy behavior are all deeply ingrained habits. Breaking life-long habits is difficult for everyone. We all have a built-in psychological resistance to making certain changes in our habits and daily routine. In addition, some people have unresolved conflicts from childhood, personality and emotional problems, and relationship problems. All of these can impact weight, daily routines, and a person's efforts to make changes. The chapter on psychological issues discusses these in more detail.

Questions You Should Ask Yourself

In making judgements about what you should do, first consider your weight. Look at the Body Mass Index chart in the prior chapter. Are you "large" and in the danger area? Are you overweight or obese? What is your age? Age matters, because the older you get, the greater the chance that you may develop an associated health problem. Do you have gallstones? Would you really be happier if you lost weight and became fit? Would it enhance the overall quality of your life? Finally, honestly assess your health risks and current health problems. Keep in mind all of the health problems associated with obesity that were discussed in this chapter. Then you have to make a real decision about what to do. As we stated in chapter 2, you should either decide to accept the condition or take charge of it so that you can manage it. Worrying about it isn't the same thing as actually doing something.

Health Costs Of Obesity

"In 1990, the Nation's health goals for the year 2000 were set forth with the release of *Healthy People 2000*, in which a national goal to reduce the prevalence of overweight was articulated. ...In 1993, the Deputy Assistant Secretary for Health (J. Michael McGinnis) and the former Director of the Centers for Disease Control and Prevention (William Foege) coauthored a journal article, 'Actual Causes of Death in the U.S.' It concluded that a combination of dietary factors and sedentary activity patterns accounts for at least 300,000 deaths each year, and, obesity was a key contributor."[15]

The August 1999 issue of the *American Journal of Public Health*[16] cites data indicating that 5.7% of direct health care costs in the United States are due to obesity. This represents $52 billion each year. Taking into account the total lifetime health costs of individuals, about 4.3% of all health care spending is due to obesity. The added costs of lost or reduced job productivity, increased insurance premiums, disability and other spending due to obesity are incalculable.

Obesity costs money in other ways, too. If you calculate your total spending on all food, snacks, fast-food, and all dietary or exercise aids for obesity you will understand how it impacts your wallet.

Chapter References & Notes

[1] Fraser, L. (1997) *Losing It: False Hopes and Fat Profits In The Diet Industry.* New York: Plume.

[2] S. C. Wooley, & O. W. Wooley (1984) Should obesity be treated at all? In: A. J. Stunkard & E. Stellar (Eds.) *Eating and its disorders.* New York: Raven Books.

[3] Consensus Development Conference (1985) Health implications of obesity. *Annals of Internal Medicine,* 103, 1073-1077.

[4] Atkinson, R. (1992) Treatment of obesity. *Nutritional Reviews,* 50, 338-345.

[5] Pamuk, E., Makuc, D., Heck, K. Reuben, C., & Lochner, K. (1998) *Socioeconomic Status and Health Chartbook. Health,* United States — 1998. Hyattsville, MD: National Center for Health Statistics.

[6] P. Ernsberger, & P. Haskew. (1987) *Rethinking obesity: an alternative view of its health implications.* New York: Human Sciences Press. This book reviews obesity-related health research up until the mid-1980s. It clearly shows how much of the older research was flawed and indicates that, at that time, there wasn't a true consensus on the health risks of obesity.

[7] Many statistics books have used smoking and health problems as an excellent example of using correlation to prove causation. Smoking has long been known to be related to health problems, but whether it actually caused them was very difficult to prove. Edward Brecher's (1972) *Licit & Illicit Drugs* (Consumer's Union) reviews the long-term history of smoking-related problems and the slow march made by science to prove causality.

[8] J. T. Doyle, et. al. (1964) The relationship of cigarette smoking to coronary heart disease. *Journal of the American Medical Association,* 190, 886-890.

[9] For those interested, the internet site maintained by the National Institutes of Health contain the complete report and other related features. The web address to access this information is www.nhlbi.nih.gov/nhlbi/cardio/obes

[10] S. K. Powers, & S. L. Dodd (1996) *Total fitness: exercise, nutrition, and wellness.* Needham Heights, MA: Allyn & Bacon.

[11] M. A. Alpert & J. K. Alexander (Eds.) (1998) *The Heart and Lung in Obesity.* Armonk, NY: Futura Publishing Co.

[12] *Dieting and Gallstones.* (1998) National Institutes of Health; National Institute of Diabetes and Digestive and Kidney Diseases Fact sheet. www.niddk.nih.gov

[13] D. G. Myers (1992) *Psychology.* New York: Worth Publ.

[14] D. W. Jones (1999) What is the role of obesity in hypertension and target organ injury in African Americans? *American Journal of Medical Science,* 317, 147-151.

[15] National Institutes of Health (1998) *Clinical guidelines on the identification, evaluation, and treatment of overweight and obesity in adults.* Washington, DC: NIH (publ. # 98-4083).

[16] Allison, D. B., Zannolli, R., & Narayan, K. M. V. (1999) The direct health care costs of obesity in the United States. *American Journal of Public Health,* 89, 1194-1199.

Chapter 6
UNDERSTANDING
THE OBESITY PUZZLE
AS A WHOLE

Society is unforgiving of the overweight individual. ... Historically,
the public has believed that weight loss is a matter of willpower.
...findings suggest that physiological and genetic factors may limit the
amount of weight that an individual can lose and maintain. These
findings have led to a new empathy for overweight individuals...
— Drew Anderson & Thomas Wadden, *Treating the Obese Patient*
Archives of Family Medicine (1999)

Chapter Summary — The visual image presented in Chapter 1 of obesity as being similar to trying to swim upstream against a strong current depicts all of the pieces of the obesity puzzle. Biological, genetic, and medical factors are symbolized by being trapped in the river. Social and psychological issues are symbolized by the influence of other people on the overweight person in the river. Exercise and diet are represented by the sustained and prolonged effort required to move up the river and maintain progress. The rapid movement back downstream each time the obese person stops swimming symbolizes the essential nature of the problem: it is a chronic, life-long disease. People with the disease never arrive or stay at the place they want to be without ongoing, life-long effort.

Medicine views obesity as a disease, yet many physicians and the majority of the public still see it as a failure of will-power or a character flaw. Even most obese people don't fully comprehend the essential nature of the disease as evidenced by their attempts to cope with it in a temporary, piecemeal manner. Obesity is not a puzzle comprised of rigid pieces as diet, exercise, and pop psychology books would have you believe. Obesity does break into understandable pieces, but the pieces aren't independent of each other. The complex puzzle that comprises obesity is actually a unified whole that only appears to be made up of pieces. When people focus their weight loss efforts on only one apparent piece of the problem, their effort is destined to fail. Looking at the puzzle in an unusual way may be helpful.

If you think of the puzzle as a star-shaped balloon you can grasp the essential problem. Each point of the star-shaped balloon represents a different aspect (or what appears to be a separate piece) of obesity. If a person squeezes one of these points, that area will seem to get smaller because air is forced into other areas of the balloon. The increased pressure in the other areas isn't noticeable to the person doing the squeezing because the balloon is so large. In addition, it's not obvious to most people that the pieces of the puzzle aren't really pieces. Instead, they are actually interconnected into a whole that is flexible. When the person quits squeezing a point of the balloon, the increased pressure in the other areas causes air to rush back in taking it back to its original shape.

What this means is that all of the areas making up the obesity puzzle have to be adequately addressed to produce the desired result. These areas are the genetics and biology of obesity, a person's diet, their activity level, underlying social and psychological factors, and an understanding that a life-long effort is necessary. People struggling with weight must have some understanding of the relevance of each of these areas to their individual situation. The most appropriate starting point is the biological and medical component.

● ● ●

In Chapter 1 we presented a visual image of the plight of obese people. If you remember that image, you know that when an obese person tries to lose weight, it's a lot like trying to swim upstream against a strong current. In addition, the further up the stream the person goes, the stronger the current can get. Small lapses in swimming, getting tired, or getting distracted usually result in being quickly rushed downstream. (These are all called relapses.) In addition, there was a social aspect to the swimming image. While other people would sometimes encourage the person in the river to keep swimming, they still somehow blamed the swimmer for every lapse. In addition, some people ridiculed the swimmer for even getting into the river in the first place. Although these other people lack a fundamental understanding of the situation, their encouragement, disappointment, blaming, and ridicule have a powerful psychological effect on the swimmer. People caught in the river's current psychologically absorb the occasional overt sarcasm directed at them as well as the more subtle taunts and looks of disappointment they constantly experience. Shame, guilt, self-esteem problems, a sense of hopelessness, and expectations of failure are a few of the psychological problems gradually developed in many, if not most, obese people. As a result of the earliest childhood taunts and cruel sayings directed at overweight children, as well as the stares and occasional mocking received in adulthood, many overweight people develop a personality style that gradually becomes self-defeating. In addition, some overweight people 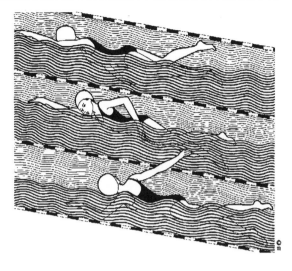 have even deeper psychological scars and issues that contribute to obesity in ways few people understand.

The Puzzle Pieces: Each Must Be Addressed

Diets Don't Work — But Diet Is Very Important

It shouldn't be surprising that the vast majority of people who diet to lose weight are destined to diet again. Virtually every text and scientific review of the results of dieting show us that at least 95% of dieters regain the weight. A person's diet represents only one piece to the remarkable puzzle of obesity. Dieting alone seldom results in permanent weight loss. Yet, one's diet (as opposed to dieting) plays a central role in permanent weight loss. Part of the problem is that people tend to see diets as temporary. Diets are an "eating restriction" a person begins with the expectation that they will eventually return to normal eating. But the truth is that people who lose weight on a temporary diet will regain the lost weight. Another part of the diet problem is that people just don't know what to eat. Dieting books give conflicting suggestions. We also believe that the generally accepted view of healthy eating (as exemplified by the USDA's Food Pyramid) gives overweight people the wrong advice.

If Exercise Make Us Feel So Good, Why Don't We Do It More?

Most people who start exercising regularly to lose weight eventually fall back into their habitual, day-to-day patterns of inactivity. This puzzle piece (exercise), although extremely important, is still just one piece of the puzzle. For both psychological and biological reasons, very few people establish a regular exercise routine after decades of relative inactivity. We are told that exercise makes us feel better. Yet lots of overweight people who start exercising don't feel better. The problem is that it takes an extended period of time with regular exercise for the "feeling good" part to kick in. In general, the more overweight a person is, the longer is this time period. Unfortunately, during the initial period of establishing an exercise routine, it can, and often does, make us feel worse. In this case, doing nothing can seem to be preferable to doing anything at all. Complicating things even more are the rigors and stresses of real-life responsibilities that always seem to be (we hope) acceptable excuses for not exercising. Despite the problems and complications of establishing exercise routines in the obese, a person's level of physical activity plays a central role in permanent weight loss.

Psychological Factors, Habits, & Attitudes

In addition to the underlying psychology of obesity briefly mentioned in the beginning of this chapter, another complicating factor revolves around the habits that have been ingrained in the individual's basic personality beginning in infancy. A person's eating style, food preferences and dislikes, times and frequency of eating, emotional eating, and even the places where a person eats all become habitual. These habits are established very early in life typically by well-meaning adults who essentially force the infant — and later the child — to adopt the same eating-related habits they have. Life-long habits established this early in life are extremely difficult to change. They stem from attitudes and beliefs that are seldom thought about — much less confronted. In addition, a person's leisure activities, exercise routines, hobbies and interests, work routines, overall level of physical activity, ways of handling stress and conflict, and style of living in a competitive world gradually establish themselves as routines. That is, they are repeating patterns of day-to-day behavior — habits — that begin to develop in early life.

Despite the importance of psychological factors, dismal outcome results are found when overweight people enter psychotherapy or counseling to deal with the underlying emotional and behavioral issues. Dealing with the psychological factors is important, but it too represents only a single piece of the puzzle. It's true that some people eat for emotional reasons and that lots of other psychological factors come into play. It's also true that basic information about diet and activity is needed and making planned behavior change is necessary. Yet most patients want to try only one approach. If a person's behavior patterns and underlying issues are not directly confronted, that person will eventually slip back into those old behavior patterns despite trying to control weight through other means (e.g., diet, exercise, medicine, etc.).

Underlying Biological & Medical Issues

People who take drugs or various "natural" diet aids also usually find that the drugs and diet aids, in and of themselves, seldom lead to the desired result over the long-term. Again, we find that attempts to deal with the underlying biological problems through drugs represent a single — though essential — piece to the puzzle. People in America have come to expect quick fixes and all of us look for easy solutions to problems. Medical science has not found a magical pill or treatment approach that results in rapid weight loss and maintenance. It may someday, but as yet there is no magic formula. What medicine does have is an array of medications that can help with the problem if the patient cooperates by complying with the physician's other suggestions. Yet most patients who come in to physician-run weight loss clinics hope (and sometimes expect) to see a rapid loss of weight from just popping a pill or two every day. The pills can be a real aid to many people. But medicines are just an aid — not a solution or cure. Patients come back and complain that the pills only helped them for a brief time. Yet these same patients will admit that they haven't done any of the other things suggested to them. They will go on to admit that they ate the same things as usual and didn't exercise because they wanted the pills to do all of the work. Many also resist attending non-threatening counseling, nutrition, or behavior change classes for lots of reasons. The most frequent excuse is lack of time.

The medications used with obese populations and on associated eating disorders are helpful in fat reduction and may be necessary to maintain weight loss. The many physical and health complications of obesity require a thorough assessment and identification of possible underlying physiological problems that contribute to the problem. Medicines can then be selected and tried based on each patient's unique needs. Medicines can address various related conditions such as diabetes and insulin disorders, binge eating, depression and stress, low metabolic rate, hormone problems, as well as targeting the absorption of fats and carbohydrates. Despite this wide range of medical interventions, patients have become accustomed to a "one size fits all" approach when they visit diet clinics.

Weight & Health Management Are Life-Long Issues

A very interesting category of patients observed in diet clinics are those who are successful at losing large amounts of weight. Some of them have lost more than a hundred pounds over a year or so while others lose lesser, but significant amounts. In general, these patients all took medicines specifically prescribed for their unique problems, developed a reasonable diet they could live with and actually enjoy, increased their activity level somewhat, and dealt with related personal issues. What's really interesting is this. After perhaps one or two years of success, many of them come in and express the desire to get off all medicines, go back to some of their old eating habits, and reduce their activity level. In addition, some say that they have resolved all of their underlying issues so it's not necessary to discuss them any more. Some of these people follow through with their expressed desire. Six months or a few years later, they reappear at the clinic guilty, ashamed, and embarrassed. We're certain you know what they look like: they regained all of the weight — and often even more.

It may be a difficult pill to swallow, but the fact is that weight and health management are life-long issues. This is true not just for the obese, but for everyone. All aspects of obesity are life-long. In this book, we have been calling each aspect a puzzle piece. But in reality, they are interconnected and so intertwined that they form a single disease — the disease of obesity. The life-long characteristic of obesity is perhaps the most difficult aspect to integrate into treatment. Yet without it, the vast majority of obese people are doomed to a repeating cycle of weight loss and weight gain.

Why We Keep Repeating
The Same Mistakes

Most people place the blame for weight problems on the over-weight person. It's his lack of will-power, his gluttony, his laziness, or his stupidity. None of this is fundamentally true. Everyone struggles with health and other issues throughout their life but these struggles are usually hidden from view. Being fat is something that can't be hidden from view. It's noticeable. The obviousness of the obese person's problem is a major factor in the discrimination, guilt and shame that accompanies it. As human beings we all struggle. We all tend to repeat some mistakes. Some people struggle with the same problems their entire life — only we don't see it.

Several factors come into play which help explain why we repeat the same health-related mistakes. First, as stated in the prior chapter, we have given other things in our lives higher priorities than we give health. We also have only so much time and energy available to deal with a particular problem. Unfortunately, that seems true with lots of impor-tant aspects of our lives — even life threatening ones. Many of you have visited a hospital or home and encountered a patient who was suffering from a smoking-related lung disease. You may have been astonished to see the patient take the oxygen tubes out of his nose in order to smoke a cigarette. This was fairly common in hospitals back in the days when smoking was foolishly permitted there. Why do some people do this? In part because smoking is a higher priority than health to lots of people. Of course, smoking is an addiction, and most addicts place their drug of choice as the highest priority in life. Some people make work a higher priority than their family. They may deny it, but when they miss one important family event after another because of extra work, their priority becomes obvious. Other people make sexual stimulation a priority over a stable marriage. Having a new car can be a higher priority than paying for good health insurance. This list could be endless.

Many of us want to take the easiest way out of our problems. That certainly doesn't seem unreasonable or stupid at first glance. But what if the easy ways fail over and over again? People want to deal with weight loss in only one way (i.e., just dieting or just taking medication). An important explanation of this is that we have been conditioned to do so.

Go into a large bookstore and look at the diet section. You'll see hundreds of diet books each touting its specific approach. Some focus primarily on protein, or fat, or carbohydrates. Some promise quick weight losses through extreme diet plans like eating nothing but cabbage soup or grapefruit. Yes, you'll lose weight quickly, but you'll put it back on even quicker. People have been conditioned to trust books, but that has been changing. It's no wonder that a backlash against the diet industry has occurred. Books with titles like *"Diets Don't Work"* sell huge numbers because most dieters have tried most diets. Books tend to focus on only one aspect of the "weight" problem. "Love Yourself Thin" books spouting pop psychology are popular, yet they miss the big picture. Exercise books are accurate, but they are ineffective for the bulk of the obese population. Exercise tapes are great, but they get old and boring after 60 or 100 viewings. People buy hundreds of thousands of copies of exercise tapes like Billy Blanks' *Tae Bo*. It's a great workout tape. In fact, one of us uses it regularly. However, it is simply unrealistic for the typical obese person to expect to start doing such stringent exercise after years of inactivity. If you don't believe this — just ask them. Yes, some obese people do manage to do it. But out of every 100 obese people who get a stringent exercise tape, how many use it and manage to lose weight? Not many. The few that do often end up on television telling others how it worked for them. The silent majority is not mentioned or acknowledged.

Obesity Is A Disease

The simple fact is that obesity is a disease. Yes, it has many other factors effecting it including a strong addiction-like aspect that we haven't yet addressed. Tell us what disease doesn't have several components. Medicine accepts obesity as a disease, yet many doctors and other health professionals can't seem to translate that knowledge into appropriate action. Most people continue to levy blame totally on the obese person for his or her fatness. "Eat less and exercise more" remains the standard response to the obese person's plight. But the reality isn't that simple. It's like telling a life-long smoker that if he quits smoking his emphysema will go away. It might get better, but it's not likely to go away. The disease of obesity cannot be treated by attending to only one or two of its components. It's simply too large and complex. Obesity is a chronic, relapsing disease and it must be viewed that way by both the patient and the health care provider in order to effectively treat it.

Why We Typically Fail To Maintain Weight Loss: Seeing The Obesity Jig-saw Puzzle As It Really Is

This chapter has briefly reviewed each of the components comprising what we call the obesity disease puzzle. The next chapters present an in-depth review of each of the specific pieces of the puzzle. Later chapters fit these pieces together and show the actions necessary for genuine, life-long fitness and weight management. But for now, we'll try to explain why the puzzle hasn't been adequately understood.

As you begin to understand the multiple factors related to obesity, you must keep in mind that all are equally important and that each one must be addressed in creating a unified, coherent plan of action that will work for you. This is why almost all people struggling to lose weight cycle through periods of momentary success followed by disappointing rapid weight gain. The fundamental problem is that these people become overly influenced by only one aspect of the obesity puzzle. For example, a person might decide to rigidly diet to lose weight. Rigidly dieting will result in weight loss — at least in the short term. But the problem is that there are many other, equally important areas that influence weight. When these areas aren't adequately addressed, they precipitate certain adjustments that result in an eventual return to the original state of obesity. This is not as difficult to understand as it may seem.

If you visualize obesity as a massive jig-saw puzzle, you can quickly grasp what's really happening. The key to understanding it is this: We usually think of such puzzles as being made of

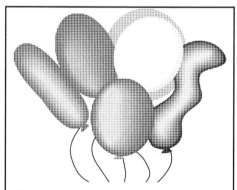

The obesity puzzle sometimes seems to be a bunch of independent pieces that don't fit together, but that is deceptive.

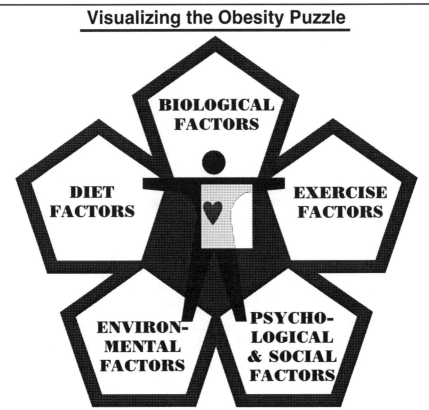

Visualizing the Obesity Puzzle

BIOLOGICAL FACTORS

DIET FACTORS

EXERCISE FACTORS

ENVIRON- MENTAL FACTORS

PSYCHO- LOGICAL & SOCIAL FACTORS

Pretend for a moment that this shape is the way the obesity puzzle actually looks. Imagine that it is large and complex — and difficult to look into — so it seems to be made of several separate, independent pieces fitted together. Now imagine that the puzzle is made out of filled balloons somehow attached together. (In fact, there are balloons made in this shape.) If you squeeze one of the 5 outer balloons, it gets smaller. But you don't realize that the air in it is actually forced out into the other balloons expanding them. When you quit squeezing, the air rushes back into the seemingly separate balloon snapping it back into its original shape. In reality, there is only one balloon with several interconnected extensions. It is almost an impossible task to deal with obesity by focusing on just one component of this complex, flexible puzzle. For example, obesity has at its core a biological, genetic basis. The genetics and biology represent just one of the interconnected puzzle pieces (it can sometimes appear to be the most important one in some people). It's debatable if the genetic and biological factor represent the most important piece, but it is certainly the area that has the greatest impact on physical health and mortality. Understanding the biological basis of obesity is the first step in solving the obesity puzzle.

rigid pieces that fit tightly together. But that's not the way it is with this puzzle. Visualize this jig-saw puzzle as being constructed of interconnected, filled balloons. These balloons are connected to each other and are flexible. Air can move from one balloon to another — but the connection isn't obvious because it can't be seen. If you focus on any one of the balloons by tightly squeezing it, it seems to get smaller—especially in the place where you are applying pressure. Because it's such a big puzzle, you can't see what's happening to all the other interconnected balloon pieces when you are putting pressure on only one of them. What happens to the balloons is easy to visualize. The balloons that aren't being squeezed are expanding, adjusting their shape and form to compensate for the pressure being applied elsewhere. In other words, the pressure in all of the unsqueezed areas increases. As soon as the pressure subsides on the other part of the puzzle, the entire puzzle snaps back to its earlier shape.

The flexible puzzle idea is a good visual representation of obesity. It explains why someone who has lost weight by rigidly dieting tends to replace all of the weight very quickly. If dieting is the only method used to lose weight, it's exactly like squeezing on only one of the puzzle balloons. The diet can seem to be working while pressure is continually applied to that one area. But when the diet is stopped dieting (because enough weight has been lost or a lapse back to old eating habits occurs) an immediate rebound effect occurs due to the increased pressure the diet has caused in all of the other areas.

During the diet underlying biological imbalances may have been created. At the same time stress and anxiety may build and relationships could become strained. The dieter might also make plans for celebration when the desired weight is achieved. These plans almost always include eating a few foods that were "forbidden fruit" during the diet. A few other real-life examples may help you understand this. Many people who go on restrictive diets will feel tired. This eventually results in less physical activity and a bodily adjustment to burn less energy. A person who suddenly starts exercising heavily tends to get hungry and will often eat more to compensate for it. The person who takes diet medications often expects that the pills, by themselves, will take off weight. Therefore, he doesn't exercise, diet, or look at underlying issues. A person who goes on a low-fat diet usually starts eating more sugar and carbohydrates. A person who goes on a low carbohydrate diet tends to eat more fat. We could probably write a book about all of these destined-to-fail weight loss attempts, but we want to focus more on what will be successful. For now, it's essential that you fully accept the fact that obesity is a genetic, physical, metabolic disease with underlying behavioral, psychological, and social factors. All of these areas have to be managed to produce a life-long desired result.

Biological Factors Are The First Piece Of The Obesity Puzzle

The next chapter presents the facts about the genetic, physical, and metabolic aspects of the disease of obesity. Biological factors represent the first piece of the obesity puzzle. Biological causes represent the underlying genesis of becoming overweight and it is one of the least understood and most denied factors. One way of understanding why biological information is so important is to go back to the mental image of being trapped in a rapidly flowing river. You might ask, "Why me?" "How did I get trapped in this situation to begin with?" Biology and genetics represent a solid beginning to answering those questions. It also represents a good beginning for understanding how to escape it.

The Issue Of Simplistic Information

One contributing factor to obesity that is seldom, if ever, discussed is nutritional oversimplification. Almost every diet and nutrition book cites the energy value in fat as 9 calories per gram, with 4 calories coming from each gram of protein and carbohydrate. This information, while easy to remember, is a rounded average. Carbohydrates contain 4.1 calories per gram, while protein essentially has 4.2 calories per gram.[1] The difference between the commonly accepted 4 calories per gram and 4.2 isn't trivial (it is 5% too low). Over a year, this 5% difference can add significant calories. Various factors influence the actual caloric value of foods and how the body responds to them. The presence of insulin resistance, for example (discussed in chapter 8), causes a reduced response to carbohydrates leading to body fat accumulation. While we address insulin resistance, nutritional oversimplification is problematical. This issue is touched upon in chapter 15 and in **Appendix F**.

[1] McArdle, et. al. (1991) *Exercise Physiology: energy, nutrition, and human performance.* Malvern, PA: Lea & Febiger.

Chapter 7
BIOLOGICAL, GENETIC, AND MEDICAL ASPECTS OF OBESITY - PART 1

The role of inherited factors in the development and
maintenance of obesity is only partially understood.
Claude Bouchard, *Obesity* — 1992

Metabolic studies using identical twins have suggested that
genetic factors determine how much food energy is converted
into lean muscle, and how much is converted into fat.
Michael R. Cummings, *Human Heredity* — 1997

The number of genes and other markers that have been
associated or linked with human obesity phenotypes
is increasing very rapidly and now approaches 200.
Perusse, et. al., *Obesity Research* — 1999

Summary — Scientific research into the biology of obesity is progressing so rapidly that it is nearly impossible for anyone but specialists to keep up with it. What is being uncovered is the understanding that an incredibly complex system of hormones, brain mechanisms, and genes are responsible for the genesis of obesity. The typical person cannot possibly comprehend all of this scientific information. However, what needs to be understood is that taking a narrow view of treating obesity will not lead to desired long-term results. There are no secret cures, miracle diets, or magical supplements that make fat disappear. Buying into the empty promises of people making these claims will make you lighter, but only in your wallet or purse.

The role genetics plays in obesity is complicated and substantial. Hereditary characteristics passed along to us through our parents' genes accounts for as much as 70% of our body mass. Research using specialized groups of people has uncovered some of the most important findings. Ongoing research begun in 1965 with the Pima Indian tribe in Arizona has shown that some obese people have a "thrifty gene" pool. This set of genes ensured the survival of the Pimas in their hunter-gatherer culture up until the early 1900s when they adopted modern eating habits. These thrifty genes allowed their bodies to easily adjust to the cyclic "feast or famine" periods common to primitive cultures. It was an excellent survival mechanism. When food was plentiful, the Pimas would easily store energy as fat. When food was scarce, their body metabolism would slow down to conserve energy stores. Until the 1900s, the Pimas weren't fat, but when ample food became available to them, they suddenly became obese and diabetes levels rapidly increased. Their bodies couldn't make adjustments to the now-abundant quantity and quality of food. Many obese people no doubt share some of this "thrifty gene" pool with the Pimas.

The current number of genes and genetic markers directly linked to obesity number over an astonishing 200. Some of these genes are directly responsible for some cases of obesity through mutations and variations. Others produce their effects by interacting with the environment. For example, when the Pima tribe's food and cultural environment changed, obesity developed because of their basic genetic predisposition to store body fat and conserve energy.

Set point theory explains a genetic and biological process through which our body maintains a predetermined body weight. If a person attempts to lose weight below his set point, the body makes physiological adjustments to regain the weight. Set point is determined by numerous factors.

The body stores fat in fat cells (adipose tissue) that are able to expand and contract depending on the needs and circumstances of the individual. Genetics plays a role in determining the number and size of fat cells. Obese adults have up to five times as many fat cells as do normal weight people. Obese children have twice as many fat cells as their normal weight peers. In addition, many obese people have abnormally large fat cells. A hormone (called leptin) that regulates fat storage in these cells was identified in 1994 and several mutated genes that can cause obesity were found shortly thereafter.

When they become full, fat cells secrete leptin into the blood stream where it is transported to the brain. A small brain structure, called the hypothalamus, has special receptors for leptin that sense the rising levels of the hormone. In response to leptin, the hypothalamus then signals other brain areas (through other hormones and transmitters) to stop eating. Initially, researchers believed that obese people didn't produce enough leptin. Various studies showed, however, that obese people had too much leptin. The problem was in the inability of leptin to produce the "stop eating signal" in the hypothalamus. Defects in the genes responsible for producing leptin receptors and the leptin itself have been found to cause the malfunction. These genetic defects contribute to both obesity and diabetes. A host of other genes which produce many other hormones and hormonal receptor sites have also been found to contribute to obesity. These hormonal defects can produce faulty signals from the hypothalamus causing increases in appetite, increased fat consumption, and emotional eating. The hypothalamus is also a direct link in the brain's center of feeling, stress, and anxiety. The hypothalamus connects eating behavior and hunger to emotion.

Several neurotransmitters (brain chemicals that transmit messages) are also involved in obesity. Low serotonin levels, associated with feelings of depression, anxiety, and stress and also with obsessive-compulsive behaviors, produce overeating and binge eating. Dopamine, the neurotransmitter employed in the brain's pleasure centers, is also implicated. The pleasure centers in the brain are directly tied into the hypothalamus. All addictions are believed to be related to dopamine release. Overeating, binge eating, and emotional eating behavior are all influenced by the brain's dopamine system. All of these neurotransmitter systems are strongly influenced by genetics.

This chapter begins our presentation of biological and genetic factors. Many other important hormones and body systems are involved in obesity. Chapter 8 continues this discussion.

•   •   •

S cience is progressing at mind-boggling speed. Knowledge is expanding so rapidly that it is nearly impossible for a scientist to keep up in his or her own speciality. Scientists today are narrowing their speciality so much that the old joke about specialists, "I am learning more and more about less and less," has a great deal of truth to it. It's not a joke anymore. College textbooks are often considered to be "out-of-date" by the time they are published. Modern textbooks publish internet sites as "references" so readers can get up-to-date reports on research findings. We are listing various internet information sites in this book for the same reason.

With so many factors influencing obesity, how can you learn everything about such a complex area? The answer is simple. You can't. If you spent every waking hour reading research reports and surfing the internet, you couldn't read it all much less remember it all. But you don't have to know everything to change things. You only have to know enough. You only have to know what to do and why you are doing it.

During our research and information gathering phase for this book, we spent countless hours accumulating and reading thousands of studies. Dr. Milnor collected the summaries of over 2,000 *recent* medical research reports on the use of medications in treating obesity. These were printed out on a neatly piled stack of 600 sheets of paper. (At least it was neat when we started.) Our offices became strewn with journals, articles, books, textbooks, and thousands of printed downloads from university web sites. Dr. Little spent approximately 900 hours searching through scientific and medical web pages and untold more hours in libraries. We had thousands of new studies from psychology, psychiatry, fitness, health, diet and nutrition, and medicine. There were times when the only area accessible in our offices were the computer screens and printers so that more information could be pulled from web sites. Long days were spent going to conferences and pharmaceutical presentations on new drugs and drugs in process. Despite all of this work, we barely scratched the surface of this topic. The truth is that no one today knows *everything* in the field of obesity. We learned a lot — but not everything.

One thing we came to understand is that researchers and health practitioners in the field of obesity tend to work in relative isolation from each other. Diet and exercise/fitness specialists usually have a good working knowledge of each other's field, but most of them have scant up-to-date information on relevant genetics or endocrinology. Endocrinologists researching obesity tend to be out-of-touch with the issues patients face in real life. Almost everyone is out-of-touch with the psychological issues. (Even many psychologists treating obese patients only focus on how to get patients to eat less and exercise more.) The pharmacologists are busy doing what they do — developing and testing new drugs in the hope of discovering a magic pill that will make fat people slim and also make a ton of money. Infomercials tout one expert or another telling us that the "secret" to permanent weight loss is a special diet, a supplement, an exercise tape, a new exercise device, to eat no carbohydrates, no fat, no sugar, or just to love yourself. The secret is only $39.95, $49.95, or whatever the market will bear (plus shipping, of course). Everybody seems to be taking a narrow view of the problem. Meanwhile, overweight people keep making the same mistakes over and over again, in part, because of lack of knowledge — but also because we are programmed to seek the simplest solution.

As we have repeatedly stressed, obesity has several components. While a very few people do manage to overcome it by focusing on one or two components, the vast majority (probably 97% or so) continue their struggle every day. Unfortunately, they seem to feel like soldiers fighting a daily battle in a war they believe they'll never win. For these people hope does exist, but only if they go at the problem by attacking all of the pieces of the disease. The biological and physical aspects of obesity are the starting point of the attack. This is true because obesity is fundamentally a disease. We have to accept this fact, because obesity not only reduces quality of life, it's a killer.

Biological Factors Are The First Piece Of The Obesity Puzzle

This chapter presents the facts about some of the genetic, physical, and metabolic aspects of the disease of obesity. However, the biological aspects of obesity are so complex, we have devoted two chapters to this massive puzzle piece. The next chapter reviews insulin resistance, metabolic syndrome, and related issues.

Biological causes represent the underlying genesis of becoming overweight. It is one of the least understood and most denied factors. One way of understanding why this information is so important is to go back to the mental image of being trapped in a rapidly flowing river. You might ask, "Why me?" "How did I get trapped in this situation to begin with?" This chapter provides a solid beginning for answering those questions. It also presents a good initial understanding of how to escape obesity's traps.

The Genetics of Obesity

The April 1998 issue of *Life Magazine* contained a rather remarkable article titled, "Were You Born That Way?"[1] The article addressed the effect that genetics has on various human characteristics. One of the areas discussed was obesity. "Twin studies show body mass to be 70 percent heritable," the article stated. What does this mean? Is our "body mass" 70% heredity?

Your height, bone structure, width, and basic overall body shape is certainly genetic to a very great extent. The amount of muscle in proportion to fat is, to some extent, determined by heredity. Body fat percentage can be changed through exercise (like weight lifting) and diet, but there is certainly a strong genetic component to it. In general, body mass tends to be somewhat consistent in families. Children *tend* to eventually attain a height and weight that is fairly similar to their parents. Of course, parental eating and exercise habits are often passed on to children through learning. So, how do we know how much of body mass is genetic? The answer lies in several ingenious types of research.

One type of important genetic research has looked at twins. For example, a 1986 study[2] evaluated the height and weight of 1,974 pairs of Monozygotic twins (identical twins from the same egg with identical genetic makeups) and 2,097 pairs of Dizygotic twins (from 2 eggs, with similar, but different genetic makeup) all of whom had been born between 1917-1927. In addition, all 8,142 of these people (4,071 twin

Obesity And Genes

"The typical adult human body has 100 trillion cells, give or take some trillions. Each cell has the entire genetic code in it, laid out in 23 pairs of chromosomes. The genetic code represents a blueprint for the entire body. The DNA creates RNA, which, in turn, produces protein structures. All of the body including its organs, cells, hormones, and various transmitters are produced according to genetic instructions. The genetic code is comprised of a strand of amino acids roughly laid out in the shape of a ladder that has been twisted repeatedly. It may seem incredible, but if this strand was untwisted and flattened, it would be six feet long."[16]

Each DNA strand is made up of three billion components. The *Human Genome Project*, begun in 1988, set the goal of mapping the entire genetic code by the year 2005. That project has almost been completed. However, the mapping of the code does not mean that we will immediately know the exact function of each component. Research that uncovers the purpose of each gene will take somewhat longer.[17]

In 1999, the journal *Obesity Research* published an update on research regarding genes that influence obesity. Almost all of the chromosomes have multiple areas that relate to obesity. The article concluded, "The number of genes and other markers that have been associated or linked with human obesity phenotypes is increasing very rapidly and now approaches 200."[18]

It is very likely that many more genes will be found to relate to obesity. This makes the problem extremely complicated and reduces the likelihood that any single medicine will be developed that will cure obesity.

pairs) had been members of the armed forces. Their armed forces induction height and weight were compared to their height and weight 25 years later. Body mass indexes were calculated for each person and cross comparisons were made between twins. If the BMIs for the Monozygotic twins were very similar, and the BMIs for the Dizygotic twins were somewhat similar, the researchers could show how much of the similarity was due to genetics. Results from the study showed that a very strong genetic component *had* to be present in obesity.

The medical text *Human Heredity* (1997),[3] summarizes the results of obesity research from twin studies. This research has looked at all types of twins — including adopted twins raised in completely different family environments. In addition, it has evaluated the influence of heredity on obesity among siblings. One of these studies looked at 3,580 adopted children and made comparisons to all of their brothers and sisters — all of whom were raised in different homes. In summarizing the research, it is stated that, "75% of obesity is explained by genetic factors." Twin studies have pointed to various clues that may explain how genetics causes obesity. For example, specific genes determine each person's ratio of lean muscle and fat.[3] The distribution of fat on a person's body (apple *vs.* pear shapes) is known to be genetic.[4] Observations of groups of individuals can show us how strong the genetic influence actually is.

The Pima Indians

In the 1950s, health specialists began noting that the rate of diabetes and obesity among the Pima Indian Tribal Reservation in Arizona was increasing to alarmingly high rates. Diabetes, accompanied by obesity, was just then being recognized as a very serious health problem. Today, nearly half of Pima Indians age 35 and over have diabetes.[3] In the 1950s, American Indian health problems were many, and the focus of research was on the national problems of heart disease, stroke, and high blood pressure.

In 1965, the National Institutes of Health moved a research team to the Pima Reservation located just north of Phoenix. The researchers arrived not to study diabetes, but to make a comparison of the Pima's rheumatoid arthritis rates with those of the distant Blackfoot tribe. The researchers' attention was quickly diverted to another Pima health anomaly: the incredibly high rate of diabetes and obesity. The original study group of 4,000 Pimas has swelled to 7,500 with comprehensive physical evaluations and interviews conducted every two years. Hundreds of research articles have been generated from this ongoing project.

The Pimas are the most obese people in all of the Americas. When compared to the entire world, only a small Western Pacific tribe has

Genetics & Environment
How Their Interaction Can Cause Confusion

During the past century, the American diet has drastically changed. We are eating more fat, more sugar, and more calories. Food is plentiful and relatively cheap. During this same time period, the overall level of physical activity has gradually declined. The average person needs less calories today than in 1900. Modern conveniences and major changes in the workplace have significantly reduced our overall activity. Many people point to increased food intake and decreased level of activity as the primary causes of increased obesity levels. It's true that these factors are important causes of overweight and obesity. However, the influence of genetics is a far more powerful factor than is generally conceded.

Research shows us that obese people tend to require less calories per day than normal weight people. That is, obese people have a lower rate of calorie burn, pound for pound, than do people of normal weight. Genetics (e.g., the "thrifty gene pool") account for at least some of this problem. In addition, type 2 diabetes and its related syndrome of insulin resistance are especially apt to develop with higher intake of sugars and simple carbohydrates. A strong genetic factor underlies diabetes, insulin resistance, and leptin resistance.

The Pima Indians exemplify how environment and genetics interact. The Pimas' underlying genetics were well suited for survival in the hunter-gatherer society in which they survived for thousands of years. But when their life-style changed, their genetics led to an immediate increase in diabetes and obesity. Suddenly, after thousands of years of a highly active life and eating foods low in fat and sugar, the Pimas didn't have to expend much energy to get food. And the foods they now consumed were drastically different. The new environment in which the Pimas found themselves interacted with underlying genetic predispositions that had once been a strength — but was now a fatal weakness.

Many obese people share some of the genetic traits seen in the Pimas as well as having other genetic traits that lead to obesity. But unless these genetic traits are matched with a particular environment, the obesity (or diabetes, etc.) may never be revealed. It is an interaction between environment and genetics that leads to problems. The chapters on exercise and diet goes into these factors in detail.

higher rates of obesity than the Pima. Obesity and diabetes run rampant even among Pima youth.[5]

In the 1970s, University of Michigan geneticist James Neel researched the Pima. He noted that the problem of obesity didn't exist in the Pima tribe until the 1900s — when the Pima abandoned its hunter-gatherer culture and began adopting American eating habits. Yet the Pimas' level of obesity and diabetes didn't just reach the level of other Americans — it far, far surpassed it. Why?

Neel found that females who developed diabetes had become reproductively mature at an earlier age and that their babies were unusually heavy. These clues led Neel to speculate that a "thrifty gene" might be responsible. That is, the underlying genetics of the Pimas was designed to adjust for the cyclical "feast or famine" periods common to hunter-gatherer societies and therefore ensure their survival. It was an excellent survival mechanism. In times when food was plentiful, the Pima's body could easily store fat in preparation for periods of starvation. This "thrifty gene" served the Pima well when they were hunters and gatherers — and they didn't get fat. The problems of rampant obesity and diabetes in the Pima only developed when food suddenly became plentiful and easy to obtain. The Pima's body metabolism and fat storage mechanism couldn't adjust to the constant supply of food or get rid of excess fat. So, their bodies just kept adding more and more fat. (See related story in box.)

Neel continued to revise his ongoing research, and in 1982 proposed that insulin responses to food intake seemed to be the central factor responsible for fat accumulation. He believed that repeated release of insulin after consumption of refined carbohydrates gradually causes a reduction in insulin's ability to have blood sugar (glucose) burned for energy — so it is turned into fat.[3] This theory is extremely relevant and will be examined more fully in the next chapter.

Set Point Theory

It has long been observed that "body weight (or body fat) is regulated at a relatively constant level in much the same manner as body temperature, blood pressure, or blood glucose levels."[6] Each of us appears to have a genetically predetermined weight level. When a person attempts to go above or below this weight level, the body makes adjustments to return to the predetermined level. This weight level is called a "set point."

A person's set point is regulated by internal body-brain mechanisms that make ongoing changes to maintain a person's weight at his set point. People who actually lose weight at levels well below their set point typically find that they regain it all more easily than they lost it. People who have a low set point find that they tend to remain slim even when they eat more. Obviously, some people have a set point that is unhealthily high.

Set point theory is a valid observation, but it's probably not caused by a single process. In truth, it is becoming a more complex issue every day as more research is released. For example, prior to the voluntary withdrawal of the diet combination fenfluramine and phentermine (fen-phen) in 1997, the neurotransmitter serotonin was the major focus of media reports on obesity. Serotonin does play an important role in hunger and feelings of well-being, but it is probably not the primary controller of set point. Serotonin is more likely a regulator of hunger, satiation, and mood. In 1998 and much of 1999, the hormone leptin was regularly in the media and many people initially believed that leptin could be the set point regulator. Now, it is known that leptin's role is extremely complicated and involves various other mechanisms. As time goes on, more and more hormones involved in regulating hunger and satiation are being found. All of them seem to play important roles in both eating and set point. For example, in July of 1999, *Nature* released a report on the newly discovered "appetite control" hormone — melanin-concentrating hormone (MCH). Given all these findings, it is likely that a combination of hormones, digestive organs, and brain areas are responsible for set point.

Various causes have been implicated in maintaining the set point. Appetite, cravings and bingeing, body metabolism and body heat, physical activity level, number of fat cells, and a host of hormones and brain neurotransmitters have all been found to have some influence on maintaining weight level.

The Influence Of Fat Cells

All of us are born with body cells specifically designed to store energy for periods of starvation. The body's main energy storage depot is fat. A person of average weight typically has between 25 to 35 billion fat cells.[7] These cells have the ability to expand in size to store additional fat as well as contract as the fat in storage is used. People who are just overweight or mildly obese tend to have about the same number of fat cells as do normal weight people. However, in the mildly obese, the fat cells are much larger and heavier. This condition is called *hypertrophy*.

As the level of obesity increases, the average number of fat cells observed also tends to increase. This increased number of fat cells doesn't result from adult obesity, but appears to stem either from childhood obesity or genetics (probably both). Obese children and adolescents typically have double the number of fat cells as do their normal weight peers.[8] In adults who have morbid obesity, the number of fat cells can number between 100 to 125 billion. This abnormally high number of fat cells is called *hyperplasia*.[9] Most of the morbidly obese have both hypertrophy and hyperplasia.

It is known that the number of fat cells cannot be decreased except through surgical removal (liposuction). However, when liposuction is employed, it is a frequent observation that all of the lost fat is regained elsewhere by expansion of the remaining fat cells.[10] The amount of fat that is stored in fat cells can be reduced through dieting, exercise, appropriate use of medications, and some counseling approaches. However, you probably already know how unsuccessful people are in using diets or exercise alone to permanently lose fat. The reasons for this are becoming more clear. Later in this chapter we will go into some depth explaining how fat cells regulate the storage of fat, and the mechanisms involved with set point.

Brain Controls

Deep within the brain lies a pea-sized structure called the *hypothalamus*. This tiny clump of brain cells is a main player in many of our body's biological functions. In addition, the hypothalamus is directly linked to the areas in the brain responsible for stress, anxiety reactions, and emotionality. (See box on emotional eating, p. 99.)

The hypothalamus is subdivided into several smaller areas, each one with a different function. The hypothalamus directly links to the body's master gland — the pituitary gland. "The hypothalamus controls eating and drinking. ... It regulates our sleep/wake cycle, basic body temperature, various emotions, many hormones, and monitors blood sugar levels, blood pressure, heart rate, and more."[7] The way researchers discovered the functions of the hypothalamus is not just interesting, but it leads to the probable complex interplay of hormones involved in maintaining set point.

In 1943, physiologists began a series of studies on the hypothalamus using rats, cats, and monkeys. They found that when they selectively destroyed a very small part of the hypothalamus (called the ventromedial nucleus) something peculiar happened. The animals ate. They ate until there wasn't any food left or the food was taken away. (This constant binge eating is called *hyperphagia*.) They all also became very large and overweight. We remember duplicating the same experiment in physiological psychology classes. It was an astonishing transformation to watch. Within two months after we had destroyed the hypothalamus in several rats, the rats got so big they couldn't turn around in their cages.

In another set of experiments on this area of the hypothalamus, researchers carefully placed small electrodes into other rats' brains so they could send weak electrical signals into it to stimulate it. When the rats were stimulated in this brain area, they would stop eating. This effect was found even if the animals were feeding after a period of starvation. Thus, this part of the hypothalamus is known to play an important role in the cessation of eating (satiation). When it is stimulated, hungry animals stop eating. If this small area of the brain is destroyed, if the animals are allowed to eat, they won't stop!

Another small area of the hypothalamus was also found to be related to eating — but it worked in opposition to the ventromedial hypothalamus. If the lateral hypothalamus is destroyed, animals simply won't begin to eat. This isn't a tempo-

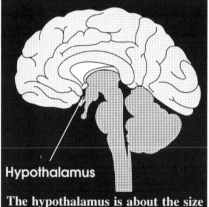

Hypothalamus

The hypothalamus is about the size of a pea. It lies deep in the brain and controls drinking and eating behavior. In addition, it is intimately involved with emotion, stress, anxiety, and feeling. Numerous hormones appear to directly influence the hypothalamus. It is the focus of intense research.

rary effect. The animals will starve to death despite the presence of food and hunger. They can be force fed, but won't start eating on their own. If this same hypothalamus area is stimulated rather than destroyed, animals will begin eating—even if they have just fed. It has been shown that this area of the hypothalamus controls the beginning of eating. If it is stimulated, animals begin to eat. If it is destroyed, they won't start eating. Other areas of the hypothalamus have been found to regulate thirst — including areas that start and stop drinking behavior.[13, 14]

If you really understand this simple review of early research, it should be apparent that at least one brain area controls the beginning of eating, its continuation, and its cessation. Lots of people on an eating binge will tell you that they aren't hungry. But at the same time, they can't stop eating. It all seems a little crazy to the person bingeing and to anyone

Emotional Eating
Emotions & Hunger Are In Your Head

The hypothalamus is a central component in a loop of brain structures called the *Limbic System*. The Limbic System is believed to be the major brain site of anxiety, stress, emotion, and other feeling. In addition, the hypothalamus is a key player in eating behaviors.

In the last chapter we wrote that the obesity puzzle is actually like a set of interconnected balloons. If a person squeezes one area of the balloon to lose weight (for example, the person goes on a rigid diet), increased pressure builds up elsewhere in the balloon. The interconnections between the balloon's components (diet, exercise, psychological factors, biological components) allow the pressure to move from one area to another.

One way to look at the hypothalamus is that it may be one of the interconnections between eating and emotion. The increased psychological pressure caused by a rigid diet often results in dreams about food, stress, anxiety, emotionality, and cravings. Eventually, so much pressure builds up in these areas that it forces its way back through. Binges can result along with rapid regaining of weight. This connection between emotional eating and the hypothalamus has been hinted at by others.[8] For example, when falling in love, many obese people find it relatively easy to lose weight. But when rejected, weight is easily regained. Some obesity researchers have suggested that emotional changes can create a fundamental change in the set point, perhaps in the hypothalamus since it is intimately connected to both emotion and weight.[8] A key point to remember is that an alteration in one area (like diet or exercise), leads to changes in other areas (such as biological and psychological processes).

who observes it. Yet it still doesn't seem to be "controllable." The same thing seems true in some cases of anorexia. Some people with anorexia report that they know they should eat. Yet they "can't." Brain mechanisms — perhaps going haywire — definitely are related to both overeating and anorexia.

Researchers have long known that some sort of hormone in the body sends signals through the blood stream that are received in the hypothalamus. The hypothalamus serves as a sort of "thermostat" that constantly monitors the temperature, level of sugar, and the levels of a host of hormones circulating in the blood. The hypothalamus, in turn, releases hormones and send signals to other areas of the body causing various behaviors — including eating.

The Search For Obesity Hormones

Leptin

In the 1940s and 1950s, researchers observed that some mice became "obese" while others stayed at normal weight despite the fact that they were fed the exact same diet. These researchers conducted a clever series of experiments connecting the bloodstreams of the obese mice with thin mice. When blood from the thin and obese mice was intermingled with each other, a startling thing happened. The obese mice eventually got thin while the thin mice stayed thin. This led scientists to suspect that some sort of substance was in the thin mice's blood that led to reduced body fat. However, scientific methods at that time did not allow scientists to identify the substance.

In 1994 and 1995, researchers funded by the National Institutes of Health isolated and identified a hormone produced by fat cells. This protein hormone was called *leptin*. Leptin is secreted by fat cells as they become full. This hormone serves as a signal to the brain to stop eating. The primary brain area where leptin exerts this effect is in the hypothalamus.

Research on mice subsequently identified several genes related to obesity through cloning. These are termed the obese gene (*ob*) and diabetes gene (*db*). The *ob* gene is responsible for producing leptin. The *db* gene is responsible for diabetes and is involved in the production of the receptor sites for leptin in the hypothalamus. At this point, six different leptin receptor site forms have been discovered. (See box on receptor sites.)

Since its discovery in mice, leptin has been found in humans. In fact, when human leptin is injected into obese mice (who have the *ob* gene mutation), the mice lose weight. The weight-loss is greatest if the leptin is injected directly into the cerebrospinal fluid of the mice. Research on the obese mice showed that leptin resistance appears to be the underlying problem. When a receptor site becomes resistant to leptin, it means that the leptin has trouble fitting into the site. In 1998, a French group of researchers reported that they had found a genetic mutation that caused

Receptor Sites

Receptor sites are small "holes" that are found on the surface of all of the cells in your body. Some cells have special areas where receptor sites are located. Receptor sites are constructed from proteins and they form into *very* specific shapes. The shape of receptors is predetermined by genes. The specific shape of a receptor site is designed to allow another substance (such as a hormone or a brain neurotransmitter) to fit snugly into it. "The typical way that this is described is that a receptor site is similar to a lock... The (hormone or) neurotransmitter that perfectly fits in it is similar to a key. When the key fits into the lock, a small door opens (on the cell itself or inside the cell). If you make a fist with one hand and cup the other, you'll notice how well the fist fits into the cupped hand. This is, in a fairly accurate sense, the way receptor sites operate. If you couldn't change the shape of your cupped hand, something like a coin couldn't fit into it snugly."[11]

Some cells in the hypothalamus have large numbers of receptor sites that are designed for the hormone leptin. When leptin is secreted by fat cells, leptin circulates in the blood stream and quickly reaches the hypothalamus. When the leptin reaches the leptin receptors located in the hypothalamus, it occupies these receptor sites. The "full" leptin receptors create a response within the cells causing the hypothalamus to send out signals. These signals are supposed to stop eating behavior. They are considered to be a "satiation" signal to the brain that stops further eating.

Researchers first thought that obese people were deficient in leptin production. Surprisingly, most obese people have *too much* leptin. Researchers now know that fat cells in obese people produce enough leptin. The problem appears to be more complex. Some people may have problems with their leptin receptors caused by an abnormal leptin receptor gene shape or insufficient numbers of leptin receptors (*db* or *Ob-R*). In addition, perhaps because of the constant high level of leptin found in obese people, the cells in the hypothalamus have become "resistant" to the leptin and leptin has trouble fitting into the receptors. Leptin receptors are also found in other areas of the brain and body including bone marrow. Leptin also seems to be involved in regulating an aspect of metabolism that increases or decreases the body's use of energy. Insulin and other hormones undoubtedly also play a role in obesity.

leptin to be mis-shaped. The faulty shape of the leptin prohibited it from fitting into the leptin receptors leading to obesity. This may be the cause of some cases of obesity. Several other factors could also cause leptin resistance.[15]

In 1998, the first scientific report on using leptin with obese humans was reported at the 58th Annual American Diabetes Association's meeting. A synthetic form of leptin was produced by the pharmaceutical firm Amgen, Inc. The leptin was injected every day under the skin of 70 moderately obese volunteers and 53 lean control volunteers. Most of the subjects were white males. In addition, all of the study's participants were placed on a diet designed to provide 500 calories under their basic daily needs. Four different levels of leptin were studied along with a placebo.

At the end of the first month, everyone in the study had lost weight. The small group of people receiving the highest leptin dosage lost the most weight (the weight loss in this group averaged just over 4 pounds). The study continued for a total of 6 months with 60 obese subjects. Subjects on the highest leptin dose showed the most weight loss after six months (they averaged 15.6 pounds weight loss). The only side effects recorded during the study were minor skin reactions at the injection site.

Many scientists have expressed disappointment with the modest results found in the first leptin study. Many other drugs in current use for treating obesity result in weight loss at similar or greater levels. Inspection of the leptin report showed that some of the study's participants actually gained weight over the six months. Only six of the study's eight subjects on the highest dose actually lost weight. Larger studies on leptin began to address its effects on blood sugar and type 2 diabetes, but in April of 1999, Amgen announced it was moving to a newer form of synthetic leptin. Various pharmaceutical firms are now attempting to develop drugs that will correct leptin receptor resistance.

We have covered leptin extensively because so much attention has been focused on it in recent years. However, many other hormones and neurotransmitters play similar roles in the brain. The complexity of hunger, eating, and satiation is exemplified by how many of these have been identified in the past year or so. A few of these other substances are briefly reviewed as follows.

Melanocyte Stimulating Hormone (MSH)

MSH is produced by the hypothalamus and is released in response to increases in leptin. When MSH is produced, food intake decreases. Leptin resistance may cause a deficiency in MSH leading to overeating. MSH may also work in harmony with another hormone reported in 1999 (Melanin-Concentrating Hormone — see below).

Enterostatin

Enterostatin is produced in the pancreas and secreted into the bloodstream. When it reaches the brain it signals the brain to stop eating. Enterostatin appears to be mostly related to fat consumption. When fat is consumed, enterostatin is released. High levels of the substance reduce fat consumption. Some researchers believe that thin people produce more enterostatin than obese people do. A number of studies are now underway on enterostatin.

Neuropeptide-Y

Neuropeptide-Y, first identified in 1983, is a brain transmitter that serves as an appetite signal to the hypothalamus. When it is secreted, hunger and eating behaviors follow. It is suspected that obese people may have too much neuropeptide-Y (or that the hypothalamus doesn't respond to its "stop eating" signals). The release of neuropeptide-Y is inhibited by leptin. If leptin resistance is present, it is possible that neuropeptide-Y levels in obese people may be too high causing overeating, cravings, and hunger. Researchers are currently trying to develop drugs that will block the effects of this neurotransmitter.

Cholecystokinin (CCK)

Cholecystokinin is found in both the brain and the gut (intestine). Eating stimulates its release. CCK has long been believed to be a signal to the brain for satiation. Research with animals showed that injections of CCK reduced food intake. However, further research showed that the effect was short-term and didn't seem to work the same way in humans. The CCK research subsequently led researchers to study leptin.

Beta-3 Receptors

Beta-3 receptors are probably responsible for the body's theromogenesis. These receptors are found in *brown fat* stores found several places in the body. Thermogenesis is caused by the burning of calories in the body's cells — thus producing body heat. By stimulating the Beta-3 receptors, it is believed that the rate of "fat-burning" would increase, leading to substantial weight loss. The next chapter will go into more detail on brown fat and Beta-3 receptors. However, (as seems to be the case in all obesity research), there is some controversy on the importance of Beta-3 receptors. For example, a 1998 study on 158 obese families in France reported that the overall effect of Beta-3 receptors on obesity was believed to be "minor."

Galanin

Galanin received a fair amount of media coverage in the mid-1990s. Galanin is a transmitter that also exerts an effect on the hypothalamus. Galanin release stimulates eating behavior especially the ingestion of fat. Research is continuing on galanin.

Orexin A & B

In 1998, two hormones (orexin A and orexin B) were isolated and identified in the hypothalamus. A gene responsible for these hormones was also found. When the hormones were injected into rats, within a couple of hours they consumed nearly 10 times their regular intake of food. Rats on starvation diets were subsequently found to have high levels of orexin. Researchers believe that the orexins serve as hunger signals in the hypothalamus. Orexin is being researched as a possible treatment for anorexia. Drugs that block the effect of orexin are also being sought.

Melanin-Concentrating Hormone (MCH)

In July 1999 another appetite stimulating hormone was reported along with the discovery of its receptor. MCH works in the hypothalamus to facilitate eating behavior, however, it is also used in various other body areas. Researchers are attempting to create drugs that would block the effects of MCH specifically in the hypothalamus.

Mahogany Gene (MG)

The MG mutation was discovered in mice and reported in 1999. However, the gene mutation appears related to maintaining thinness in spite of eating a high fat diet. Mice with a normal MG were fed high fat diets — they gained significant amounts of weight. Mice with the MG mutation who were also fed the high fat diet showed no weight gain. MG is believed to exert control over metabolism and the rate of energy expenditure (i.e., glucose burning). Although the gene has not yet been identified in humans, it is highly probable that it will be soon. Researchers are currently trying to find the product of the MG mutation and assess its possible use as a means to raise body metabolism.

Neurotransmitter Involvement In Obesity

Serotonin

Many obesity experts believe that a dysfunction in the serotonin system in the brain is a primary causal factor in obesity.[19] When serotonin is injected into animals' hypothalamus, eating behavior is reduced and suppressed.[20] In addition, many drugs that increase serotonin levels available to the brain lead to a reduction in total food intake. The drugs fenfluramine (Pondimin) and dexfenfluramine (Redux) (half of the drug combination commonly called fen-phen) resulted in many obese people losing significant amounts of weight prior to the voluntary removal of them in 1997. Many of these patients simply stated that they weren't as obsessed with food as they had been prior to taking the drug. In addition, once they began eating, their impulsive overeating habits just seemed to evaporate. A significant comment was, "this must be how normal people feel." Unfortunately, once they stopped taking the drug, their prior obsessions with food and compulsive eating usually returned.

Pondimin and Redux caused a release of brain serotonin as well as inhibiting the reuptake of serotonin. (See box on reuptake, p. 106.) It is interesting that several serotonin selective reuptake inhibitors (SSRIs) like Celexa, Prozac and others result in a significant weight loss in a fair percentage of people. These drugs are typically given to relieve depression, anxiety, and stress. The SSRIs also reduce obsessive-compulsive behaviors and can be an aid to binge eaters and compulsive eaters. Some physicians treating obese patients prescribe both an SSRI and phentermine. Phentermine is the safe half of fen-phen. Results are mixed, but many patients show significant weight loss, lowered obsessive thinking about food, less compulsive and binge eating, as well as depression and anxiety relief. Stress-induced eating behaviors, confirmed in both humans and animals, are also reduced by drugs that cause serotonin levels to increase.[20]

The chapter on drugs used for obesity will review more results regarding serotonin. One other finding is worth noting in this section however. Neurotransmitters are typically molecules that the body constructs from simpler substances such as amino acids. The substances used to construct neurotransmitters are called precursors. The precursor for serotonin in the body is 5-hydroxytryptophan. Taking 5-hydroxytryptophan (or tryptophan) results in an increased serotonin level. Unfortunately, research shows that obese people who take the serotonin precursors don't lose weight.[21]

Dopamine

The "reward" system in the brain is comprised of an interconnected set of brain structures that have high levels of the neurotransmitter dopamine as well as dopamine receptors. The reward system's brain structures also control some of the most evolved, "higher" human functions. For example, impulse control, planning, and thinking are located

Reuptake

When a brain transmitter substance like serotonin is released into the space where it can occupy a receptor site on an adjacent cell, what happens to it once it completes its mission? The answer is interesting. Each molecule of serotonin can move back and forth, into and out of receptor sites. To prevent this from happening, the brain uses several methods to remove the serotonin from the area. One of these methods is called reuptake. Reuptake occurs so that some of the serotonin can be reused again and again. But before it is reused, it is taken back to the site where it came from. This method is accomplished by small brain structures solely designed for that purpose. Once the serotonin is taken back to its original site, it is stored and readied for release again. Reuptake inhibitors greatly reduce this transportation process. SSRIs (Selective Serotonin Reuptake Inhibitors) such as Celexa and Prozac specifically inhibit the reuptake of serotonin. The result is that more serotonin is available and in use at the receptor site enhancing the effects of serotonin.

within these areas. This "reward system" connects to the limbic system as well as the hypothalamus. Remember that the hypothalamus is directly related to eating behaviors and that the limbic system is the main brain system involved with our feelings, emotion, anxiety, and pleasure.[11] Cocaine, a highly addictive drug because of its intense, rapid reward to users (the feelings and energy burst), gains it primary effect from dopamine. It is believed today that all drugs of abuse must somehow influence the dopamine system.

The relationships between dopamine and eating behavior are complex. Research on animals has shown that when hungry animals eat, dopamine is released in several reward centers in the brain.[19] In addition, food deprivation tends to lower dopamine levels.

Dopamine's involvement in eating and the pleasures derived from eating lend credence to the idea that an addictive component may be present in binges and overeating. As cocaine users repeatedly use the drug for its high, some binge eaters report pleasurable sensations during the binge. At the *same time*, the person can suffer anxiety and distress. The exact same mixed sensations are found in most drug users. For example, many drug users acknowledge the pleasant high. However, they often have thoughts of shame, guilt, and anxiety while they are using. Yet, just like binge eaters, they will tell you that during a drug binge they just can't seem to quit.

In an earlier section in this chapter on the hypothalamus, you may have gotten the idea that we can sometimes respond like robots when one area or another in the hypothalamus clicks on or off. That is only part of the picture. The dopamine reward system is viewed as a link between the "lower" brain centers that basically respond without thought and the "higher" brain centers in humans that permit us to think, plan, exert control, and make decisions. It may well be that, once a person with a predisposition toward obesity or binge eating (or drug addiction for that matter) ingests a "forbidden" or "tempting" food (or a drug for the addict), the reward centers so activate the hypothalamus that the person does, indeed, begin to respond like a robot to the commands to "eat, eat, eat." We will return to the connection between overeating and addictions in other chapters.

Chapter References & Notes

[1]Colt, G. H. & Hollister, A. (April, 1998) Were you born that way? *Life Magazine*, Pp. 39-50.

[2]Stunkard, A. J., Foch, T. T., & Hrubec, Z. (1986) A twin study of human obesity. *Journal of the American Medical Association*, 256, 51-54.

[3] M. R. Cummings (1997) *Human heredity*. Belmont, CA: Wadsworth.

[4] Bouchard, C. et. al. (1990) The response to long-term overfeeding in identical twins. *New England Journal of Medicine*, 322, 1477-1482.

[5]Malcolm Gladwell (1998) The Pima Paradox. *The New Yorker*, Feb. 2, 44-57.

[6] Brownell, K. D., & Wadden, T. A. (1991) The heterogenity of obesity: fitting treatments to individuals. *Behavior Therapy*, 22, 153-177.

[7] Leibel, R. L., Berry, E. M., & Hirsch, J. (1983) Biochemistry and development of adipose tissue in man. In: *Health and Obesity*. New York: Raven Press.

[8] Knittle, J. L., Timmens, K., Ginsberg-Fellner, F., Brown, R. E., & Katz, D. P. (1979) The growth of adipose tissue in children and adolescents. *Journal of Clinical Investigation*, 63, 239-246.

[9] Hirsch, J., & Knittle, J. L. (1970) Cellularity of obese and nonobese human adipose tissue. *Federation Proceedings*, 29, 1516-1521.

[10] Sjostrom, L. (1980) Fat cells and body weight. In: *Obesity*. Philadelphia: Saunders.

[11] Little, G. (1997) *Psychopharmacology*. Memphis: Advanced Training Associates.

[12] Stunkard, A. Obesity. (1975) In: *Comprehensive Textbook of Psychiatry - II*. Baltimore: Williams & Wilkins.

[13] Bjorntorp, P., & Brodoff, B. N. (1992) *Obesity*. Philadelphia: Lippincott.

[14] Isaacson, R. L., Douglass, R. J., Lubar, J. F., & Schmaltz, L. W. (1971) *A Primer of Physiological Psychology*. New York: Harper & Row.

[15] Lots of information sources exist on leptin. The Howard Hughes Medical Institute internet site has an updated feature by one of the primary researchers, Jeffrey M. Friedman of The Rockefeller University. The address is: www.hhmi.org/science/genetics/friedman.htm

[16] Little, G. L. (1998) *Psychopharmacology 2*. Memphis: Advanced Training Associates.

[17] Fox, S. I. (1996) *Human Physiology*. New York: McGraw-Hill.

[18] The human obesity gene map: the 1998 update. (1999) *Obesity Research*, 7, 111-129.

[19] Hernandez, L., Murzi, E., Schwartz, D., & Hoebel, B. G. (1992) Electrophysiological and neurochemical approach to a heirarchical feeding organization. In: *Obesity*. Philadelphia: Lippincott.

[20] Leibowitz, S. F. (1992) Brain neurotransmitters and hormones in relation to eating behavior and its disorders. In: *Obesity*. Philadelphia: Lippincott.

[21] Strain, G. W., Strain, J. J., & Zumoff, B. (1985) L-tryptophan does not increase weight loss in carbohydrate craving obese subjects. *International Journal of Obesity*, 9, 375.

Chapter 8
BIOLOGICAL, GENETIC, AND MEDICAL ASPECTS OF OBESITY - PART 2

In the past, obesity has been treated as an acute disorder. Many patients still appear to believe that 10 to 20 weeks of treatment should be enough to "cure" obesity or at least control it for several years. This view of obesity is often encouraged by the commercial diet industry, which promises miraculous results with little or no effort. The results of such an approach are clear; if treated as an acute disorder, obesity will return.
Anderson & Wadden —1999 — *Archives of Family Medicine*

Since the pathophysiology of type 2 diabetes virtually always includes significant insulin resistance, there is good reason to hypothesize that the treatment of insulin resistance could prevent or delay the onset of type 2 diabetes.
American Diabetes Association — 1997[1]

Summary—Type 2 diabetes is one of the most common diseases of obesity. As with type 2 diabetics, almost all obese people have a related condition called insulin resistance. In insulin resistance, insulin's ability to move glucose into cells is impaired. Most cells in the body use glucose (sugar) for energy and insulin plays the key role in getting glucose into the cells. In response to insulin resistance, the pancreas secretes even more insulin in an attempt to overcome the problem. This leads to high insulin levels (called hyperinsulinemia).

Insulin not only helps transport glucose into cells, but also promotes fat storage and prevents fat stored in the body from being used as energy. Insulin release is markedly increased in response to consumption of sugar and simple carbohydrates (starch). High insulin levels, therefore, promote increased fatness. For this reason, many new, best-selling diet books propose low or zero carbohydrate diets.

The pancreas secretes another hormone, called glucagon, when blood sugar levels fall. Glucagon signals the liver to produce glucose from its energy stores and ultimately leads to the conversion of body fat to energy. But glucagon also causes muscle protein to break down into amino acids. The amino acids are then converted into glucose. The actions of glucagon explain why many people who lose large amounts of weight within a brief time also lose substantial muscle tissue.

Leptin (discussed in the prior chapter) is related to insulin. Leptin appears to inhibit insulin's effectiveness (and perhaps is a causal factor in insulin resistance). High leptin levels are found in obese people. Predictably, high insulin levels are also found in the obese. Ongoing research on the Pima Indian tribe has shown that insulin resistance and obesity usually precede diabetes. Several genetic links have been identified that may produce insulin resistance.

There is no doubt that high insulin levels are directly related to obesity. Treatment of insulin resistance is now standard with type 2 diabetes and is being used with some obese patients. Current research shows that the successful treatment of insulin resistance with several new classes of medications may prevent diabetes and even some related diseases. For example, 80% of diabetics eventually die of cardiovascular diseases. Since the delay or prevention of diabetes can reduce the development of heart disease, the treatment of insulin resistance should be addressed in all obese people — even those without diabetes.

The cluster of symptoms that surround insulin resistance are collectively known as *syndrome x* (also called metabolic syndrome). Syndrome x includes high levels of insulin, decreased levels of good cholesterol (HDL), increased levels of bad cholesterol (LDL), high blood pressure, and high levels of upper and middle body fat storage. Gout, heart disease, and other diseases are also related to it. Syndrome x is a significant risk factor for the development of cardiovascular heart disease. The syndrome is believed to stem from genetic predispositions coupled with certain behavioral and life-style factors.

One important causal factor in syndrome x is high alcohol consumption. While moderate drinking (3-4 drinks per day) appears to have a beneficial effect on cardiovascular disease, exceeding the moderate level of alcohol consumption rapidly escalates the risks. A significant genetic research finding has linked obesity to both drug addiction and alcoholism. The neurotransmitters dopamine and serotonin are both associated with obesity and addiction. This finding appears especially strong in young females. Anxiety and depression are also linked to these neurotransmitters and researchers believe that many overweight women (and men) are unconsciously trying to "medicate" unpleasant mood states with food.

Another important biological link to obesity relates to weight cycling (the cycle of weight loss and regain typical in "yo-yo" dieters). While a "return to old habits" appears to be the obvious cause of these relapses, several genetic mutations have been found that are important contributing factors. In addition, the body's ability to generate heat when a person eats (called "diet-induced thermogenesis") is strongly related to genetics. When the heat generated by food ingestion is low, fat tends to be more rapidly stored leading to weight gain.

All of the biological factors related to obesity interact with environmental, life-style, and psychological factors present in an individual. This complex interplay makes it unlikely that a single drug will be developed in the near future which effectively treats obesity. Thus, a combination of appropriate medications should be developed for each obese person depending on specific individual characteristics. At the same time, obese people attempting to manage fat loss should understand that obesity has to be viewed as a life-long issue. The biological influences of set point, leptin and insulin, and other hormonal and neurotransmitter mechanisms make setting realistic weight loss goals critical. Medical treatment and personal vigilance over diet, activity level, and psychological factors have to be understood as never-ending concerns.

• • •

The development of type 2 diabetes (also known as adult onset diabetes) is one of the most frequent health related consequences of obesity. Diabetes is strongly genetic and is linked to obesity as well as leptin and insulin. Almost everyone with type 2 diabetes has a condition known as *insulin resistance*. (This is true even in type 2 diabetics who are of normal weight.[2]) Insulin resistance can be described as a reduced tissue sensitivity to insulin. In other words, in insulin resistance, insulin doesn't work as well.

A few minutes after food is ingested, the pancreas begins to se-

Clarifying Diabetes Types

In 1998, the National Institutes of Diabetes and Digestive and Kidney Diseases accepted a recommended consolidation of diabetes names to stop the confusion caused by multiple terminology. Two primary types of diabetes exist:

type 1 diabetes
    The type of diabetes formerly known as Type I, juvenile onset diabetes, or insulin dependent diabetes (IDDM) is now *type 1 diabetes*.

type 2 diabetes
    The type of diabetes that was known as Type II, noninsulin-dependent diabetes (NIDDM), or adult-onset diabetes is now *type 2 diabetes*.

crete insulin into the bloodstream. The amount of insulin released is directly linked with the amount and type of food consumed. Sugar and carbohydrates produce the largest insulin release. Insulin plays a crucial role in moving blood sugar (glucose) into the body's cells so that the glucose can be used as fuel. The pancreas secretes insulin after a meal is digested in response to the rising level of glucose in the blood. Insulin gradually lowers blood sugar levels. The pancreas also secretes other hormones with its essential function being to maintain blood sugar levels within the "normal" range. (The "normal" ranges of blood sugars are typically described as a glucose plasma concentration of no higher than 170 mg. per 100 ml after a meal and no lower than 50 mg. per 100 ml

Diagnosing Diabetes

In 1998, the National Institutes of Diabetes and Digestive and Kidney Diseases created new guidelines in diagnosing diabetes. Fasting plasma glucose levels above 126 mg. per 100 ml indicate diabetes. (Two tests are used to verify the diagnosis.) Glucose intolerance is defined as a fasting plasma glucose value between 110-125.9 mg. per 100 ml.

Diabetes in the United States

- Approximately 16 million Americans have diabetes
- 6% of the United States population has diabetes
- Each year, 800,000 Americans are diagnosed with the disease
- 8.2% of men & 8.2% of women have diabetes
- 123,000 children and teens have diabetes
- Yearly cost of diabetes in America is $98 billion

Who Is At Risk In The United States?

Percentage of Race/Ethnic Groups With Diabetes (over age 20):
- 7.8% of Whites (non-Hispanics)
- 9% of Native Americans
- 10.6% of Mexican-Americans
- 10.8% of African-Americans

Risk Of Diabetes By Age

- 18.4% of people over the age of 65
- 8.2% of people over the age of 20
- 0.16% of people under the age of 20

Source: National Diabetes Information Clearinghouse. *Diabetes Statistics* (March, 1999)

between meals.) Abnormally low blood sugar levels are harmful — especially to the brain. Dizziness, weakness, changes in personality, coma, and even death can result from low blood sugar. High blood sugars are also harmful. Uncontrolled high blood sugar levels (called *hyperglycemia*) can result in blindness, kidney failure, and serious circulation problems. Many people refer to diabetes as "having sugar" because some of the excess sugar is sometimes excreted in urine and can be detected. Type 2 diabetes is diagnosed when blood sugar levels don't fall sufficiently and exceed established limits. In some cases of type 2 diabetes, the pancreas may not be producing enough insulin. In other cases, the pancreas may be producing more than enough insulin — but the insulin fails to work properly due to insulin resistance.

When insulin resistance develops, the body's cells have a reduced ability to move blood sugars to their interior. In response to the sustained high levels of blood sugar, the pancreas secretes even more insulin in an attempt to lower the levels. The sustained presence of abnormally high levels of insulin is called *hyperinsulinism* or *hyperinsulinemia*. The constant "flogging" of the pancreas to produce insulin can eventually reduce the pancreas's ability to make insulin necessitating routine insulin injections.

Insulin resistance was recognized over 50 years ago.[4] At the same time, it was recognized that higher levels of insulin were closely associated with increases in weight and body fat.[5] Thus, obesity, diabetes, and insulin resistance are intimately linked.

Insulin's Effects

In addition to moving blood glucose into cells for use as energy, insulin also acts to transform glucose into triglycerides and promotes fat storage. At the same time, insulin prevents fat already stored in the body from being used as energy. High levels of insulin, a condition usually associated with insulin resistance, tends to lead to increasing fat stores — i.e. weight gain. Popular diets touting low or zero carbohydrate consumption are based upon these insulin effects. Insulin release is especially stimulated by eating sugar and simple carbohydrates. Current thinking is that, by reducing the amount of insulin released by the pancreas, the body will not store fat and may begin to burn fat stores. This reasoning is generally true.

Insulin & Pancreatic Hormones
Weight Gain, Weight Loss, & Low Carbohydrate Diets

The pancreas is a soft organ located just under and behind the stomach. A cluster of three types of cells (in the *islets of Langerhans*) produce and secrete three major hormones into the bloodstream in response to glucose levels. The *delta* cells produce *somatostatin*. Somatostatin is also produced in the intestines and in the hypothalamus and is a growth regulator hormone. The exact function of pancreatic somatostatin is not completely understood.

The *beta* cells produce *insulin*. Insulin moves blood glucose into most body cells so the cells can use the glucose as energy. Insulin also promotes fat storage and prevents stored fat from being used as energy. Thus, high levels of insulin tend to facilitate weight gain.

The pancreatic alpha cells produce *glucagon*. Glucagon serves to increase blood glucose levels and is released when blood sugar levels are low. Glucagon signals the liver to produce glucose from its own energy stores and also from amino acids it obtains from muscle tissues.

Hormones are molecules produced by endocrine glands, including the hypothalamus, pituitary gland, adrenals, gonads, thyroid, and pancreas. The term "endocrine" implies that the hormones are produced in response to specific stimuli and then released into the bloodstream. For example, insulin is produced in response to the stimulus of carbohydrate ingestion and released into the bloodstream to move glucose into cells.

From: *Alcohol Health & Research World* (1998) 2, 154.

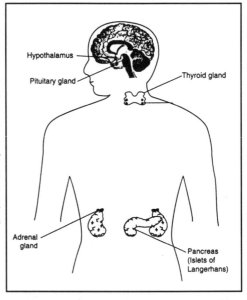

Many dieters who lose weight rapidly on very low calorie diets find that much of their weight loss comes from loss of muscle mass — not just fat. This happens because proteins from muscle fibers are broken down and converted into glucose. Glucagon signals the liver to perform this function. Very low calorie diets attempt to counter-act the muscle loss by making their formulas high in protein.

So, how does the body consume its own fat stores under these conditions? During a carbohydrate restrictive diet, people tend to have low insulin release. This can produce ketosis (see end of story). Remember that insulin is necessary for glucose uptake into muscle cells. When insulin levels are low, the body uses any glucose available for life-sustaining brain cell function. The body's muscles and most organs, then must use free fatty acids as an energy source. Glucagon activates an enzyme in fat cells (called hormone sensitive lipase) that ultimately leads to the release of free fatty acids into the bloodstream so they can be used as energy by muscles and organs. Thus, body fat is consumed. Unfortunately, at the same time, muscle tissue can be lost aggravating the underlying obesity problem. As muscle and lean-body mass decline, the body's basic energy require-ment lowers. After the dieter goes off the diet, the body's setpoint mechanism causes rapid weight regain. The vast majority of this weight is typically fat.

Ketosis — When a typical person consumes less than 100 grams of carbohydrates a day, protein in muscles is consumed. Due to the high glucagon levels present during a carbohydrate restrictive diet (or diets less than 800 calories a day), the liver converts some free fatty acids into ketones. Ketones are used by skeletal muscles for energy. However, abnormally high levels of ketones can cause ketosis. This creates a rapid weight loss during the first few days of the diet — but the weight loss is primarily water.[3] Virtually all low carbohydrate diets and low calorie, protein supple-mented diets stimulate ketosis-related water loss. As long as the person remains on the diet, the dehydration continues.[3] Ketosis causes fatigue and headaches, bad breath, elevated uric acid levels, leaves a stale taste in the mouth, and strains the kidneys.

Understanding Insulin & Insulin Resistance

Insulin is a lot like a key designed to fit into a lock. The lock is called a receptor site. When insulin occupies the receptor site, it causes a complex reaction in the cell which releases a special glucose transporter. The transporter, acting somewhat like a truck, picks up glucose and brings it into the cell. Once inside the cell, glucose can be converted to usable energy. A calorie is a specific amount of energy that is "burned" by the cell to maintain its life functions. Calories are extremely important in weight control and weight loss. If insulin has trouble doing its job (because of insulin resistance) the pancreas continues to "jack up" the level of insulin. This ultimately leads to enhanced fat storage and is a factor in the development of type 2 diabetes.

Insulin Resistance may be caused by several factors. One factor may be a genetic defect in how the receptor site is shaped. A small distortion in the shape of an insulin receptor could prevent insulin from entering the receptor. It's as if the lock has altered shape so that the key won't fit. Note that insulin won't fit this distorted (smaller) hole.

Outside of Cell

Glucose (sugar) in fluid surrounding cell is brought to the site by the bloodstream

Insulin

Insulin Receptor (unoccuppied)

Cell Wall (Membrane)

Glucose Transporter

This glucose transporter was released from the receptor (above) when insulin entered the receptor site. The transporter brings glucose into the cell. Once it deposits the glucose in the cell, it reattaches to the base of the receptor site until more insulin enters the receptor site.

Glucose Transporter

Interior of Cell

As blood glucose levels fall, insulin is no longer secreted by the pancreas. In response, another hormonal system comes into play to produce energy from fat. The "fat burning" is caused by a second pancreas hormone, *glucagon*, released when blood sugar levels are low. Glucagon serves as a counterbalancing hormone to insulin. Glucagon signals the liver to produce glucose from its own energy stores and release it into the blood to maintain normal levels. Glucagon also causes a breakdown of muscle protein to amino acids so they can be converted into glucose. The brain is the primary recipient of the released glucose. The body's muscles and most organs then use fat (free fatty acids) as their energy source. Glucagon activates an enzyme in fat cells that ultimately leads to the release of free fatty acids into the bloodstream so they can be used as energy by muscles and organs.

Since insulin promotes fat storage, conditions that cause high insulin levels are implicated in obesity. Insulin resistance is the main culprit suspected of causing sustained, high levels of insulin. In addition, consumption of high carbohydrate foods and sugars are definitely related to high insulin levels and fat storage.

Is The Food Pyramid Wrong?

The United States Department of Agriculture has established a "healthy eating guide" for Americans called the "Food Guide Pyramid." (See box, p. 118.) It is described as a good visual representation depicting the building blocks for a healthy diet. Foods at the bottom of the pyramid (the largest part of the pyramid) represent the basic foundation of the recommended daily diet. As you go up the pyramid, foods are to be consumed at lower levels. The base of the pyramid recommends 6 to 11 servings each day of breads, cereals, rice, and pasta. The second level of the pyramid recommends 2 to 4 daily servings of fruits and 3-5 servings of vegetables. The third level recommends 2-3 servings of protein rich foods (meats, nuts, etc.) and 2-3 daily servings of milk products. Fats and sweets are to be eaten very sparingly.

For a "normal" weight, healthy person, the Food Guide Pyramid may be appropriate. But there are serious, valid questions about whether it is healthy for the obese (all of whom probably have insulin resistance), others with insulin resistance, and type 2 diabetics. The Food Guide

Pyramid's daily eating suggestions are anchored heavily by carbohydrates. About 70% of daily calories come from carbohydrates (starch). When digested, carbohydrates are converted into sugar (glucose) and stimulate the release of insulin. Excess carbohydrate calories (in the form of glucose) are converted into fat and the insulin prevents the conversion of body fat into usable energy. The frequent consumption of carbohydrates (based on the Food Pyramid's guidelines) may be counterproductive to weight loss in obese people and those with insulin resistance.

Many popular diet books focus on this issue. Barry Sears' book, *Enter The Zone*, proposes that carbohydrates should make up no more than 40% of daily calories. He proposes that a favorable balance between insulin and glucagon can be created by proper diet. Each meal should be 40% carbohydrate, 30% protein, and 30% fat. Staying in this balanced state is the "Zone." The elementary book *Sugar Busters!* is also based on

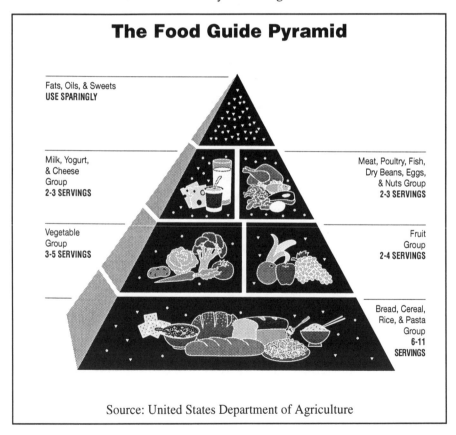

The Food Guide Pyramid

Fats, Oils, & Sweets
USE SPARINGLY

Milk, Yogurt,
& Cheese
Group
2-3 SERVINGS

Meat, Poultry, Fish,
Dry Beans, Eggs,
& Nuts Group
2-3 SERVINGS

Vegetable
Group
3-5 SERVINGS

Fruit
Group
2-4 SERVINGS

Bread, Cereal,
Rice, & Pasta
Group
**6-11
SERVINGS**

Source: United States Department of Agriculture

lowering sugar and carbohydrate intake — especially avoiding foods that are rapidly taken into the bloodstream. Examples of these forbidden foods are pasta, white bread, carrots, and bananas. Other popular diet books proposing that excess carbohydrates lead to insulin resistance and obesity are *The Carbohydrate Addict's Diet*, *Protein Power*, and Adkin's *New Diet Revolution*.

We believe that the vast majority of obese people have insulin resistance and many are moving down the road toward diabetes. Certainly, almost all obese patients treated at medical clinics manifest symptoms of insulin resistance. Treating the insulin resistance with appropriate medications would be prudent. On the other hand, following the Food Guide Pyramid or going on an extremely low carbohydrate diet would both be counterproductive. This is because the Food Guide Pyramid is too heavily based on carbohydrates while on the other extreme, the zero carbohydrate diet leads to mostly water weight loss and relies on high amounts of unhealthy dietary fat.

In principle, we agree that the evidence clearly shows that insulin-related factors are a cause of obesity in some people. In others, insulin resistance may manifest as a consequence of obesity caused by a multitude of factors. But either way, insulin is an issue and an ongoing diet should address it. A fundamental problem with the drastic diet approaches (such as zero carbohydrate diets) presented in many best-selling diet books is that they **are drastic**. They are often unrealistic and simply cannot be taken seriously as a life-long diet for the majority of people. They reinforce the mistaken idea that diets are something we go on to eventually go off. A more balanced, reasonable approach to eating is required. In chapter 15, we will present a life-long alternative.

The Leptin-Insulin Connection

Diabetes has long been recognized as having a strong genetic basis and recent research has uncovered several genes believed responsible for its development. These genes are also related to the hormone leptin. An excess insulin level (hyperinsulinemia) is a primary defect present in mice that have variations in leptin genes as well as the diabetes gene. Hyperinsulinemia is considered a component in the eventual development of type 2 diabetes.

In 1996, not long after leptin's discovery, it was proposed that leptin played a role in insulin release. You will recall from the last chapter that leptin is a hormone released by fat (adipose) cells in response to "fullness." Leptin signals a site in the hypothalamus that triggers a feeling of satiation. In 1998, a group of Brazilian researchers reported on a series of studies that attempted to clarify the leptin/insulin relationship.[6] They found that leptin produced by fat cells inhibited the effects of insulin on glucose. That is, the ability of insulin to move glucose into cells is *lowered* by leptin. This, in turn, produced an increase in insulin levels. In addition, they found that leptin increased the transformation of body fat into usable energy — free fatty acids for use in skeletal muscle tissue. Leptin and insulin appear to work together in a complicated interaction designed to regulate overall body weight. But leptin resistance (demonstrated in both mice and humans) leads to obesity and may lead to hyperinsulinemia, insulin resistance, and diabetes development.

The Pima Indians: Diabetes, & A Genetic Link

In chapter 7, the ongoing research on the Pima Indian tribal reservation in Arizona was reviewed. From 1983 to 1993, researchers gathered genetic samples from nearly 300 non-diabetic Pimas. Detailed measurements of insulin functioning were repeatedly gathered on the volunteers. Some of the volunteers developed diabetes over the course of the study and scientists were able to find a number of important factors that could predict the development of the disease. Insulin resistance and obesity were the first factors found in the Pimas that predicted diabetes.

In 1993, the scientists studying genetic samples from the Pimas

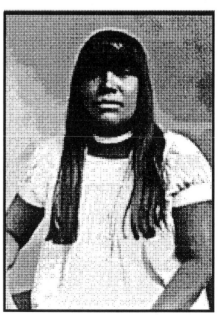

19th Century Pima.

found a gene that appears to produce insulin resistance. Called FABP2, "the gene makes an internal Fatty Acid Binding Protein using one of two amino acids. When the gene makes the protein with threonine, one of those amino acids, the body seems to absorb more fatty acids from the fat in meals. NIH (National Institutes of Health) scientists think that could lead to a higher level of certain fats and fatty acids in the blood, which could contribute to insulin resistance."[9]

Other factors present in insulin resistance are related to enzymes. Researchers have identified three protein phosphatase enzymes (remember, enzyme actions are controlled by genetics) that determine how cells respond to insulin. A study is currently underway to compare the three enzyme genes in Pima groups.

There is no doubt that insulin resistance, at least partly genetically controlled, plays a crucial role in obesity and diabetes. Controlling insulin resistance should, perhaps, be a major consideration in obesity treatment approaches.

Treating Insulin Resistance

Research has confirmed that insulin resistance is associated with obesity, various diseases (including diabetes), and early death.[7] For this reason, there is no debate in medicine regarding whether or not insulin resistance should be treated *in diabetics*. Insulin resistance is lowered within a few days after a low-calorie diet is initiated. Weight loss beneficially effects insulin resistance. Vigorous exercise also lowers insulin resistance. However, both exercise and low-calorie diets help with insulin resistance only as long as they are maintained. For example, within 5 days after exercise cessation, insulin resistance levels return.

Several new medications have become available to treat insulin resistance. Rezulin (*troglitazone*) and Glucophage (*metformin*) both greatly reduce insulin resistance. These medications will be discussed in more detail in the next chapter, but many patients lose weight more easily after starting them. Xenical (*orlistat*) is a fat-enzyme blocker that reduces the absorption of 30% of dietary fat. While Xenical produces a modest to moderate weight loss in patients, it appears that when Xenical is combined with other medications, it enhances lower insulin and cholesterol levels. All three of these medications are useful in diabetic treatment.[8]

Another class of medications has been introduced that is useful for diabetes and insulin resistance. Precose and Glyset both slow the absorption of ingested sugar and carbohydrates. Some sugar passes through the intestinal tract and is excreted. However, sugar that is absorbed enters the bloodstream slowly and doesn't stimulate a massive insulin response.

Should Insulin Resistance Be Treated In The Non-Diabetic Obese?

There is some medical debate on whether insulin resistance should be treated to *prevent* diabetes and other diseases. Unfortunately, almost no research exists on this issue. The reason for this is simple. Medications that treat insulin resistance have been available for less than three years. We simply don't know what the long-term effects of insulin resistance treatment will be on the subsequent development of disease. The American Diabetes Associations' 1997 conference on insulin resistance[7] concluded that diabetes *may* be prevented or delayed by treating insulin resistance. This conclusion is based on a host of research findings

Diabetic Treatment Changes

Until 1997, the only oral treatment option for diabetes was a class of drugs called sulfonylureas. These drugs (there are about 6 generic types of sulfonylureas used) "flog" the pancreas to secrete more insulin and help the cells better utilize the insulin. Unfortunately, increased cardiovascular disease and higher mortality rates were shown in some research. In addition, the drugs were associated with weight gain.

Since 1997, a host of new diabetic drugs have been approved. One of these drugs is glucophage which reduces the liver's production of glucose and lowers insulin levels by impacting insulin resistance. Many "controlled" type 2 diabetics and patients with only insulin resistance lose weight on Glucophage and have lower blood fat and cholesterol levels. Another drug, Rezulin lowers insulin resistance — especially in skeletal muscles.

Two new sugar enzyme inhibitors (called alpha-glucosidase inhibitors) block the digestion of starch and sugars and lead to a slower increase in blood glucose levels after meals. Precose blocks mainly on starch-based carbohydrates and Glyset blocks sugar. The fat blocker Xenical should also be used in treating type 2 diabetics. Xenical blocks the absorption of 30% of dietary fat and results in modest weight loss.

showing "that insulin resistance/hyperinsulinemia usually precedes the diagnosis of type 2 diabetes by years to decades."[8]

Another major issue that should be considered by patients contemplating medical treatment for weight control, obesity, or insulin resistance is cardiovascular disease. You probably recognize that heart disease and obesity overlap and, also, that many obese people eventually develop diabetes. You may not be aware that 80% of people with diabetes eventually die of heart disease.[8] The reasons for this are exceedingly complex and it is now realized that the **traditional** treatment of diabetes (managing blood glucose levels) has no effect on the high heart disease mortality rate.

In the past decade, treatment approaches for diabetes have drastically changed. (See related story in box, p. 122.) In addition to the management of glucose levels, diet and exercise are recognized as genuinely helpful. More significant are the many new medications available to type 2 diabetic patients that make the management of this disease more effective. All of these medications beneficially impact some physiological processes in the chain of events that lead to obesity and cardiovascular disease. Many physicians will, no doubt, recommend the use of some of these newer medicines to patients for insulin resistance, obesity, and management of heart disease. We would urge you to discuss these options with a physician who will both understand and be sensitive to the needs of patients saddled with the disease of obesity.

Syndrome X: Metabolic Syndrome

Syndrome x is a term sometimes applied to a cluster of obesity-related diseases and physical problems. The core of syndrome x is insulin resistance. Hyperinsulinemia, impaired glucose tolerance, increased blood levels of bad cholesterol (LDL), decreased blood levels of good cholesterol (HDL), high blood pressure, and upper and middle body fat distribution (central adiposity) comprise the cluster of symptoms in syndrome x.[10] Syndrome x is also known as *metabolic syndrome* and is a significant risk factor for the development of cardiovascular disease. Cardiologists also use the term syndrome x to describe patients who have angina pectoris and specific (heart) stress test results — but who do not have significant constriction of coronary arteries. It has been suggested that the cardiologists' syndrome x and metabolic syndrome (syndrome x) may be different aspects of the same problem.[11, 19]

Metabolic syndrome is believed to be based on a combination of insulin resistance, individual genetic predispositions, and behavioral and life-style factors.[11] The general consensus of the medical literature is that obesity is a strong diagnostic indication for metabolic syndrome.

The major behavioral and life-style factors involved with metabolic syndrome are overconsumption of fats and sugars, physical inactivity, and consumption of alcohol.[12] The effects of alcohol on metabolic syndrome are complicated. Many recent media reports have cited research showing the "protective" effects of moderate alcohol consumption on the heart. Some of the beneficial effect of moderate alcohol consumption may simply be stress reduction. The key to this is the word **moderate**. Moderate alcohol consumption does appear to lead to lower cardiovascular risk and help with insulin resistance. But once a drinker exceeds moderate levels, the risk increases. At the 1999 annual meeting of the Society for Epidemiological Research, a University of Buffalo researcher (Jian Liu) reported on a study of nearly 22,000 Italian men and over 16,000 Italian women. The study correlated syndrome x with alcohol consumption. Non-drinkers had a higher rate of syndrome x than drinkers. However, this effect was true only for moderate drinkers consuming three or four drinks a day (this is a maximum of 4 oz. of alcohol). As the number of drinks increased, the risk for syndrome x increased exceeding the rates in nondrinkers.

Alcohol, Syndrome X, & Obesity: An Addictive Component

Alcoholism and drug addictions have a strong genetic component.[13] In 1990 the first gene was found that was clearly related to alcoholism. This gene, encoding receptors for the neurotransmitter dopamine, was later found to be linked to polydrug abuse and cocaine addiction. In 1996, the same gene was linked to obesity — especially in women. The dopamine receptor gene was found to interact with the leptin obesity gene (ob).[14] It has been suggested that the dopamine gene variation leads to cravings and the experience of pleasure derived from food consumption. This effect is especially strong when anxiety and depression are "medicated" by food. The study found that leptin and dopamine genes combined accounted for 22% of obesity variation in young women.

As discussed in the last chapter, we know that serotonin levels play a role in food consumption. The popular book, *The Serotonin Solution* (by J. Wurtman, 1997), proposes that many people overconsume carbohydrates and sugars to cope with stress. The high levels of insulin that occur because of increased blood sugar leads to a rapid utilization of all amino acids in the bloodstream by muscle tissue — except the amino acid tryptophan. The tryptophan selectively enters the brain where it is rapidly synthesized into serotonin. The increased serotonin levels are believed to improve mood. (See box on stress defeat syndrome, p. 126.)

Many behavioral aspects of obesity mimic addiction. Overeating and binge eating occur with the knowledge of detrimental effects, matching the behavior seen in alcoholics and drug addicts. Alcoholics and drug addicts will use their drug of choice to the extreme — even when they realize it is harmful and want to stop. Brain systems controlling pleasure have been implicated in both addiction and obesity. The dopamine system in the brain controls pleasure sensations and links to the hypothalamus. In addition, many foods commonly consumed by binge eaters have been shown to enhance the release of the endorphin neurotransmitters.[15] The endorphins (short for *endogenous morphine*) exert a calming, pleasant sensation. Current genetic research shows that over 200 genes contribute to obesity suggesting to us that syndrome x, diabetes, and obesity are related in an incredibly complex interplay involving most major hormonal and brain systems. The overlap of gene mutations in both obesity and substance addictions should not be surprising and simply confirms the long-term observations of people afflicted with obesity as well as many health professionals.

Body Fat Distribution & Syndrome x

Evidence has accumulated indicating that body fat distribution is a key to understanding insulin resistance and syndrome x (metabolic syndrome). Android obesity (also called central obesity — the apple shapes seen most often in men) is both a trigger for metabolic syndrome and an accelerator of metabolic syndrome once it develops.[11] Abdominal body fat is more active than fat that accumulates in lower body areas.[20] The "activity" in upper and middle body fat renders it a higher risk for the development of various cardiovascular diseases and other metabolic syndrome symptoms.

Insulin resistance is worsened by inter-abdominal body fat (the fat located on the intestines). The metabolic turnover rate in abdominal fat storage areas is greater leading to increased levels of free fatty acids in the bloodstream. This leads to increased insulin resistance. Numerous other differences have been found between abdominal fat and lower body fat. Taken in total, the risk of developing metabolic syndrome (and a higher mortality rate) is increased by abdominal fat.[20]

In chapter 7, we reviewed research showing the overall influence genetics exerts on body mass. Up to 70% of body mass is directly linked

Stress Defeat Syndrome

A relatively new idea related to obesity and serotonin has been coined *stress defeat syndrome*. The idea is being discussed at some drug information workshops and the initial physiological basis of it is in the book *Enter The Zone*. We live in a stress-producing, stress-filled society. The work world is filled with competition. Our social lives are stressful and competitive. Managing bills, family, friends, health, school, children, and work produce stress in the best of us. Stress produces genuine emotional and physical changes. How we respond to stress — and the outcome we expect — can play a role in the development of insulin resistance, obesity, and overall health.

During times of stress, epinephrine (adrenaline) levels increase as do levels of cortisol. The increased cortisol leads to insulin resistance and increasing insulin levels. High insulin levels, of course, result in weight gain and are a step toward the development of both insulin resistance and metabolic syndrome.

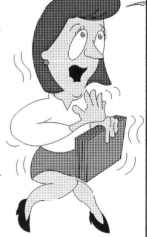

The increased epinephrine level also produces a more difficult-to-see reaction. Epinephrine decreases the levels of an enzyme responsible for converting one of the essential fatty acids (linoleic acid) into gamma linolenic acid (GLA). GLA is an activated form of essential fatty acid that enables the body to utilize other fatty acids. The low levels of GLA that occur as a result of a stress produced epinephrine release can trigger a chain-reaction that cascades through the body. Chronic fatigue can result. Increased viral illnesses occur. Bad cholesterol levels increase. Fat storage increases and the utilization of fat decreases. Epinephrine also causes the heart to beat faster and blood vessels to constrict increasing the heart's work load.

— Continued on next page —

to genetics. Genetics also plays a large role in determining where fat tends to distribute on the body. Research on this question tells us that genetics appears to control between 25% to 30% of body fat distribution.[20]

Genetic Weight Cycling & The Beta-3 Adrenaline Gene

A consistent observation made about many chronic dieters is that they often lose weight and quickly regain it. This is referred to as *weight cycling* or yo-yo dieting. Once again, this finding is similar to the chronic relapse shown in drug addicts and alcoholics after treatment.[13] While this phenomenon is partly explained by "a return to old habits," something biological is clearly at work. As related in earlier chapters, it is generally conceded that 95% of dieters who lose weight eventually regain the

It is believed that some people respond to stress by confidently overcoming stress-producing events. Such people expect success and master the situation. When the goals they have set appear unreachable, they simply switch goals — but they don't become depressed or feel defeated. They see it as an object lesson in reality and learn from it. These people appear to function as if they believe they have reasonable control over the outcomes of stress-filled situations. Such people are believed to have a lower adrenaline response to stress as well as lower corticol levels. The result is that they don't suffer from increased insulin levels and tend to be healthier. They also don't gain weight.

On the other hand, some people seem to respond to stress as if they expect defeat. This expectation could occur because of their past experiences in competitive situations. These people tend to respond to stress with a quiet desperation and a belief that they can't overcome the situation. Because of this, their response to stress is an exaggerated release of adrenaline and cortisol. Depression, anxiety, fatigue, and illness will occur in higher levels in such people. They are described as having *stress defeat syndrome*. Weight gain and obesity are related to stress defeat syndrome because of the unique body chemistry produced by the expectation of defeat in stressful situations.

The genesis of stress defeat syndrome is like the chicken and the egg question. Which comes first? Does the genetically programmed physiological reaction cause the expectation of defeat, or does the "stress defeat" mentality cause the physiological reaction? Either way, it become a vicious cycle — a self-perpetuating cycle that alters the body's chemistry and may very well lead to obesity, decreased activity level, and increased anxiety, more emotional eating all of which, in turn, lead to more stress with the expectation of failure.

weight. The same relapse rates are typically observed in addicts and alcoholics.

In 1998, researchers in Finland studied weight cycling in 77 young, obese women.[16] The women were placed on very low-calorie diets for 12 weeks followed by a 40-week maintenance diet. The women were placed in four groups. One group had gene mutations in both the Beta-3-adrenergic gene and the UPC-1 gene (called the uncoupling protein). The other groups consisted of obese women with only one gene mutation or neither gene mutation. The women with both gene mutations lost an average of 20 pounds during the initial 12 weeks. All of the other groups were more successful with weight loss. Also significant was weight regain. Women with both gene mutations regained significantly more weight (nearly 13 pounds) during the maintenance period than any of the other three groups. The authors concluded that a strong genetic component appeared to be present in both the ability to lose weight as well as the propensity to regain it.

Brown Fat & Body Heat

Many obesity experts believe that the Beta-3-adrenergic receptors (B3A) may be the key to genuine weight loss in the obese — without the weight regain. B3A is tied to brown adipose tissue (BAT) — brown fat. Brown fat was identified as distinct organ tissue 300 years ago. Its function is to produce body heat and it has been found in hibernating

The *fat* and *tubby* Genes
Fat Cell Hormones Can Produce More Fat Cells

In 1996, researchers at the Jackson Genetics Laboratory in Bar Harbor, Maine cloned two genes related to obesity and insulin in mice which they oddly dubbed *fat* and *tubby*. The *fat* gene produces an enzyme responsible for insulin production. Mutations in it lead to "creeping obesity" in mice. This is similar to the gradual obesity that occurs in humans as they age. The *tubby* gene is a mystery. While both *fat* and *tubby* appear to cause late-onset obesity and insulin resistance in mice, it is still not known what function the *tubby* gene serves other than to worsen insulin resistance. The scientists believe that linkages between *fat* and *tubby* and several other genes are probable genetic causes of obesity and type 2 diabetes.[23]

In addition, in 1995, researchers at the Salk Institute discovered an additional hormone secreted by fat cells. Dubbed 15d-PGJ$_2$, this hormone produces an increase in the body's number of fat cells leading to obesity.[23]

mammals.[17] BAT appears to serve as a control mechanism for the body's energy expenditure and it is linked to the hypothalamus as are almost all of the other hormones and neurotransmitters we have discussed.

One by-product of body cells burning calories for energy is heat. All of the metabolic reactions that take place in the body generate heat. (The normal average of this heat in humans is 98.6°F.) This is called *obligatory thermogenesis* — the amount of energy necessary to keep the cells and body alive. A related term you may have frequently heard is *resting metabolic rate*. It is the amount of energy your body continually has to consume just to keep you alive. Several later chapters address resting metabolic rate.

A term you may not have heard is *facultative thermogenesis* — but you probably will recognize what it means. When you exercise, your body generates more heat because some cells become more active. As muscles work, more energy is burned. This is the basis of the idea, "eat less and exercise more." If you burn more energy than you take in, your body will burn its own fat for energy. The energy used above the level necessary to keep you alive is facultative thermogenesis.

Brown fat plays a key role in basic body temperature maintenance and what is called *diet-induced thermogenesis*. The amount of food consumed and its digestive properties produce diet-induced thermogenesis. Brown fat is stimulated by low temperatures and high energy diets. (This is one reason why we get hot after eating a big meal.) Brown fat is deposited in small amounts around the heart, in the chest, near the kidneys and in several other areas. When it becomes active (through low temperature or eating) it tends to have a high blood flow rate. Adrenaline and neuropeptide-Y are both found in brown fat.

The uncoupling protein (mentioned earlier as a key factor in weight cycling) is found in brown fat. It is used by the small organelles in the cells (called mitochondria) that produce energy. Brown fat cells use fatty acids for fuel, and the uncoupling protein directs energy use toward producing heat. The Beta-3 adrenaline receptors in brown fat start the process of energy generation.

Both exposure to cold and eating tend to stimulate brown fat via the release of adrenaline. This stimulation, in turn, increases the number of brown fat cells. On the other hand, when brown fat isn't stimulated, it tends to reduce in size. Researchers are focusing on ways to stimulate brown fat to burn energy through the generation of body heat. This line of research may be one of the most promising in obesity treatment. In fact, the most effective obesity drug ever used — fenfluramine (combined with phentermine) — gained some of its effectiveness from thermogenesis in brown fat.[17]

Obese animals tend to have defective BAT functioning. Research on humans has shown that both of the key components related to brown fat — Beta-3 adrenaline receptors and the uncoupling protein — can have defects that are related to obesity. In many cases of obesity, the brown fat cells are small, unreactive to adrenaline, and are insulin resistant. In addition, lower body temperature may be present.

In general, obese people have a lower thermic effect (lower heat production) in response to eating than do people of normal weight. Many studies show that the resting metabolic rate (energy use) of obese people is significantly lower than in nonobese. When the obese lose weight, their energy use is even lower. Research tends to affirm that the lower metabolic rate is a contributor to obesity rather than a cause of it.[18]

A frequent observation among people who lose significant amounts of weight is chronic chills. It is probable that this effect is often due to defects in their brown fat's ability to generate body heat. In addition, these defects may also be related to a lowered metabolic rate after weight loss — making it easier to regain the weight.

A Brief Review

If we had decided to write a comprehensive review of *all* of the genetic, physical, and biological variables that directly relate to obesity, it would have taken as many as 5,000 pages. Countless research studies have been published on obesity, diabetes, metabolic syndrome, brain and neurotransmitter involvement, endocrinology, metabolic factors, and every other associated area. Current research on genetics is progressing at a mind-boggling speed and no matter how comprehensive we make this book, by the time you read it, something new will have been discovered and released. But we never intended to do a comprehensive review. Our intention in chapters 7 and 8 is to give you a quick overview of where obesity research is and to show the incredible complexity of the problem. The development of obesity is not caused by a weak character. The genesis of obesity lies in genetic predispositions.

Obesity itself (fatness) represents a single, totally visible characteristic of a complex, genetic disease that is multi-factorial in nature. Acceptance of obesity as a disease has been slow within the medical community but even slower among the general public. In view of the current findings implicating 200 separate genetic components in obesity, how can anyone scientifically deny that many biological predispositions set the stage for the development of the disease?

Recent mainstream medical articles cite the more empathic attitudes medicine has assumed toward the obese patient.[21, 22] Increased understanding of the plight of the obese may be present in some physicians, but many vocal physicians continue to argue against long-term treatment of the obese patient and some argue against any treatment. Meanwhile, media reports continue to highlight each new discovery that could finally "lead to a cure." Unfortunately such reports only serve to falsely raise the hopes of people who must continue a day-by-day struggle with weight, prejudice, and feelings of hopelessness.

Obesity clearly involves psychological, life-style, environmental, diet, and exercise variables in addition to inherited, biological factors. The following chapters detail these other important variables. However, from the information presented in these two chapters on the biological and genetic influences on obesity, we'd like to end with a few positional and speculative statements based on current research findings:

1. Patients have to understand that obesity treatment is long-term.[22] (Obesity, like diabetes cannot be cured, only managed. It should be stressed that life-long management of obesity-related factors is required.)

2. Obesity is a chronic (life-long), relapsing disease. Only long-term treatment will produce prolonged, beneficial changes. (Note that this view is also proposed in the 1998 Position Statement of the American Association of Clinical Endocrinologists/American College of Endocrinology[21] and in a 1999 article in the Archives of Family Medicine.[22])

3. It is unlikely that one medication will be developed in the near future that results in significant weight loss in the bulk of obese patients. (This appears to be true because of the involvement of so many hormonal, neurotransmitter, and brain systems in obesity.)

4. The goal for sustained weight loss in the obese should be set at a realistic level: the initial goals should be a loss of 5% to 15% of starting body weight.[22] (Unrealistic weight loss goals can be in direct conflict with the body's set point. Losing too much weight sets in motion physiological processes designed to regain the weight and even add excess weight.)

5. Medical treatment for obesity should involve a combination of drugs tailored to each patient's unique profile. (The one-size fits all strategy commonly employed leads to unrealistic expectations and failure. It also ignores research findings and observations of what actually works with specific patients.)

6. Medications for insulin resistance, neurotransmitter deficits, low metabolic rate, fat and sugar/starch blocking, metabolic syndrome symptoms, and psychological problems should be in the potential drug treatment arsenal of physicians treating obesity. (Each patient would typically be placed on several drug combinations.)

7. Medical treatment for obesity should always include additional components stressing diet, exercise, management of personal and psychological issues, and the provision of ongoing support. (Patients have to understand that a medication only approach seldom leads to a sustained or satisfactory weight loss. Medication can make weight loss efforts more effective, but only if the patient becomes actively involved.)

8. Ultimately, reducing body fat percentage is the main focus of treatment. (Weight loss, while being one measure of treatment success, is not the primary goal. A reduction in fat "fluffiness," sometimes measured objectively in waistline and subjectively in the fit of clothing, should be suggested as a goal.)

Chapter References & Notes

[1] American Diabetes Association (1997) Consensus development conference on insulin resistance. *Diabetes Care*, 21, 2, 310.

[2] Fox, S. I. (1999) *Human Physiology*. New York: McGraw-Hill.

[3] Dwyer, J. T. (1992) Treatment of obesity: conventional programs and fad diets. In: P. Bjorntorp & B. N. Brodoff (Eds.) *Obesity*. New York: Lippincott.

[4] Himsworth, H. P., & Kerr, R. B. (1939) Insulin-sensitive and insulin-insensitive types of diabetes mellitus. *Clinical Science*, 4, 119-152.

[5] Bray, G. A. (1992) An approach to the classification and evaluation of obesity. In: P. Bjorntorp & B. N. Brodoff (Eds.) *Obesity*. New York: Lippincott.

[6] Ceddia, R. B., William, W. N., Lima, F. B., Carpinelli, A. R., & Curi, R. (1998) Pivotal role of leptin in insulin effects. *Brazilian Journal of Medical and Biological Research*, 31 (6), 715-722.

[7] American Diabetes Association. (1997) Consensus development conference on insulin resistance. *Diabetes Care*, 21 (2), 310.

[8] O'Keefe, J. H., Miles, J. M., Harris, W. H., Moe, R. M., & McCallister, B. D. (1999) Improving the adverse cardiovascular prognosis of type 2 diabetes. *Mayo Clinic Proceedings*, 74, 171-180.

[9] National Institute of Diabetes and Digestive and Kidney Diseases (1999) The Pimas: Genetic Research. web: nih.gov/health/diabetes/pima/genetic/genetic.htm

[10] Ferrannini, E. (1993) Syndrome X. *Hormone Research*, 39, 107-111.

[11] Krone, W., & Meinertz, T. (1995) Metabolic syndrome as a cardiovascular risk factor. *Herz*, 2, 4.

[12] Wirth, A. (1995) Non-pharmacological therapy of the metabolic syndrome. *Herz*, 20, 56-69.

[13] Little, G. L. (1996) *Psychopharmacology*. Memphis: Advanced Training Associates. A discussion of the genetics for each type of drug addiction and alcoholism is included in this text. A genetic "craving" is believed to be set up by several neurotransmitter deficiencies and receptor site abnormalities.

[14] Comings, D. E., Gade, R., MacMurray, J., Muhleman, D. Johnson, P., Verde, R., & Peters, W. R. (1996) Genetic variants of the human obesity (OB) gene: association with body mass index in young women, psychiatric symptoms, and interaction with the dopamine D_2 receptor (DRD$_2$) gene. *Molecular Psychiatry*, 1 (4).

[15] Milkman, H., & Sunderwirth, S. (1987) *Craving for ecstasy: the consciousness and chemistry of escape*. Lexington, MA: Lexington Books.

[16] *Journal of Endocrinology and Metabolism* (1998) 88, 4246-4250.

[17] Himms-Hagen, J. (1992) Brown adipose tissue. In: P. Bjorntorp, & B. N. Brodoff (Eds.) *Obesity*. New York: Lippincott.

[18] Nelson, K. M., Weinsier, R. L., James, L. D., Darnell, B., Hunter, G., & Long, C. L. (1992) Effect of weight reduction on resting energy expenditure, substrate utilization, and the thermic effect of food in moderately obese women. *American Journal of Clinical Nutrition*, 55, 924-933.

[19] Goodfellow, J., Owens, D., & Henderson, A. (1996) Cardiovascular syndromes X, endothelial dysfunction and insulin resistance. *Diabetes Research and Clinical Practice*, 31, 163-171.

[20] Lonnroth, P., & Smith, U. (1992) Intermediary metabolism with an emphasis on lipid metabolism, adipose tissue, and fat cell metabolism: a review. In: P. Bjorntorp & B. N. Brodoff (Eds.) *Obesity*. New York: Lippincott.

[21] Obesity Task Force (1998) *AACE/ACE Position statement on the prevention, diagnosis and treatment of obesity*. American Association of Clinical Endocrinologists/ American College of Endocrinology. web: www.aace.com/clin/guides/obesity/obesity.htm

[22] Anderson, D. A., & Wadden, T. A. (1999) Treating the obese patient. *Archives of Family Medicine*, 8, 156-167.

[23] *The Jackson Laboratory: scientific report 1998-1999*. (1999) Jackson Laboratory: Bar Harbor, ME. This massive report is a summary of ongoing genetic research with speculative science indicating possible research directions. *Scientific American's* August, 1996 issue contained a commentary on the Jackson research and the Salk Institute. W. Gibbs, "Gaining on fat."

Chapter 9
MEDICATIONS FOR MEDICAL & BIOLOGICAL FACTORS

It isn't enough to cut down on calories and exercise more to lower excess weight. The most effective way to reduce obesity and its related risks for the long term is to combine drug intervention with behavioral changes...
David Loshak — 1999 — *Doctor's Guide Medical News*[1]

Summary—The failure rate of diet and exercise is phenomenally high for the obese. At least 95% of people who lose weight through diet and exercise regain all of that weight within 5 years. This high relapse rate is usually blamed on one factor: obese people eventually return to old eating habits and prior levels of inactivity. Diets are usually touted as a temporary fix for weight loss — they are something to be endured (a sacrifice) until the desired amount of weight is lost. Exercise routines are also viewed in a similar temporary way. In short, diets and exercise are thought of as *something to go on to eventually go off.* Usually overlooked in this explanation is the strong underlying genetic and biological basis of obesity.

In previous chapters, we have described the obesity puzzle as a complex, interconnected whole with several seemingly separate components: biological, psychological, environmental, diet, and exercise. All of the puzzle pieces have to be comprehensively addressed in order to permanently impact obesity. This requires an ongoing effort on the part of the individual who must make sustained changes in almost every area of day-to-day living. These efforts can be experienced as merely uncomfortable to downright painful. Medication can help to *reduce the pain of reducing* and should be deemed as a critical component in obesity treatment.

One of the most important issues that you must consider in making a decision to take medication involves your level of health risk. If you have obesity related diseases, the loss and maintenance of only 5% to 10% of body weight frequently results in substantial health improvements. A comprehensive health assessment is the starting point in making this decision. Then you must balance the risks of the medications against the risks associated with obesity. You must understand that all medications, including aspirin, carry risks. In 1994, for example, over 100,000 people died from reactions to properly prescribed medications and another 7% of hospitalized patients had drug reactions. With appropriate and frequent medical monitoring, medications that assist obese and overweight people have satisfactory safety profiles and should be strongly considered — especially if the health risks associated with obesity are high.

Many people were alarmed, frightened, and angered by the voluntary withdrawal of Pondimin and Redux (the fen half of phen-fen) from the market. Prior to this withdrawal, the most important side-effect described for Pondimin (fenfluramine) and Redux (dexfenfluramine) was Primary Pulmonary Hypertension (PPH). PPH is a serious medical problem from which 45% of those afflicted die, and, those that survive may have significant disability. However, the incidence of PPH is estimated to be 1 case per every 22,000 to 44,000 people taking these drugs. Most physicians describe this problem as occurring in *one* patient per 33,000: a remote possibility for most of us. But, in July of 1997 a report was released which described an unusual heart valve problem in 24 female patients who had taken phen-fen. The problem was traced to Pondimin and Redux. Further research determined that the heart valve problems were occurring in 5% to 30% of people who took these medications. Some of the most recent research indicates that, perhaps 16% of "fen-phen" users who took the drug over three months, has some identifiable heart valve lesion. A. H. Robbins, the manufacturer, voluntarily recalled both Pondimin and Redux in September of 1997.

The appropriate use of medications can greatly aid obese people in fat reduction efforts. Combined with a comprehensive program that includes food plans, increased activity, life-style changes, and attention to personal issues, obese patients almost always achieve marked improvements in health as well as decreased body fat percentage. Current categories of drugs that are used for obesity treatment include appetite suppressants, fat blockers, diabetes treatment drugs that reduce sugar and starch absorption, drugs that reduce insulin resistance, and, lastly, the medications that increase the level of serotonin in the brain (SSRIs).

Phentermine remains the most effective "appetite suppressant" drug. This drug gives a feeling of satiation because it increases the level of neurotransmitters in the brain that signal fullness. It remains a fairly safe drug with few side effects. Other "appetite suppressants" in use are diethylpropion, mazindol, and phendimetrazine. Meridia (sibutramine) is the only "appetite suppressant" approved by the FDA for use up to a year. However, many physicians treating obesity prescribe drugs for much longer periods under terms called "off-label" use. *Off-label use is not inappropriate use.* The chronic nature of obesity frequently warrants long-term use of medications.

The blocking agents are Xenical (orlistat), Precose (acarbose), and Glyset (miglitol). Xenical blocks the absorption of approximately 30% of the fat ingested during a meal. Patients on Xenical usually experience a slow, but steady, weight decline of about 5-10% of total body weight. (This drug is very useful in treating obese diabetics.) Precose and Glyset delay the absorption of sugar and starch from the intestines, producing decreased insulin blood levels in response to the stable absorption of glucose.

Obesity is almost always aggravated by a condition known as "insulin resistance." When the body needs higher and higher levels of insulin to attempt to keep blood sugars in the normal range, the person is said to be insulin resistant. Glucophage (metformin) and Rezulin (troglitazone) decrease insulin resistance (by increasing insulin sensitivity) and reduce the amount of insulin circulating in the blood stream. Fat is burned as fuel much more rapidly when insulin levels decline.

Another diabetes medication, Prandin (repaglinide), is helpful for some obese type 2 diabetics. Prandin results in lower blood sugars by causing a quick, but brief, release of insulin just before meals.

The last category of helpful medications is the SSRIs. SSRIs are serotonin specific reuptake inhibitors. We know these drugs raise serotonin levels in the brain, treating depression and obsessive-compulsive behavior. Studies have shown that obese people tend to have low levels of serotonin in the fluid surrounding the brain. Also, obese people tend to obsess about food, and many, if not most, are sub-clinically depressed. Thus, the antidepressants Celexa, Prozac, Paxil, Zoloft, and Luvox may be helpful. We find Celexa the most effective of these with Prozac coming in second.

• • •

Simply trying to reduce fat (weight) through diet and exercise overwhelms the vast majority of obese people. Diet and exercise are typically viewed as temporary behavior changes by the person losing weight. As a result, there is a staggering rate of failure in maintaining weight loss through diet and exercise alone. This failure indicates that this two-pronged approach is insufficient. At least 95% of people who lose weight through diet and exercise regain all of the weight within five years.[2] At the same time, medication *alone* is rarely successful in long-term weight loss and maintenance.[3, 4, 5] "Today, patients who complete traditional programs designed to produce short-term weight loss lose approximately 10% of body weight but tend to regain two-thirds of it within 1 year and almost all of it within 5 years. This relapse occurs because treatment of obesity does not *cure* the condition. When treatment stops, weight is regained."[5] This view has been echoed frequently in the obesity treatment community. "There is a growing perception among investigators that obesity should be treated as a chronic illness and subjected to long-term pharmacologic intervention, much as other chronic illnesses such as hypertension and diabetes."[6]

Why Medication?

As stated in the prior paragraph, obesity programs that stress diet and exercise often lead to temporary weight loss. The weight loss is seldom maintained over time. The question of *why relapse occurs* seems to have a simplistic answer. The obvious answer is that people return to the "way they were." Since the diet is seen as a temporary sacrifice (lasting only until the weight is lost), it is abandoned as soon as possible by the patient. Old eating habits, as well as the former weight, return. Exercise plans show a similar relapse pattern. Many dieters rigidly exercise during the weight loss phase. At some point, the exercise begins to taper off and there is a return to prior habits of inactivity. The observation of relapse back to prior habits is valid. But an important factor is missed by these simplistic — yet true — answers: It is the role the multitude of genetic and biological factors play in the disease of obesity.

Since the prior two chapters reviewed the many biological issues involved with obesity, we won't review them here. But a review of the two mental images we employed previously in this book may be helpful in understanding the deeper biological problems involved in obesity treatment that are unaddressed by diet and exercise. In the first image you will recall that the obese person is in a never-ending struggle to swim up a river against a strong current. The genetic and biological situation imposed on the obese person tends to push him or her down river (adding fat). When this natural flow is resisted by an attempt to actively swim against the current (as with diet and exercise), some progress can be made. But a single small behavioral lapse in the effort causes a rapid rush back downstream (relapse causing weight regain). The river's current makes progress in weight loss increasingly difficult. The more progress the person makes in swimming against the current, the stronger the current working against the person becomes (the more you lose, the more difficult it becomes to lose more).

In analyzing this first image, it should be obvious that being successful (making it all the way up the river — and staying there) is nearly impossible for the vast majority of people. What is required is simply more than human nature permits. In short, to be successful in this scenario, a person has to permanently change almost *every* habit and behavior. This change has to be complete and absolute with no backsliding or lapses. The individual has to learn to cope with constant hunger, food obsessions and dreams, stress-induced eating situations, holiday eating, and yet must keep on exercising regardless of feelings or obligations. Virtually every text and scientific article examining basic human nature, personality, and behavioral change gives us the same message about the probability of success in making *total* life-style change. It is seldom accomplished. We should not be surprised that only 5% of people seem to be successful in permanently losing fat through diet and exercise. Perhaps we should be surprised that 5% actually do it. We can learn important facts from those who are successful, but for the 95% who can't make such a total change other help is needed. This help can be provided by medication.

The second mental image we have employed is the representation of obesity as a gigantic, flexible balloon puzzle with five seemingly separate pieces. Except the pieces aren't separated — they only appear to be. In reality, they are interconnected. Pressure applied to one or two pieces of the balloon (i.e., diet & exercise) seems to result in progress. The problem is that, since the puzzle is an interconnected whole, the pressure applied in one area produces increased pressure in other areas. When your attention wavers, the air forces its way back in. The example we gave in the river image works well to explain what happens in the balloon. If you acted to change everything in your diet and increased your physical activity level, you would lose body fat. But chances are that you'd also begin to dream about food and eating. You'd also probably become obsessed with thoughts about food. Why? The answer is that your self-imposed behavior change produces massive psychological pressure. Your biological systems also would experience increased pressure from the self-induced diet and exercise. Your metabolism might begin to slow down and your overall energy expenditure would decrease. Hormonal signals may change, leading you to crave certain foods and encourage binge eating.

We hypothesized that the hypothalamus was the area in the brain connecting biological and psychological processes. Imagine the pressure applied to the hypothalamus' eating centers from both hormones and the psychological stress created by rigid diets. Do you recall the research with animals showing how they would continually binge eat when a specific area in the hypothalamus was stimulated? If the person on the rigid diet/exercise routine loses concentration, she can begin eating like a robot responding to an electrical impulse. This happens to a lot of yo-yo dieters. During the lapse, large quantities of food can be quickly consumed. She knows she should stop eating, but for some unclear reason she just can't. In this situation the hypothalamus seems to be overriding conscious control and she is, indeed, responding a lot like a robot. All of this occurs because of pressure moving from one component of the obesity puzzle to another. Medication is probably the most important, and maybe the only effective way, to cope with this complex brain-body signaling problem.

Potential Benefits of Medication Treatment

The primary role of medication in the treatment of obesity is to help reduce the pain of reducing caused by the body's genetic makeup. When body fat goes down, biological "speed bumps" are encountered that can result in quick weight regain. Remember, over the short term, weight loss in obese individuals may reduce a number of health risks. Studies looking at the effects of medical treatment on obesity-related health risks have found that some agents lower blood pressure, blood cholesterol, triglycerides (fats) and decrease insulin resistance (when insulin doesn't work well in handling blood sugar) over the short term. However, long-term studies are needed to determine if weight loss from appetite suppressant medications can improve health. The use of other obesity medications (such as orlistat) prevents the absorption of some dietary fat (leading to weight loss) and sometimes results in lower cholesterol levels. Other drugs can lessen insulin resistance, improve glucose tolerance, block or slow the absorption of some sugars and starches, and improve mood. All of these effects can lead to weight loss and improved health.

Coping With The Obesity Puzzle:
Medical Interventions Are Usually Necessary To Treat Underlying Biological Factors

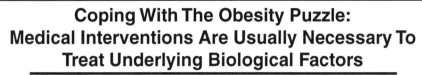

Biological factors that contribute to obesity can be greatly aided with medications. These include a wide range of possible problems including:

Uncontrollable appetite
Low metabolic rate
Lack of satiation
High fat diet
Insulin resistance
Glucose intolerance
Depression & anxiety
Obsessive-compulsive eating

If the biological puzzle piece is adequately addressed, it makes coping with the other pieces easier. It can reduce the pain of reducing.

BIOLOGICAL FACTORS

DIET FACTORS

EXERCISE FACTORS

ENVIRON-MENTAL FACTORS

PSYCHO-LOGICAL & SOCIAL FACTORS

Potential Risks and Areas of Concern When Considering Medication Treatment

The decision to take obesity treatment drugs lies with you. All medications appropriate for obesity treatment should be safe, but all medications carry risks. You must weight the potential benefits of taking the drugs against the potential risks. A frank and open discussion with a physician knowledgeable in obesity is strongly encouraged. When considering long-term medication treatment for obesity, you should consider the following areas of concern and potential risk.

• Potential for Abuse or Dependence

Currently, all appetite suppression medications used to treat obesity are controlled substances, meaning doctors have to follow more stringent state and federal guidelines when prescribing them. Although abuse and dependence are not common with non-amphetamine appetite suppressant medications, doctors should be cautious when they prescribe these medications for patients with a history of alcohol or other drug abuse.

• Development of Tolerance

Most studies of weight control medications show that a patient's weight tends to level off after 4 to 6 months while still on medication treatment. While some patients and physicians may be concerned that this shows tolerance (a diminished effect) to the medications, the leveling off may mean that the medication has reached its limit of effectiveness. It is not clear if subsequent weight gain (or failure to continue to lose weight) with continuing medication treatment is due to drug tolerance of reaching the treatment limits of the drug.

• Reluctance to View Obesity As a Chronic Disease

Obesity is often viewed as the result of a lack of will-power, weakness, or a life-style "choice" — the choice to overeat and underexercise. The belief that people choose to be obese adds to the hesitation of health professionals and patients to accept the use of long-term medical treatment to manage obesity. Obesity, however, is a chronic disease — not a life-style choice. Other chronic diseases, such as diabetes and high blood pressure, are managed by long-term drug treatment, even though these diseases also improve with changes in lifestyle, such as diet and exercise. Although this issue may concern physicians and patients, social views on obesity should not prevent patients from seeking medical treatment to prevent serious health risks that can cause illness and death. Medications useful in treating obesity are not "magic bullets," or a one-shot fix. They cannot take the place of improving one's diet and becoming more physically active. The primary role of medication in the treatment of obesity is to help *reduce the pain of reducing*. Much of the discomfort and many of the other problems that accompany efforts to reduce fat are primarily caused by genetic factors.

• Side Effects

Because medications useful in treating obesity are used to treat a condition that affects millions of people, many of whom *appear* healthy, side effects are less acceptable than when treating other diseases (e.g., cancer). Most side effects of obesity medications are mild and usually improve with continued treatment. **Serious or fatal side effects are rare.**

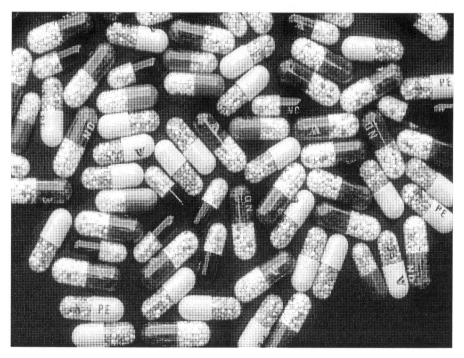

Medication Considerations

The starting point when considering the use of medications for obesity treatment is a thorough medical evaluation. A review of your personal health history, health problems, physical condition, current medications, and other factors by a qualified physician is essential so that an individualized plan of action can be devised. In addition, your body mass index and body fat percentage should be assessed to determine your degree of obesity.

Next, your personal level of health risk related to obesity is considered. Family history is often used as a way of estimating some future risks. For example, as discussed in chapter 8, diabetes is a major health complication of obesity with a strong genetic component. Current

Off-Label Use

While the FDA regulates how a medication can be advertised or promoted by the manufacturer, these regulations do not restrict a doctor's ability to pre-scribe the medication for different conditions, in different doses, or for different lengths of time. The practice of prescribing medication for periods of time or for conditions not approved is known as "off-label" use. You should understand that "off-label" use does not mean unsafe or improper use. While such use often occurs in the treatment of many conditions, you should feel comfortable about asking your doctor if he or she is using a medication or combination of medications in a manner that is "off-label." The use of more than one appetite suppressant medication at a time (combined drug treatment) is an example of an off-label use. Using currently approved appetite suppressant medica-tion for more than a short period of time (i.e., more than "a few weeks" is also considered off-label use. However, as stated above, off-label use can be quite appropriate and necessary.

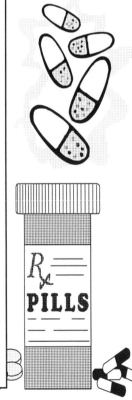

medical conditions such as high blood pressure, heart disease, high cholesterol levels, breathing problems, and insulin resistance also directly influence the appropriateness of medication.

In general, the higher your level of obesity, the more you will be encouraged to take medication. If you have central obesity (the apple shape) you will be strongly encouraged to consider medication. The presence of current health risks will also increase the likelihood that medication will be prescribed. A strong family history of some health problems, such as heart disease and diabetes, will probably result in the recommended use of medication to prevent or delay the onset of these diseases.

Stress and psychological issues that impact weight and eating can often be helped by medication. Your personal behavioral pattern of eating, the types of food you eat, the presence of obsessive-compulsive eating, and depression and anxiety all have a direct bearing on what medications may be best for you.

In all likelihood, more than one medication may be suggested to treat different aspects of this disease. At the same time, life-style changes, food plans, and an exercise plan are typically devised. Counseling or support groups may also be recommended. All of these "nonmedical" obesity treatment components will be explored in subsequent chapters.

The best obesity treatment providers will want to work closely with your primary care physician to assure that you receive a comprehensive treatment plan that helps solve your obesity puzzle and doesn't adversely interfere with any other medical problems. *Appendix A* contains a summary and evaluation of widely available commercial programs that purport to treat overweight and/or obesity. But choosing the right — or best — specialist for you is your responsibility. You should look for programs and providers who offer comprehensive and individualized services rather than a one-size-fits-all approach. Medication is most effective when it is employed in conjunction with a carefully crafted food plan, exercise, and professional psychological services with counseling and support. We offer a few hints below to help in the search:

* Make certain your individual medical and health history is addressed.

* Understand that, the higher your level of obesity, the more appropriate it will be for medications to be suggested to you. The presence of some family

health problems increases the appropriateness of medications. The more current health problems you have — especially those related to obesity — the greater the likelihood that you will be encouraged to take medications.

* Have a full understanding of why any medication is being prescribed. Each medicine has an intended purpose and you should know how that purpose fulfills your needs.

* Understand the risks and benefits of each drug you take. You must realize that there is no such thing as a completely safe drug. Even aspirin can have serious side effects and risks. On the other hand, you have to understand that the many current drugs used to treat obesity have a safe profile and that few people experience serious side effects. You must balance the risk of the disease (obesity) against the potential problems associated with the treatment. In almost all situations with obese patients, we believe that medication is an appropriate adjunct if it is combined with a comprehensive plan and regular medical assessments.

* Accept only eating plans that are permanent and healthy. Ask yourself, "*can* I eat like this the rest of my life?" Then ask, "*should* I eat like this the rest of my life?"

* Accept only fitness routines that account for your age, condition, and life-style. Make gradual increases in physical activity until you reach a level acceptable to you.

* Look for a program that emphasizes permanent life-style changes and offers some sort of life-long support and relapse prevention component.

* Avoid the one-size-fits-all approach typical of some programs and providers.

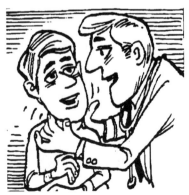

Medications Appropriate In Obesity Treatment

(Note: Portions of this section are adapted from *Prescription Medications for the Treatment of Obesity*, published by the National Institute of Diabetes and Digestive and Kidney Diseases [1998])[7]

The medications most frequently employed in the management of obesity are commonly known as "appetite suppressants." Appetite suppressant medications (also called *anorexiants*) promote weight loss by decreasing appetite or increasing the feeling of being full. These medications cause a decline in appetite by facilitating an increase in the appetite suppressing neurotransmitters serotonin, dopamine, and norepinephrine. It is important that a person taking an anorexiant reports side effects to the provider and that they do, in fact, take only one of these drugs.

Primary Pulmonary Hypertension

Primary pulmonary hypertension (PPH) is a rare but potentially fatal disorder that effects the blood vessels in the lungs and results in death within 4 years in 45% of its victims. PPH is a significant risk in morbidly obese patients and with patients with sleep apnea whether they take appetite suppressant drugs or not. However, patients who use certain appetite suppressant medications for more than 3 months have a greater risk for developing this condition, estimated at 1 in 22,000 to 1 in 44,000 patients per year. It should be noted that the vast majority of cases of PPH have occurred in patients who were taking fenfluramine or dexfenfluramine, either alone or in combination with phentermine. There have been only a few case reports of PPH in patients taking phentermine alone. No cases of PPH have been reported with sibutramine, but it is not known whether or not sibutramine may cause this disease. While the risk of developing PPH is very small, physicians and patients should be aware of this possible complication when considering the risks and benefits of using appetite suppressant medications in the long-term treatment of obesity. (But remember that some obese patients will develop the disease anyway!) Patients taking appetite suppressant medications should contact their doctors if they experience any of the following symptoms:

shortness of breath,
chest pain,
faintness,
or swelling in lower legs and ankles.

Combined Drug Treatment: The Fen-Phen Fiasco

In July 1997, researchers at the Mayo Clinic reported a case series of 24 women, identified as fen-phen users, who developed an unusual form of disease involving the heart valves. The disease primarily affected the left side of the heart, and five patients required valve replacement. In cases where samples of valve tissue were obtained, there was an unusual appearance of the heart valves generally only seen with a serotonin-producing tumor called carcinoid or with excessive amounts of medications containing ergotamine. Following these initial case reports, the Food and Drug Administration (FDA) continued to receive a number of reports of similar valve disease from physicians. Some of these cases involved patients who were taking fenfluramine or dexfenfluramine alone. **No cases were reported in patients taking phentermine alone.** In addition, physicians at five sites provided information to the FDA regarding patients, most of whom did not have signs or symptoms of valve disease. About 30% of patients at these sites showed some evidence of damaged valves, usually mild or moderate. The findings were of enough concern to prompt the FDA to ask the manufacturers of fenfluramine and dexfenfluramine to voluntarily recall the drugs. This withdrawal took place on September 15, 1997. Patients who were on fenfluramine or dexfenfluramine were advised to discontinue the drug, and to contact their physicians in order to be evaluated for signs and symptoms of heart disease and to determine the need for an echocardiogram. Two small studies looking at relationships between sibutramine and valvular heart disease did not find any increased incidence in valvular lesions in patients taking sibutramine compared with placebo. Combined drug treatment using fenfluramine and phentermine ("fen/ phen") is no longer available or suggested because the adverse reaction rate encouraged the manufacturer to take fenfluramine and dexfenfluramine off the market voluntarily. As related in the following paragraphs, we now know much more about the actual incidence of heart valvular lesions attributed to this drug combination.

How Bad Was Fen-Phen?

On July 8, 1997, the FDA issued an advisory to health providers regarding fenfluramine and dexfenfluramine. By September 30, 1997, the FDA had received a total of 132 complete reports from physicians of possible heart-valve problems in patients possibly caused by fenfluramine or dexfenfluramine.

Continued on next page—

These reports included the 24 cases reported by the Mayo Clinic. Analysis showed that 86% of these cases met the definition criteria. The average age of the patients was 44 years and 98% of them were female. All of the patients had used fenfluramine or dexfenfluramine either alone or in combination with other drugs. "None of the cases used phentermine alone." The average length of drug use was 9 months. Cardiac valve replacement surgery was performed on 24% of these patients.[8]

In September of 1998 three studies were published in the *New England Journal of Medicine* on fenfluramine and dexfenfluramine related heart valve problems. One study performed in Minnesota compared the echocardiograms of a control group to 257 patients who had taken the drugs. Mild abnormalities were found in 22.7% of the patients and 1.3% of the controls. Another study in Washington, D.C. made comparisons between 718 patients who took dexfenfluramine an average of 70 days and 354 patients who were on a placebo. This study found only a slight increase in the level of heart valve problems in the dexfenfluramine patients. The third study evaluated the medical records of nearly 10,000 United Kingdom patients who had taken fenfluramine or dexfenfluramine to a control group of patients who took other drugs. There were no cases of heart valve problems in the control group or in any patients who had taken phentermine only. A total of 11 cases of heart valve problems (.0011%) were found in the fenfluramine and dexfenfluramine group.

A July 1999 study published in *Obesity Research*[9] reported that the estimated number of people who took fenfluramine or dexfenfluramine in the United States was between 1.2 to 4.7 million people. Results regarding the actual incidence of heart valve problems in these patients are inconsistent ranging from about 5% to 30%. However, the rate of heart valve problems present in patients prior to taking the drugs is unknown, as is the percentage of these people who would have developed the problems even if they hadn't taken the drugs. The Framingham Heart Study reported that middle aged adults typically show a 10.5% rate of heart valve problems. The 1999 study[9] was the first to report on echocardiogram results both prior to taking fenfluramine or dexfenfluramine and after. Results on the 86 patients in the study showed that just over 6% had heart valve problems prior to taking the appetite suppressant drugs (beginning in 1995). In late 1997, about 23% of the total patient group showed heart valve problems. The patients had taken the drugs an average of 17 months. Thus, about 16-17% of the patients developed heart valve problems while taking the drug combination.

How Safe Are Any Drugs?

On April 15, 1998, the *Journal of the American Medical Association* published an article on the risks of medicines that are properly prescribed. The study estimated that in 1994, over 100,000 people died from various prescribed drug reactions or from complications arising from the drugs. An additional 7% of all hospitalized patients experienced drug reactions requiring medical attention. Narcotic painkillers, antibiotics, antiviral drugs, heart medications, and even aspirin caused some deaths. Adverse drug reactions represent the fifth leading cause of death. In comparison, few deaths have been attributed to fenfluramine and dexfenfluramine and even fewer to other obesity medications.

Several appetite suppressant medications are available to treat obesity. In general, these medications are modestly effective, leading to an average weight loss of 5 to 22 pounds above that expected with non-medical obesity treatments. People respond differently to appetite suppressant medications, and some people experience more weight loss than others. Some obese patients using medication lose more than 10 percent of their starting body weight — an amount of weight loss that may reduce risk factors for obesity-related diseases, such as high blood pressure or diabetes. Maximum weight loss usually occurs within 6 months of the start of medication treatment.

Transparency of Drug Effects

"Obesity is a chronic, relapsing disease and some patients are probably going to need pharmacological assistance indefinitely. Therefore, as a physician, I want my medical treatment to be as transparent as possible. In other words, I want my patients to feel healthy, happy, and not feel drugged; neither drugged up or down. To me, patients on the correct medications say, 'I don't feel a thing, but I do notice weight loss.'"[10]

Prescription Appetite Suppressant Medications	
Generic Name	Trade Name(s)
Diethylpropion	Tenuate, Tenuate dospan
Mazindol	Sanorex, Mazanor
Phendimetrazine	Bontril, Plegine, Prelu-2, X-Trozine
Phentermine	Adipex-P, Fastin, Ionamin, Oby-trim
Sibutramine	Meridia

Phentermine (trade names: Adipex-P, Fastin, Ionamin, Oby-trim)

"Phentermine is almost the prototypical weight loss drug. It is a second cousin to amphetamines, but, in the large majority of people, it has no significant long-term side effects. It has been used since the 1960s and has a good track record. Phentermine increases brain levels of dopamine and norepinephrine. This increase in neurotransmitters seems to increase the efficiency with which signals are sent to the hunger center telling it to shut down. Also, the increased dopamine and norepinephrine levels raise the body's basal metabolic rate slightly. Thus, not only is there a diminution of hunger, there is a slight increase in the metabolic rate. So people will lose some weight on the drug."[10]

Phentermine is usually taken in the morning and early afternoon and should always be used in conjunction with an eating and exercise plan. While the greatest weight loss typically occurs in the first six months of use, weight loss can be maintained and continued with long-term use. However, because of the development of tolerance and lack of understanding of obesity, many physicians and the FDA have been very cautious about continued use of the drug.

Tolerance is a form of physiological accommodation to a drug's effects. "Because this drug (phentermine) causes a person to feel a little bit more active for a short amount of time, people think the medicine is not working when that feeling goes away. Yet, the drug is still working. If the phentermine is discontinued, weight typically returns."[10]

Studies have evaluated the use of phentermine (without the use of other weight loss drugs) for periods of 36 weeks. "No case reports have been published of heart valve abnormalities with the use of phentermine alone. Few reports of PPH (primary pulmonary hypertension) have been associated with the use of phentermine alone."[11]

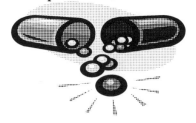

Contraindications To Phentermine

If you have any of the following conditions, be certain to tell your provider because phentermine may not be appropriate for you:

- Pregnancy (possibly breast feeding)
- Allergy to phentermine or amines that stimulate the sympathetic nervous system
- Advanced atherosclerosis
- States of agitation or mania
- Glaucoma
- Hyperthyroidism
- Moderate/severe hypertension
- Symptomatic cardiovascular disease
- History of drug abuse
- Use of antidepressants called MAO-I
- Age over 60 or under 12

Common Symptoms &
Side Effects With Phentermine

During the first few days on phentermine, patients typically experience more energy and loss of appetite. These feelings gradually dissipate and most patients experience few side effects. In those patients who do have some side effects, the most common symptoms can be wide-ranging and include:

- Drowsiness
- Dry mouth
- Tiredness
- Depression
- Nervousness
- Irritability
- Sense of well-being
- Increased blood pressure

Less common side effects include:

- Skin rash, itching
- Nausea
- Diarrhea
- Stomach pain
- Unpleasant taste in mouth
- Headache
- Dry mouth
- Blurred vision
- Confusion
- Dizziness
- Irregular heartbeat

Overdose can be indicated by:

- Fever
- Stomach cramps
- Irregular heartbeat
- Confusion
- Nausea, vomiting, diarrhea
- Irregular blood pressure
- Restlessness, panic, or tremors
- Hallucinations, irrationality

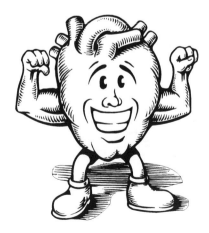

Diethylpropion (trade names: Tenuate, Tenuate dospan)

In patients with mild hypertension, diethylpropion is considered to be one of the safest anorexiants.[11] Its effects on neurotransmitters is similar to phentermine. It can greatly aid in short-term weight loss, but a large percentage of patients discontinue the drug due to side effects that occur in greater frequency than with phentermine.[11]

Contraindications To Diethylpropion

If you have any of the following conditions, be certain to tell your provider because diethylpropion may not be appropriate for you:
- Pregnancy (possibly breast feeding)
- Allergy to diethylpropion
- Advanced atherosclerosis
- States of agitation or mania
- Glaucoma
- Hyperthyroidism
- Severe hypertension
- Cardiovascular disease
- History of drug abuse
- Use of antidepressants called MAO-I
- Age over 60 or under 12
- Epilepsy
- History of arrhythmias

Common Symptoms & Side Effects With Diethylpropion

During the first few days on diethylpropion patients typically experience more energy and loss of appetite. These feelings typically gradually dissipate. The most common symptoms include:
- Irritability and nervousness
- Insomnia

Less common side effects include:
- Anxiety
- Hypertension
- Rash
- Nausea
- Constipation or diarrhea
- Headache
- Blurred vision
- Euphoria or dysphoria (sense of uneasiness)
- Dizziness
- Irregular or pounding heartbeat
- Tremors
- Changes in sex drive

Overdose can be indicated by:
- Insomnia
- Mood changes, restlessness, irritability
- Irregular, rapid heartbeat
- Trembling
- Nausea, vomiting, diarrhea, fever
- Irregular blood pressure
- Panic states, confusion
- Stomach or heart pain
- Hallucinations, confusion, coma

Mazindol (trade names: Sanorex, Mazanor)

Mazindol is related to a class of antidepressants called tricyclics.[11] It achieves its appetite suppressant effects by releasing dopamine and blocking the reuptake of norepinephrine. It has been shown to produce enhanced weight loss in obese patients in some studies lasting up to a year. While some of its side effects are similar to amphetamines, it has little abuse potential and does not cause euphoria.[11] However, the drug does produce withdrawal symptoms when it is discontinued and should be tapered off rather than simply stopped.

Contraindications To Mazindol

If you have any of the following conditions, be certain to tell your provider because mazindol may not be appropriate for you:
- Pregnancy (or breast feeding)
- Allergy to mazindol
- Glaucoma
- Severe hypertension
- Symptomatic cardiovascular disease
- History of drug abuse
- Use of antidepressants called MAO-I
- Age over 60 or under 12

Common Symptoms
& Side Effects With Mazindol

During the first few days on mazindol patients typically experience more energy and loss of appetite. These feelings typically gradually dissipate. The most common symptoms include:
- Irritability and nervousness
- Insomnia
- Dry mouth
- Irregular or pounding heartbeat

Less common side effects include:
- Rash or hives
- Nausea or vomiting
- Constipation or diarrhea
- Headache
- Blurred vision
- Dizziness
- Changes in sex drive
- Hair loss
- Unpleasant taste in mouth
- Breathing difficulty
- Increased sweating
- Nightmares
- Urgency or difficulty in urination
- Weakness or cramps

Overdose can be indicated by:
- Insomnia
- Mood changes, restlessness, irritability
- Irregular, rapid heartbeat
- Trembling
- Fever
- Stomach or heart pain
- Hallucinations, confusion, convulsions

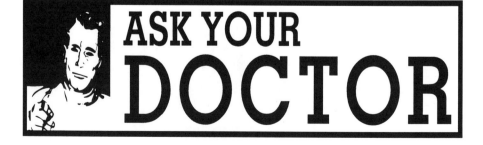

Phendimetrazine (trade names: Bontril, Plegine, Prelu-2, X-Trozine)

Phendimetrazine is chemically similar to amphetamine and has an abuse potential. It suppresses appetite by stimulating norepinephrine and dopamine release. Tolerance and psychological dependence can develop to the drug and cessation of the drug may require a gradual reduction in dosage. Extreme caution is advised.

Contraindications To Phendimetrazine

If you have any of the following conditions, be certain to tell your provider because phendimetrazine may not be appropriate for you:

- Pregnancy (possibly breast feeding)
- Allergy to phendimetrazine
- Glaucoma
- Hyperthyroidism
- Hypertension
- Cardiovascular disease
- History of drug abuse
- Use of antidepressants called MAO-I
- Adults over 60 & children/adolescents
- History of arrhythmias

**Common Symptoms
& Side Effects With Phendimetrazine**

During the first few days on phendimetrazine patients often experience more energy and loss of appetite. These feelings, typically, gradually dissipate. The most common symptoms include:

- Irritability and nervousness
- Insomnia
- Dry mouth

Less common side effects include:

- Rash or hives
- Nausea
- Constipation or diarrhea
- Headache
- Blurred vision
- Euphoria or dysphoria (sense of uneasiness)
- Dizziness, weakness, or cramps
- Hair loss
- Irregular or pounding heart rate
- Breathing difficulty
- Nightmares
- Unpleasant taste in mouth
- Urgent or difficult urination
- Changes in sex drive

Overdose can be indicated by:

- Insomnia or overactivity
- Mood changes, restlessness, irritability
- Rapid heart beat
- Trembling
- Fever
- Disorientation or confusion
- Hallucinations or coma

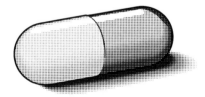

Sibutramine (trade name: Meridia)

Sibutramine is the only appetite suppressant approved by the FDA for long-term use (one year). However, "off-label use" for much longer time periods is typical with all of the appetite suppressants. Sibutramine inhibits the reuptake of norepinephrine and serotonin, and, to a lesser extent, dopamine.[12] Research shows that patients taking the drug typically lose 7% to 8% of their weight with most of the weight loss occurring during the first 6 months. Continuation of the drug for another 6 months has shown that maintenance of the weight loss was enhanced. There is no data on the effects of the drug beyond 12 months and no cases of heart valve problems have been reported.[12]

Contraindications To Sibutramine

Sibutramine is not considered appropriate for patients with a history of seizures, stroke, coronary artery disease, congestive heart failure, uncontrolled hypertension, or severe renal or hepatic function impairment. The drug has been shown to markedly increase blood pressure in some patients so frequent blood pressure monitoring is required. Drugs that should not be used with sibutramine include antidepressants, lithium, and several over-the-counter drugs: cough suppressants, decongestants, or migraine drugs. If you have any of the following conditions, be certain to tell your provider because sibutramine may not be appropriate for you:

- Pregnancy (possibly breast feeding)
- Allergy to sibutramine
- Congestive heart failure
- Uncontrolled hypertension
- Coronary artery disease or stroke
- Irregular heart beat
- Severe renal or hepatic failure
- Use of antidepressants called MAO-I
- Adults over 60 and adolescents under 16
- Anorexia nervosa

Common Symptoms & Side Effects With Sibutramine

Because of its possible effects on blood pressure, frequent monitoring is required — especially in the beginning of treatment. The most common symptoms include:

- Constipation
- Insomnia and headache
- Dry mouth

Less common side effects include:

- Rash or allergic reaction
- Nausea or vomiting
- Abdominal, chest, back, or stomach pain
- Weakness, depression, and anxiety
- Dizziness and coughing
- Muscle and joint pain
- Inflammation of nasal membranes
- Sleepiness
- Increased blood pressure, irregular or fast heart rate
- Sweating, blood vessel dilation
- Edema (fluid accumulation)
- Liver enzyme elevations

Overdose can be indicated by:

- Seizures
- Increased heart rate
- Increased blood pressure
- Heart arrhythmias

Fat Blockers - Lipase Inhibitors

With the FDA approval of orlistat (trade name Xenical) in 1999, a new class of antiobesity drugs has become available. Orlistat doesn't enter the blood stream, instead, it works by partially inhibiting the enzymes in the intestines responsible for digestion and absorption of dietary fat (these enzymes are called *gastrointestinal lipases*). When it is taken with meals, orlistat effectively blocks the absorption of 30% of fat calories. For example, a McDonald's meal of a Quarter-Pounder with cheese, large fries, and soda has 1,166 calories with 51 grams of fat. Taking orlistat with the meal would block the absorption of about 15 grams of fat and reduce the calories by 135 (each fat gram has 9 calories). (We don't suggest you eat this way.)

The fate of the unabsorbed fat leads to the primary side effects experienced with orlistat. The fat moves rather quickly through the intestines and can cause gas, bloating, and sudden bowel urges. People who eat high fat meals especially experience these effects and can even have occasional "accidents" with uncontrollable "leakage" of oily fecal matter.

For some people, orlistat has a psychological deterrent effect that is very similar to the way antabuse affects alcoholics. People who take antabuse experience very unpleasant physical effects after drinking alcohol. Those on orlistat pay a price for consuming too much fat in a meal. This can result in less fat being consumed.

It is recommended that those who take orlistat consume no more than 30% of their daily caloric intake in fat. This aids in reducing side effects and helps with weight reduction. A multivitamin at bedtime is also recommended because orlistat blocks the absorption of some vitamins.

Research shows that obese people who take the drug with a daily 1,500 to 1,800 calorie diet lose 50% more weight than through diet alone. Other significant findings have shown that patients on orlistat have lower cardiovascular risks including lower cholesterol levels, lower blood pressure, and lower blood sugar levels. Research with type 2 diabetics has shown that the drug can produce substantial improvements in symptoms.[13, 14]

Our experience with the drug shows that it appears to be safe and effective for obese patients and can be used in combination with other weight loss drugs. One of its major drawbacks is its high expense.

Contraindications To Orlistat (Xenical)

The implications of using orlistat with pregnant or nursing mothers are not known and the use of the drug with children has not been studied. Eating a balanced diet and taking a multivitamin are recommended. People with problems causing an increase in urinary oxalate should not take this drug. If you have any of the following conditions, be certain to tell your provider because orlistat may not be appropriate for you:

- Allergy to orlistat
- Gallbladder disease
- Chronic malabsorption syndrome

**Common Symptoms
& Side Effects With Orlistat**

The most common symptoms include:

- Gas with discharge
- Fatty, oily stool
- Frequent bowel movements
- Oily evacuation and "spotting"

Less common side effects include:

- Abdominal pain
- Nausea or vomiting
- Tooth disorder
- Headache, dizziness, and anxiety
- Ear inflammation
- Fatigue, muscle or back pain, menstrual irregularities
- Dry skin, skin rash
- Respiratory disorder

No symptoms of overdose have been reported

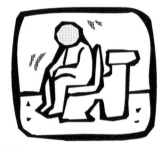

Drugs Approved For Use With Diabetics That Can Be Useful In Obesity Treatment

During the past three years, several new classes of drugs have been developed and approved by the FDA for use with type 2 diabetes. These include drugs that inhibit the absorption of dietary sugar and simple carbohydrates and insulin sensitizers. These drugs are very helpful in the treatment of type 2 diabetes and should be considered in obese patients who show insulin resistance.

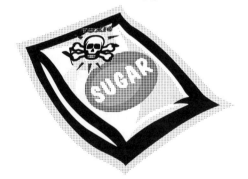

Sugar & Starch Absorption Inhibitors

Two drugs, trade names Precose (acarbose) and Glyset (miglitol), are used to slow the absorption of simple sugars and starch consumed in diet. By decreasing the absorption of sugar and starch, insulin release is less stimulated. This is helpful for insulin resistance. The class of drugs they represent are called alpha-glucosidase inhibitors. As with orlistat, the drugs block intestinal enzymes, but these block the enzymes responsible for sugar absorption: alpha-glucosidase.

Acarbose (trade name: Precose)

Acarbose was developed to keep glucose levels from rising after a meal in type 2 diabetics when diet and other diabetes medications are insufficient. The dosage of acarbose depends on the individual patient's response. Acarbose is taken with the first bite of a meal and alcohol should be avoided. The drug can increase liver enzymes, thus, liver function tests are recommended.

Contraindications To Acarbose

Acarbose is not considered appropriate for patients with several types of preexisting conditions. In addition, it can cause hypoglycemia (low blood sugar) in some diabetics, especially when infections, fever, or physical trauma occur. If you have any of the following conditions, be certain to tell your provider because acarbose may not be appropriate for you:

- Pregnancy (unknown effects; possibly breast feeding)
- Allergy to acarbose
- Diabetic ketoacidosis
- Cirrhosis of the liver
- Inflammatory bowel disease
- Colonic ulceration
- Intestinal obstructions (or history of)
- Severe renal function impairment
- Infants, children
- Chronic intestinal digestion/ absorption disorders

Common Symptoms & Side Effects With Acarbose

Because acarbose blocks the absorption of some starch and simple carbohydrates, the primary side effects are intestinal. Hypoglycemia can occur when acarbose is used with other diabetic medications. The most common symptoms of acarbose include:

- Diarrhea
- Bloating, feelings of fullness
- Abdominal pain
- Gas

Less common side effects include:

- Anemia, pale skin
- Heart palpitations, shortness of breath, fatigue
- Low blood sugar
- Elevation of liver enzymes

Overdose can be indicated by:

- Diarrhea
- Stomach pain
- Gas

Miglitol (trade name: Glyset)

Miglitol was also developed to keep glucose levels from rising after a meal in type 2 diabetics when diet and other diabetic medications are insufficient. It works to inhibit the absorption of sugars (sucrose) consumed in diet. The dosage of miglitol depends on the individual patient's response. Miglitol is taken with the first bite of a meal. This drug, unlike acarbose, does not appear to increase liver enzymes. Diabetics who have low blood sugar reactions should understand that when taking miglitol, table sugar products are ineffective in raising blood sugar and glucose (honey, not table sugar) should be used.

Contraindications To Miglitol

Miglitol is not considered appropriate for patients with several types of preexisting conditions. If you have any of the following conditions, be certain to tell your provider because miglitol may not be appropriate for you:
- Pregnancy or breast feeding
- Allergy to miglitol
- Diabetic ketoacidosis
- Inflammatory bowel disease
- Colonic ulceration
- Intestinal obstructions (or history of)
- Severe renal function impairment
- Infants, children
- Chronic intestinal digestion/ absorption disorders

Common Symptoms & Side Effects With Miglitol

Because miglitol blocks the absorption of sucrose, the primary side effects are intestinal. Hypoglycemia can occur when miglitol is used with other diabetic medications. The most common symptoms of miglitol include:
- Diarrhea
- Bloating, feelings of fullness
- Abdominal pain
- Gas
- Rash

Less common side effects include:
- Anemia, pale skin
- Heart palpitation, shortness of breath, tired
- Low blood sugar
- Elevation of liver enzymes

Overdose can be indicated by:
- Frequent urination
- Hunger, thirst
- Unexplained weight loss

Insulin Sensitizers: Drugs That Lower Insulin Resistance

Two new classes of insulin sensitizers are used to treat insulin resistance. The drugs have a low rate of serious side effects, however, both have an incidence of potentially life-threatening complications. Thus, monitoring of kidney and liver functioning is required. Metformin (trade name Glucophage) is in the class of medications called *biguanides*.

Metformin lowers blood sugar levels by decreasing sugar (glucose) production in the liver and increasing tissue responsiveness to insulin. Troglitazone (trade name Rezulin) is in a class of drugs called *thiazolidinediones*. Troglitazone decreases insulin resistance by increasing tissue responsiveness to insulin. Many patients experience weight loss from lower insulin levels when taking insulin sensitizers. Since obese patients typically have some insulin resistance, the drugs should possibly be considered for use in obesity treatment. (As we were finishing this book, two new medications in the same family as troglitazone (Rezulin) were released. They are touted as having fewer side effects.)

Metformin (trade name: Glucophage)

Prior to metformin therapy, kidney function should be evaluated with blood levels of creatinine. After the drug is initiated, those tests should be repeated several times the first year and at least annually thereafter. Abnormal kidney function tests contraindicate the use of the drug. The drug can also produce anemia and reduced absorption of folic acid and some amino acids. Routine checkups should be made.

Contraindications To Metformin
Metformin is not considered appropriate for patients with several types of preexisting conditions. If you have any of the following conditions, be certain to tell your provider because metformin may not be appropriate for you:
- Pregnancy (possibly breast feeding)
- Allergy to metformin
- Kidney dysfunction
- Inflammatory bowel disease
- Severe liver disease
- Acute or chronic metabolic acidosis
- Infants, children, adults over age 60

Common Symptoms
& Side Effects With Metformin
The most common symptoms of metformin include:
- Anorexia, nausea, or vomiting
- Bloating, stomach pain, gas

- Headache
- Unpleasant taste in mouth
- Weight loss

Less common side effects include:
- Skin rash, itching
- Anemia
- Lactic acidosis (diarrhea, weakness, cramps)
- Low blood sugar

Overdose can be indicated by:
- Lactic acidosis
- Low blood sugar

Troglitazone (trade name: Rezulin)

Prior to troglitazone therapy, a liver function test should be performed. After the drug is initiated, liver function tests should be monitored monthly the first year and every three months thereafter. Abnormal liver function results contraindicate the use of the drug. Rare cases of liver failure sometimes requiring transplants (and even death) have been reported with troglitazone. Any suggestion of liver injury or dysfunction requires discontinuation of the drug. Nausea, stomach pain, anorexia, and dark urine can indicate liver problems.

Contraindications To Troglitazone

Troglitazone is not considered appropriate for patients with several types of preexisting conditions. If you have any of the following conditions, be certain to tell your provider because troglitazone may not be appropriate for you:
- Pregnancy or breast feeding
- Allergy to troglitazone
- Diabetic ketoacidosis
- History of liver disease
- Evidence of liver dysfunction
- History of alcohol abuse
- Severe renal function impairment
- Infants, children
- Chronic intestinal digestion/ absorption disorders

Common Symptoms & Side Effects With Troglitazone

Despite the serious warnings of rare liver problems that occur with troglitazone, the drug has only one common side effect:
- Headache

Less common side effects include:
- Swelling of extremities
- Diarrhea, nausea, dizziness
- Weakness, back pain
- Inflammation of nasal membranes or pharynx
- Urinary tract infection
- Jaundice (yellowing of eyes or skin)

Overdose can be indicated by:
- Signs of liver failure

Repaglinide (trade name: Prandin)

Prandin is in a separate class of oral diabetic medications called *meglitinides*. Prandin is taken prior to each meal of the day and causes insulin release with meals, rather than keeping insulin levels elevated all day like the sulfonoreas do. This is more natural, and the lower insulin levels between meals causes less hypoglycemia, and allows more effective burning of fat.

Contraindications To Prandin

If you have any of the following conditions, be certain to tell your provider because Prandin may not be appropriate for you:
- Breast feeding
- Allergy to Prandin
- Diabetic ketoacidosis
- Liver or kidney impairment

Common Symptoms & Side Effects With Prandin

The most common side effects with Prandin include:

- Hypoglycemia
- Headache, back or joint pain
- Nausea, diarrhea
- Bronchitis, sinusitis

Less common side effects include:

- Skin rash

- Vomiting, indigestion, constipation
- Chest pain, heart rhythm irregularities
- Tingling
- Urinary tract infection
- Blood clotting reduction
- Low white blood count

Increased blood pressure

Overdose can be indicated by:

- Heart rhythm abnormalities
- Coma or convulsions

Antidepressants & Drugs For Obsessive Compulsive Disorder

Not long after its release in 1988, psychiatrists noted that the then unique antidepressant Prozac did not stimulate weight gain like the older antidepressants did and some patients actually lost weight. Studies have confirmed that a proportion of patients taking Prozac actually lose weight.[15, 16, 17]

By the time fen-phen was voluntarily withdrawn in September 1997, some physicians had already begun using a combination of Prozac and phentermine to treat obesity. Perfectly timed with fen-phen's withdrawal, the book *Safer Than Phen-Fen* was released in September 1997. In the book, Harvard-trained physician Michael Anchors suggested that Prozac should be combined with phentermine to produce a safe weight loss drug.

Prozac has been called a "miracle" drug, a "killer" drug, and a "personality transformation" drug since its release. The major advantage of Prozac and related antidepressants is that, unlike older antidepressants, they produce few side effects. The decreased number of side effects with Prozac is due to the fact that it only effects the brain's serotonin system. The older antidepressants essentially effected all of the brain's major neurotransmitters thus producing a wide variation in side effects. This new class of serotonin antidepressant drugs are not killer drugs, but some patients do find them to be miraculous. (See related story in box.)

We have reviewed Prozac and many of the similar drugs. Paxil and a few other related antidepressants are not reviewed, although their effects and side effects are similar.

Many physicians do, in fact, combine phentermine with Prozac or substitute newer antidepressants such as Celexa that have a similar mechanism of action as Prozac. The combination appears to be safe and, to our knowledge, no reports of heart valve problems have emerged. Many patients do, indeed, appear to lose weight on the combination, and, food obsessions and compulsive eating are diminished. Prozac and related antidepressants work by inhibiting the reuptake of serotonin in the brain (Selective Serotonin Reuptake Inhibitors — SSRI drugs). Since low serotonin levels are genetically linked to obesity and addiction, as well as obsessive-compulsive disorder, it is not surprising that obese patients can be helped with SSRIs.

Fluoxetine (trade name: Prozac)

Prozac was the first of the selective serotonin reuptake inhibitors. Its major uses are to treat depression, obsessive-compulsive disorder, binge eating, and for some cases of bulimia. All of the SSRI antidepressants can take a few weeks before they begin to become effective.

A Miracle Antidepressant?

A brief media-fed controversy in the early 1990s developed over the possible violence producing effects of Prozac. However, there is no valid, reliable evidence that Prozac or other drugs that produce their effects in the same manner as Prozac produce violence or increase the risk of suicide. In 1993 psychiatrist Peter Kramer published the book, *Listening To Prozac*. In it, Kramer proposed that Prozac was able to accomplish in a month or two what normally takes years of psychotherapy: it could transform personality for the better. Wallflowers could be become social extroverts, timid people could have confidence, and passive people could be assertive. In addition, people who were easily angered would show a much lessened response. Can these antidepressants produce such a transformation in personality? The answer is yes — but the greatest effects occur only in a small, but quite noticeable, minority of patients. About 10% of those who take Prozac or related antidepressants show remarkable improvements, but almost everyone who takes the drugs improves.[18]

In 1996, "serotonin syndrome" was first reported by hospital emergency room staff. Symptoms can be potentially life threatening and include irregular heart rate, stiffness, high temperature, fluctuating blood pressure, confusion, and possible hallucinations. Serotonin syndrome usually results from a drug interaction between Prozac (or other SSRI drugs) and LSD, cocaine, ecstasy, or other abused drugs. In addition, combining an SSRI antidepressant with MAO-I antidepressants, imipramine, or demerol can produce serotonin syndrome.

Contraindications To Prozac

Prozac is tolerated well by most patients. If you have any of the following conditions, be certain to tell your provider because Prozac may not be appropriate for you:

- Severe insomnia
- Allergy to Prozac
- Use of MAO-I antidepressants
- Very low weight
- Infants, children
- Breast-feeding

**Common Symptoms
& Side Effects With Prozac**

The most common symptoms of Prozac include:

- Skin rash, itching
- Loss of appetite, tiredness
- Nausea, headache, drowsiness
- Increased sweating
- Restlessness, tremor, insomnia
- Change in sexual functioning

Less common side effects include:

- Constipation, stomach pain
- Dry mouth
- Chills, fever, muscle pain
- Low blood sugar
- Facial flushing, vision changes
- Intense dreams
- Fast or irregular heartbeat
- Mania

Overdose can be indicated by:
- Serotonin syndrome
- Seizures, agitation
- Nausea, vomiting
- Heart rate increase

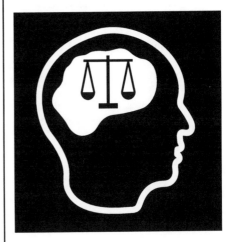

Citalopram (trade name: Celexa)

Celexa, a relatively new SSRI, is rapidly becoming one of the most often prescribed antidepressants. Although Celexa has a similar mechanism of action as Prozac, it produces less side effects, and, for most patients, we have had a better outcome with this drug.

Contraindications To Celexa

Celexa is well tolerated by most patients and produces minimal side effects. If you have any of the following conditions, be certain to tell your provider because Celexa may not be appropriate for you:

- Pregnancy (possibly breast feeding)
- Allergy to Celexa
- Use of MAO-I antidepressant
- Breast feeding
- Seizure disorders
- Liver, heart, or kidney disease

Common Symptoms
& Side Effects With Celexa

The most common symptoms of Celexa include:

- Dry mouth
- Rash
- Loss of appetite, tiredness
- Nausea, headache, drowsiness
- Diarrhea
- Increased sweating, upset stomach
- Restlessness, tremor, insomnia
- Change in sexual functioning
- Cough, runny nose

Less common side effects include:

- Stomach pain, vomiting
- Decreased appetite
- Chills, fever, muscle pain
- Leg cramps
- Low blood sugar
- Change in taste, ringing in ears
- Anxiety
- Fast heartrate
- Increased liver enzymes
- Low sodium levels in blood

Overdose can be indicated by:

- Serotonin syndrome
- Seizures, agitation
- Confusion, coma
- Nausea, vomiting
- Heart rate increase
- Dizziness, sweating, tremor
- Excessive sleep

Sertraline (trade name: Zoloft)

Zoloft was the second SSRI antidepressant. Zoloft is cleared from the body quicker than Prozac. Thus, if a patient developed side effects from Zoloft, they would disappear faster than they will if the patient had taken Prozac.

Contraindications To Zoloft

Zoloft is well tolerated by most patients and produces minimal side effects. It is approved to treat children age 6 and over as well as adults. If you have any of the following conditions, be certain to tell your provider because Zoloft may not be appropriate for you:

- Pregnancy (possibly breast feeding)
- Allergy to Zoloft
- Use of MAO-I antidepressant
- Breast feeding
- Seizure disorders
- Liver, heart, or kidney disease

Common Symptoms
& Side Effects With Zoloft

The most common symptoms of Zoloft include:

- Dizziness
- Gas, abdominal pain
- Loss of appetite, tiredness
- Insomnia
- Nausea, headache, drowsiness
- Diarrhea
- Increased sweating, tremor
- Change in sexual functioning
- Weight loss

Less common side effects include:

- Skin rash, itching
- Vision changes
- Increased appetite, vomiting
- Agitation, confusion, mania
- Facial flush, abnormal bleeding
- Change in taste, ringing in ears
- Restlessness
- Fast heartrate
- Involuntary muscle movements

Overdose can be indicated by:

- Serotonin syndrome
- Seizures, agitation, anxiety
- Nausea, vomiting
- Heart rate increase
- Dilated pupils
- Drowsiness
- Changes in electrocardiogram

Commonly Asked Questions About Treating Obesity With Medication

Q: Can medications replace physical activity or changes in eating habits as a way to lose weight?

A: No. The use of medications to treat obesity only solves part of the obesity puzzle. You still must address physical activity, food, environment, and stress issues.

Q: Will I regain some weight if I stop taking medications?

A: Probably. Most studies show that the majority of patients who stop taking obesity medications often regain the lost weight. Maintaining healthy eating and physical activity habits will increase your likelihood of keeping weight off.

Q: How long will I need to take medications to treat obesity?

A: The answer depends upon whether the medication helps you to lose and maintain a new lower weight, and whether you have any side effects. Because obesity is a chronic, relapsing disease, any treatment, whether medical or nonmedical, may need to be continued for years, and perhaps a lifetime, to improve health and maintain a healthy weight. There is little information on how safe and effective appetite suppressant medications are for more than 1 year of use.

Q: What medications are right for me?

A: There is no one correct combination of medications. Your doctor will decide what works best for you based on his or her evaluation of your medical condition and response to treatment.

Q: I only need to lose 10 pounds. Are medications appropriate for me?

A: Medications may be appropriate for carefully selected patients who are at significant medical risk because of obesity. They are not recommended for use by people who are only mildly overweight unless they have related health problems that are worsened by increased body fat. **Medications are not appropriate for cosmetic purposes only.**

Appropriate Treatment Goals
For Using Obesity Medications

If you and your doctor believe that the use of medications may be helpful for you, it is important to discuss the goals of treatment. Improving your health and reducing your risk for disease should be the primary goals. For most severely obese people, achieving an "ideal body weight" is both unrealistic and unnecessary to improve health and reduce the risk for disease. Most patients should not expect to reach an ideal body weight using the currently available medications, but even a modest weight loss of 5 to 10 percent of your starting body weight can improve your health and reduce the risk factors for disease. Use of medications for cosmetic purposes is not appropriate. Medications should be used with a program of behavioral treatment, nutritional counseling, exercise and life-style changes designed to help you make long-term alterations in your diet and physical activity. You should see your physician regularly so that he or she can monitor your response to the medications, not only in terms of weight loss, but how it effects your overall health. Again, if any new or unusual medical symptoms appear (shortness of breath, chest discomfort, fatigue) contact your physician.

Chapter References & Notes

[1] Loshak, D. (1999) Drugs needed to reinforce dietary, lifestyle measures in obesity management. *Doctor's Guide To Medical News*, June 4, 1999. www.pslgroup.com

[2] Powers, S. K., & Dodd, S. L. (1996) *Total fitness: exercise, nutrition, and wellness.* Boston: Allyn and Bacon.

[3] Anderson, D. A., & Wadden, T. A. (1999) Treating the obese patient. *Archives of Family Medicine*, 8, 156-167.

[4] Dalen, J. E. (1997) The treatment of obesity. *Archives of Internal Medicine*, 157, 602-604.

[5] American Association of Clinical Endocrinologists and The American College of Endocrinology (1998) *Position statement on the prevention, diagnosis and treatment of obesity.*

[6] Brodoff, B. N., & Nathan, C. (1992) Pharmacologic treatment of obesity. In: P. Bjorntorp, & B. N. Brodoff (Eds.) *Obesity.* New York: Lippincott.

[7] National Institute of Diabetes and Digestive and Kidney Diseases (revised 1998) *Prescription medications for the treatment of obesity.* Washington: National Institutes of Health publication number 97-4191.

[8] U. S. Department of Health and Human Services. (1997) Cardiac valvulopathy associated with exposure to fenfluramine or dexfenfluramine. *Morbidity and Mortality Weekly Report*, 46, November 14.

[9] Ryan, D. H., Bray, G. A., Helmcke, F., Sander, G. Volaufova, J., Greenway, F, Subramaniam, P., & Glancy, D. L. (1999) Serial echocardiographic and clinical evaluation of valvular regurgitation before, during, and after treatment with fenfluramine or dexfenfluramine and mazindol or phentermine. *Obesity Research*, 7, 313-322.

[10] Pettit, J. (1999) Interview with Pervis Milnor, III, M.D.: pharmacological interventions for obesity. *Addictive Behaviors Treatment Review*, 1 (2), 10-11.

[11] American Association of Clinical Endocrinologists and the American College of Endocrinology. (1998) *AACE/ACE Position Statement on the Prevention, Diagnosis, and Treatment of Obesity.* AACE/ACE Task Force.

[12] Anderson, D. A., & Wadden, T. A. (1999) Treating the obese patient. *Archives of Family Medicine*, 8, 156-167.

[13] Davidson, M. H., et. al. (11 authors) (1999) Weight control and risk factor reduction in obese subjects treated for 2 years with orlistat. *Journal of the American Medical Association*, 281, 235-242.

[14] Hollander, P. A., et. al. (15 authors) (1998) Role of orlistat in the treatment of patients with type 2 diabetes. *Diabetes Care*, 21 (8) 1288.

[15] Harlo, N. E., Spera, K. F., & Branconnier, R. J. (1988) Fluoxetine-induced reduction in body mass in patients with major depressive disorder. *Psychopharmacological Bulletin*, 24, 220-223.

[16] McGuirk, J, & Silverstone, T. (1990) The effect of the 5-HT re-uptake inhibitor fluoxetine on food intake and body weight in healthy male subjects. *International Journal of Obesity Related Metabolic Disorders*, 14, 361-372.

[17] Michelson, D., et. al. (9 authors) (1999) Changes in weight during a 1-year trial of fluoxetine. *American Journal of Psychiatry*, 158, 1170-1176.

[18] Little, G. L. (1998) *Psychopharmacology 2*. Memphis: Advanced Training Associates.

Chapter 10
OBESITY, PREJUDICE, & PSYCHOLOGICAL ISSUES: THE SECOND PUZZLE PIECE

The thin, narrow-shouldered ectomorph who was yesterday's
spinster librarian is today's high fashion model; the plump
and buxom endomorph who was a Victorian romantic ideal
today is eating cottage cheese and grapefruit, and
weighing in every Tuesday at Weight Watchers.
— **Phyllis Bronstein-Burrows (1981)**

I hate being fat; not just because it affects my health,
but also because I know I am stigmatized by my
body shape. "I am certain that some people look at me
and judge me," to paraphrase Dr. Martin Luther King, by
the shape of my body, "not by the content of my character."
— **Dr. Pervis Milnor, III**

Chapter Summary — Overweight people in America face deep prejudice. Many people deny that they judge others based on their looks, but psychological research shows otherwise. It has been demonstrated that people form initial impressions of others based almost solely on physical appearance. This fact can be upsetting to overweight people once they become aware of how much they have been judged by their body shape. This happens when a person loses a lot of weight and begins to get many compliments from others. The compliments are initially appreciated, but can ultimately disturb the person who lost the weight as she begins to understand how negatively she was viewed prior to the weight loss. Overweight Americans are stigmatized and discriminated against in almost all life areas. They tend to have lower education, lower income, and are less likely to be married. Studies show that obese people are usually judged by others to be lazy, ugly, cheaters, stupid, and morally defective. These prejudgments have been found to cause discrimination.

Overweight adults do not have higher levels of *diagnosable* psychological disorders than normal-weight adults. However, higher levels of depression, anxiety, and fear are observed in obese people — especially in adolescent females seeking treatment. Self-esteem issues also occur frequently in overweight people. Dissatisfaction with body image increases as weight increases. Overweight young females are especially distressed by their body image. By the time they enter the first grade, overweight children already show low self-esteem and body image problems. American children come to believe that thin people are healthy and smart while fat people are unhealthy and stupid. These beliefs contribute to the prejudice and discrimination experienced by the obese.

Almost all people who are overweight would decide to be thin if they had a real choice. But many come to believe that they are weak, lazy, inferior, and inadequate. "If you weren't," they have been told, "you'd be thin." Thus, self-esteem and self-concept are negatively effected and the person may accept that he or she is weak and inferior. But obesity is caused by a combination of biology and environment — not personal inadequacy. *In fact, obese people have to be much more resilient and disciplined than others to cope with the problem.*

Modern research shows that levels of emotional pathology are the same for obese people and people of normal weights. Yet overweight people do show low self-esteem, elevated depression and anxiety, and poor body image. Researchers believe that obese people suffer chronically from these problems at a subclinical level. This means that the suffering is not at a diagnosable level, yet it is constantly endured by the individual. One consequence of this suffering is the development of shame and guilt as the person begins to feel inferior to others.

One childhood factor that may cause some people to become overweight, is abuse — both physical and sexual. It is estimated that about 33% of women and 14% of men experience some form of sexual abuse before age 18. Some researchers and treatment professionals have speculated that childhood sexual abuse may be a major factor in the development of all addictions: drugs, alcohol, gambling, workaholism, eating, etc. The personal issues observed in obese people are often similar to the issues observed in other addictions as well as in victims of childhood sexual abuse. These can include low self-esteem, shame, guilt, anxiety, depression, poor self image, and suspicion. Some people — especially women abused sexually during their childhood — may become obese to form a physical barrier isolating them from others. There is little research investigating this, however, one important study found several childhood event differences between obese people and others.

Obese adults experienced the death of a parent in their childhood at more than double the rate seen in others. In addition, obese patients had more than twice as many alcoholic parents, twice the rate of childhood physical abuse, and four times the rate of childhood sexual abuse.

In many ways, overeating and obesity parallel other addictive disorders. The concept of codependency is often applied to obese people. Codependency is an unhealthy pattern of behaviors that develops because of a relationship. Codependents have problems with intimacy because of distorted feelings, underlying anger, resentment, shame and guilt. Codependent people tend to have a poor idea of self and overly respond to other's standards of appearance. Low self-esteem and self-blame occur when the codependent is unable to live up to these standards. Eating disorders and obesity are listed as codependent problems by virtually all books on the subject.

Overeating and obesity are also related to life-long habits that become deeply ingrained. Unconscious eating in front of the television, using food as a form of self-medication (numbing oneself by stuffing oneself), eating in response to boredom, stress, anxiety, or rejection are all dysfunctional habits that become very difficult to break.

• • •

Prejudice wounds deeply. Racism, sexism, cultural and religious hatreds are all recognized as universally destructive. However, the prejudices against the overfat and obese often go unchecked and unacknowledged by society.

We are taught that beauty is only skin deep and that appearances can easily fool us. Yet it is clear that people form their first impressions of others **by physical appearance**. Psychologists who have conducted hundreds of carefully controlled research studies investigating this fact have consistently shown the profound influence of physical appearance. Women are only slightly less likely than men to be influenced by attractiveness. However, women tend to be judged initially by men based *almost solely* on their appearance.[1] The appearance factor is so profound that researchers have evaluated how improving one's physical appearance effects the individual who made the improvement. For example, people who have had cosmetic surgery can actually be deeply *disturbed* by the complimentary reactions they receive from others.

Researchers believe that this happens because other's reactions confirm the extent to which we are judged by appearance.[2] This effect is frequently encountered by the person who loses a substantial amount of weight. Others' praise and comments, while initially perceived as positive, can have a reverse effect as the person begins to realize how negatively he or she was viewed by others *prior* to the weight loss. The underlying psychological framework of a yo-yo dieter (who cyclically loses weight and then regains it) is also bound to be negatively affected by the cycles of praise and shame-producing comments coming from others.

Myers' introductory text *Psychology*[1] simply concedes, "Being obese can affect how you are treated and how you feel about yourself. Many people think fat people are gluttons. ...If being obese signifies either a lack of self-discipline or a personality problem, then who would want to hire, date, or associate with such people? And if obese people believe such things about themselves, how could they feel anything but unworthy and undesirable."

The profound influence of culture, personality, social interactions, and emotional issues on obesity is often discounted. But, in actuality, the biological functioning of the brain is intimately tied to psychological processes. Our emotion affects our biological processes and our biological processes affect our emotions. Feelings, beliefs, behavioral patterns, and social pressures are perhaps the most unaddressed areas in obesity treatment. Psychological issues represent the second piece of the obesity puzzle and, if they are not properly understood and addressed, the probability of successful treatment is low.

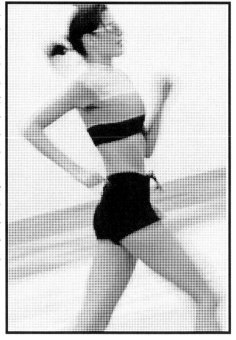

Thin is always associated with health.

Obesity Stigmatization Results in Discrimination

Obesity is stigmatized in America. Fat Americans are in a separate, negative class by themselves. A 1993 study[3] of 10,039 people who were between the ages of 16-24 years in 1981 showed that, seven years later, overweight women had lower education, lower income, and were less likely to be married. Overweight men showed the same basic results, although in men the trends were less pronounced. The study also concluded that *obesity resulted in subsequent discrimination* leading to lower socioeconomic status. Recent (1998) data from the National Center for Health Statistics[4] confirms that obesity is associated with income and socioeconomic status. In general, as weight increases, income and socioeconomic status decreases.

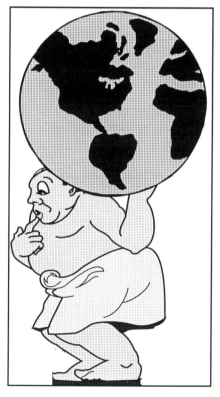

Studies published over the last 30 years consistently show that as a person's weight increases, he or she is less liked and judged less favorably by others. Obese people are labelled as morally deficient, lazy, ugly, cheaters, and stupid.[5] Discrimination against the obese has been confirmed by research in employment[6], housing[7], and even college admissions.[8] *America is a society that condemns overweight people and places the blame for obesity squarely on the shoulders of the overweight person.* In truth, there is little compassion for overweight people in America from family, friends, co-workers, neighbors, **doctors**, and sometimes even themselves. Shame, guilt, feelings of alienation, and feelings of weakness can run rampant in fat people.

Cultural Influences, Sex Differences, & Media Influences

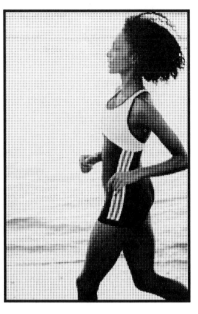

Culture plays a role in discrimination against obesity. The feminine ideal among American whites tends toward the very thin, low body-fat, athletically-fit model. "For those who internalize this ideal, and who come to equate body shape with self-worth, rigorous dieting and compulsive exercise can be the consequence."[9] African-Americans tend to subscribe to the thin female ideal much less than whites. But this appears to be changing in response to a powerful media influence. (See box on Fiji.) Bulimia nervosa (a pattern of binge eating and purging) tends to be far more frequent in white females and is seen most often in women who are perfectionistic,

How Powerful Is The Influence Of Television On Body Ideals?

Natives of the Fiji Islands have traditionally viewed obesity as a positive body characteristic. (Chapter 3 detailed how various cultures view thinness and obesity.) Harvard's Anne Becker has been studying America's rate of eating disorders and investigating the role of the media in influencing women — especially minority women — in the development of bulimia. Fiji has long been one of Becker's focal points because of its positive view of obesity. For centuries, eating well has been a status symbol in Fiji. Becker studied 129 Fiji females in 1995 and found the rate of bulimia (purging after eating) to be 3%. In 1999, Becker found the rate of bulimia had increased to 15%. Interestingly, Becker reported that in 1995 American television shows began to be shown in Fiji for the first time on its sole television station. Becker believes the super-slim actresses on these shows rapidly became role models for Fiji's young females leading to the increase of bulimia.

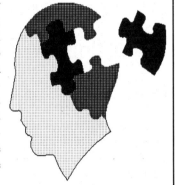

have negative self-evaluations, and a vulnerability to obesity.[10]

The influence of media-driven sex-based body ideals probably plays a crucial role in the development of serious eating disorders especially among women. For example, of all people with eating disorders, only 10% are men.[11] Women in America definitely experience a greater obsession with thinness than do men, and obese women face more discrimination than do obese men. But all overweight people experience some level of discrimination because of their weight.

The influence of the media on the development of eating disorders has long been suspected. Harvard University medical anthropologist Anne Becker has been researching the genesis of eating disorders for nearly 20 years. A 1999 forum sponsored by Harvard's Eating Disorders Center ("Culture, Media, and Eating Disorders") concluded that women are encouraged by the media to look like fashion models. The fact that fashion models and magazines represent entertainment rather than news or factual reporting is overlooked. Studies of female immigrants show a tendency to develop higher rates of eating disorders after exposure to American body-ideals. As a result, overweight minority

Emotional Eating

Chapters 7 & 8 outlined a connection between limbic system emotionality and eating. The hypothalamus appears to be the brain site that directly connects emotions, stress, and anxiety with various eating disorders including binge eating. Depression and anxiety are related to low levels of serotonin. The added stress placed on overweight people — especially women — may serve as a sort of driving force for some stress-related eating because of the influence of stress on the hypothalamus. Eating may relieve stress because many foods stimulate the production of serotonin and dopamine. Dopamine is a pleasure-producing neurotransmitter. William Vayda's (1995) book, *Mood Foods*, outlines how specific foods are often used for the pleasure they produce by releasing neurotransmitters such as dopamine, serotonin, and endorphins. Endorphins are the body's natural pain reliever and feelings of well-being and even bliss can result with their release. In addition, the consumption of carbohydrates, especially sugars, can create drowsiness in some people. Thus, some people who consume large amounts of carbohydrates prior to bedtime may be "self-medicating" stress with food in order to sleep. The issue of stress is directly linked to a person's inability to control eating because of a biological link.

women experience double doses of discrimination as rates of eating disorders among all minority groups continues to increase.

Obesity & Psychological Problems

Overweight people often have lower self-esteem and feelings of self-worth than do people of "normal" weight. In addition, certain social deficits (the ability to interact with others) and minor psychological difficulties have long been observed in the overfat. But which comes first is not always clear. Does obesity cause psychological problems or do psychological problems cause obesity? Research on this question has shown inconsistent and occasionally contradictory results.[5] For example, while the obese show the same basic levels of psychopathology as observed in normal weight people, subtle differences between obese males and females do occur.

Do Overweight People Have More Psychopathology?

In general, most research shows that *overweight adults do not have higher levels of diagnosable psychopathology* than adults with "normal" weight. Levels of psychological disorders like schizophrenia, psychotic depression, mania, alcoholism, and drug addiction are similar for normal weight people and overweight people. Depression and anxiety levels are generally similar for the obese and nonobese.[5]

Women who compare their body image to this amazingly thin model are destined for disappointment.

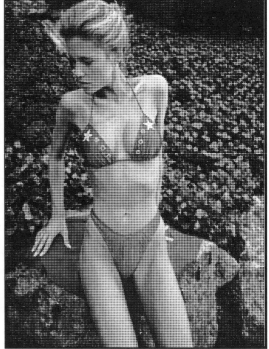

But some significant differences between obese males and females have been uncovered. Some research shows that obese women may be more *susceptible* to depression than obese men.[12] Adolescent females who are overweight **and** seek treatment do show elevations in emotional complaints when compared to overweight females who do not seek treatment. Among the significant findings with obese adolescent females seeking treatment are higher levels of depression, elevated levels of paranoia, and elevated anxiety and obsessions.[13]

Despite findings that adult obese populations do not have higher levels of diagnosable disorders than nonobese adult populations, depression is frequently observed in adults who enter weight-loss treatment. Studies[14,15] have shown that people who volunteer for obesity treatment have significant levels of depression. Other research points out that *morbidly obese* females who have gastric restriction surgery have higher phobia (fear-based) anxiety levels, more depression, more

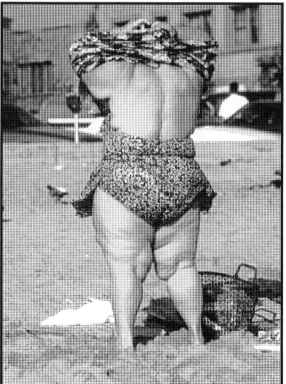

physical concerns and complaints, and are harder on themselves as compared to nonobese females.[16,17]

This woman certainly does not reflect the American ideal. How does a woman this size feel when she's compared to a model? How many people would immediately make fun of her? Youth and thinness are many people's highest values in America. You have to give her credit and admire her. She has enough self-esteem and inner strength to go to a public beach and reveal her body. How many obese people would be willing to risk doing this?

In summary, research on the levels of psychopathology in obese samples shows that overweight adults tend to have the same basic level of diagnosable pathology as seen in normal weight people. Yet, in general, when given standardized tests, the obese *usually* show more depression, anxiety, and concern about physical problems. Adults who seek medical treatment for obesity tend to show even more depression, anxiety, fear, and physical concern and are very self-condemning. This effect is even greater for obese adolescent females who seek treatment. Both fear of being overweight[18] and a greater stigmatization of obesity[19,20,21] in females have been proposed as reasons that adolescent females have more pathology.

Body-Image Problems

Self-Esteem & Self-Concept

Self-esteem can be defined as how a person *feels* about herself. Much research has been conducted on the self-esteem of overweight people. Both men and women who seek treatment for weight loss have high levels of emotional distress caused by body image.[22] Researchers believe that *levels of distress increase as the difference between a person's actual body and ideal body increases*. Research results comparing self-esteem in obese and nonobese groups are sometimes conflicting but, nevertheless, suggestive of a relationship between obesity and low self-esteem.[5]

Female adolescents, young adults, and women are particularly more dissatisfied with body shape as obesity increases.[23,24,25,26,27,28] This effect has been shown to begin as early as the first grade for both sexes.[29,30] In both children and adults, self-esteem related to body image decreases as body weight and fat increases.

Self-concept (what a person *thinks* about herself) studies tend to show that obese adults have poor self-concept. Studies with obese children have produced conflicting results, but the trends indicate that obese children tend to have poor self-concept.[19] In addition, people with binge eating disorders tend to have negative self-esteem as measured by self-evaluations.[10]

Self-concept and self-esteem form early in life. They develop as a result of what children are taught about themselves and others. For example, very early in life, children are influenced by the media, parents, and peers to believe that "thinness" is healthy and being overweight is unhealthy. They are surrounded by stereotypes that depict thin people as smart and fat people as stupid. These stereotypes are further employed as children judge others and themselves based on body size. Prejudice (prejudging based on appearance) and discrimination against "fat" people results from these comparisons and judgements. Research shows that this effect can be measured in children by age 8 or 9[31] and begins as early as the first grade. Furthermore, this research demonstrates how self-concept and self-esteem interact. Our self-concepts are based on the things we have come to believe. If a child believes that fat people are stupid and lazy — and he becomes fat — the logical step is to begin to think, "I must be stupid and lazy, or else I wouldn't be fat." Next, self-esteem plummets as he begins to feel bad about himself.

What are the effects of low self-esteem and poor self-concept?[32] When people with low self-esteem feel responsible for their condition, they tend to engage in behaviors that confirm the low self-esteem. For the obese individual, this could mean that he or she might engage in binge eating. A comparison may be helpful here. Some drug addicts and alcoholics have been told again and again that they are **weak**, are **no good**, and **want** to be addicted. "If you weren't," they are told, "you'd stop." In truth, if given a genuine choice, few (if any) addicts and

Understanding Self-Esteem & Self Concept

The technical distinction between self-esteem and self-concept is that esteem relates to feelings, and, concepts are beliefs. Researchers have developed various tests that measure self-esteem and self-concept. The way you *feel* about yourself (esteem) differs from what you *think* or *believe* about yourself (concept). For example, you might say, "I feel bad about my overall performance at work, but I believe that I did a really good job on that report." Self-esteem and self-concept are intertwined and obviously feed off one another. One negative feeling about yourself in a single important area can override all the positive beliefs you have about yourself. For example, an adolescent girl can have positive beliefs about herself (by getting good grades, being good at sports, and being a good, helpful person) but still have very poor self-esteem (because she's overweight). This is a complicated issue. The most important thing to keep in mind is that one important negative belief about yourself can override all of the other positive beliefs causing low self-esteem.

alcoholics would consciously choose to be addicted. But in view of their frequent relapses, broken promises, and the disparaging remarks of others, the addict shrugs it off by saying, "well, you said I'm weak and no good, what'd you expect?" This sort of thinking process is known as a "self-fulfilling prophecy." If we believe something is true, we act in ways to make it true.

Although there might be a few exceptions to this statement, *no one who is fat would consciously choose to be fat if he or she had a genuine choice*. But when the overweight individual has heard time and again that it is completely her fault, she comes to accept a set of beliefs about her personality. These beliefs can include ideas of personal weakness, gluttony, laziness, inferiority, and inadequacy. Once some of these beliefs are accepted, the way the individual feels about herself adapts to the beliefs. Self-esteem then tends to become poor. Due to learning and life experiences, many overweight people come to believe they are weak. If they accept this concept about themselves, they are likely to engage in behaviors that confirm these beliefs. Their behavior, in turn, reinforces negative self-concept and low self-esteem. This self-reinforcing cycle is

American society has almost no compassion for overweight people and pokes fun at them at nearly every opportunity. The blame for the disease is placed squarely on the shoulders of the obese. People believe the obese are weak, lazy, and stupid. Yet the obese continually suffer because of the condition and often see no way out. Diets don't work for them. They are told that one "miracle" substance or another will magically burn the fat off (it doesn't), and they are given conflicting information by the many "experts" promising them "quick fixes." As Dolly Parton has stated, we should be compassionate. It's a heartbreaking condition. Obesity isn't caused by weakness, laziness, or stupidity. It isn't caused by defective character. Ironically, to truly escape the condition, the obese person has to have much stronger will-power and self-discipline than other people.

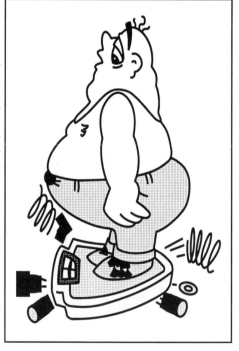

extremely difficult to break. And if underlying genetics predisposes the person to overeating or binge eating, it is even more difficult to break.

People who have low self-esteem tend to have deep-seated feelings of personal inadequacy — they feel personally incompetent in some life areas they believe are important. In times of stress, they often turn to the only coping methods they know. Some people turn to work-a-holism focusing all of their attention on keeping busy. This defense shields the person from having to face his personal inadequacy. For the addict, it's drugs. For the alcoholic, it's alcohol. For the obese, it's food.

It is critical that you come to realize that obesity and staying overweight are *influenced* by your behavior, your feelings, and the ideas you believe about yourself. But obesity is *not caused* by these. Obesity has a strong genetic, biological component that sets up the development of the related psychological factors. Obesity is caused by biology *plus* environment. As you may recall, research shows us that overweight children begin to have feelings of inadequacy, low self-esteem, and poor self-concept early in life. Where do these ideas come from? The answer is through social interactions with others where taunts, ridicule, and subtle discrimination are often first experienced.

Overcoming Obesity Requires Much Higher Than Normal Levels Of Will-Power

There is another important issue to keep in mind regarding psychological factors of obesity. In truth, *overweight and obese people have to have much higher than average levels of will-power and self-discipline to cope with this burden.* The normal weight person who has never experienced genetic-based weight gain has no real idea of the extreme deprivation and will-power that overweight people have to exert over themselves. The genetic influence working on the obese person is a profoundly difficult factor to deal with in itself. Add to that the effects of societal discrimination, belief systems imposed on the obese, the media influence, and the nature of the American environment with its stresses, work and family responsibilities, and food availability and the result is that dealing with obesity becomes a nearly impossible task. But America remains uncompassionate towards the obese — rejecting and blaming the sufferer for the suffering.

The lack of compassion shown to overweight people by others stems from a nearly complete lack of understanding of the plight the overweight person struggles with every day. In televised interviews, singer Dolly Parton has detailed her struggles with weight gain and loss. She says that every time she sees someone who is overweight her heart aches because she knows what that person is going through. Other people just can't seem to comprehend the problem.

It's not our intention to oversimplify this brief discussion on self-esteem and obesity. However, the impact of self-esteem on obesity — especially the ability to lose and keep off unwanted weight — is apparent. A 1991 study[33] found that obese women with high or medium levels of self-esteem were the ones most likely to be successful at losing weight and keeping it off. Those with low self-esteem were least likely to lose weight in the 10-week program. "If being overweight in a culture that values thinness affects any aspect of well-being, self-concept is a logical candidate."[5]

Your Beliefs Are An Important Factor

Your beliefs about yourself and the way you feel about yourself are important components to your overall health. They are also keys to losing weight and maintaining the loss. In later chapters, we will detail how these issues can be addressed in self-help groups, cognitive-behavioral groups, and in counseling. **But, at this point, it is critical that you begin to challenge some of your negative self-beliefs about being overweight.** If you are overweight, you must come to understand that the primary reason for it most likely lies in your genetics and physiological processes — it is simply not your fault. Obesity is a health condition not a character condition. It is nevertheless true that *you and only you* can do what's necessary to deal with it. And that means you either come to accept it as "the way you are" or exert much greater than average will-power and discipline to change it.

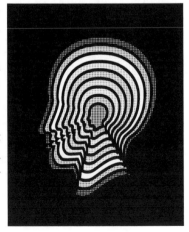

Obesity & Chronic Suffering

As related earlier, obese people tend to have levels of diagnosable psychopathology that are similar to nonobese populations. However, depression, anxiety, low self-esteem, poor self-concept, body image distortions, physical concerns, and obsessions *are* found in elevated levels in overweight people. But these trends are not to the extent that they are diagnosable psychopathology. They are defined as "problems" rather than pathology. What are the implications of this?

Researchers now believe that most overweight people *suffer chronically* from the psychological and social impact of being overweight. This "suffering" is endured by the person at a subclinical level.[5] In simple terms, the depression and anxiety is there, but it's not at the level at which the individual would be diagnosed with a depressive disorder. Many doctors don't perceive this suffering, especially when the patient is avoiding or denying it. Some medications (especially SSRI's like Prozac and Celexa) can greatly aid overweight people who are suffering at this subclinical level.

As the personalities of obese individuals develop, they attempt to learn ways of coping with the ridicule, discrimination, and taunts they experience from others. Some overweight people learn to cope by joking about themselves, showing off how much they can eat, and sometimes by even ridiculing other overweight people. Others cope by turning inward, avoiding social contact, avoiding competition, or becoming shy. A consequence of these coping styles of personality can be the development of shame, guilt, feelings of inadequacy, and a host of negative self-concepts.

As briefly discussed in the prior section, the music star Dolly Parton has spoken rather candidly about her struggles with weight. She talks about the constant suffering endured by the person who is overweight. The suffering begins when the person first comes to believe that he or she is different in size and shape from "others" and is made to feel somehow inferior. You probably remember the 1969 book title, *I'm OK, You're Ok*. The title described one of four "life positions" taken by people in their day-to-day life-style. I'm OK, You're OK is the best position — everyone wins with it. People who are depressed, feel inadequate, and have low self-esteem usually have the "I'm Not Ok, You're OK" position.

In comparing themselves to others, they feel inadequate or inferior. Regarding overweight people, most normal weight people send the message, "I'm OK, You're FAT!!"

Obesity is one of only a few life problems that can't be hidden. It's visible for all to see. We forget that everyone has some sort of ongoing problem. Some thin people don't feel thin enough. But that's not visible to others. Thin people may have disastrous relationships or a host of other difficulties, but they aren't easily observed. Most of us tend to hide our problems from other's view, but obesity is a problem that can't be hidden.

Every time the overweight person eats, she is confronted with her self-image, self-concepts, and self-esteem. Eating in the presence of others amplifies these feelings — usually for the worse. Every time the overweight person puts on clothing, tries on new clothes, or looks into a mirror, she is confronted with her ongoing problem. Television programs, infomercials on exercise/weight, magazine articles, and posters on telephone poles are a constant reminder to the obese person. What results from this constant bombardment is chronic, constant, low-grade suffering with shame, guilt, and self-disparaging feelings.

In speaking with their physicians about weight concerns and problems, the obese are given little solace. "Push away from the table and exercise more" is the standard refrain. Of course, there is some truth to the

Obesity can begin in childhood in response to various forms of abuse. Physical abuse and violence, sexual abuse, and emotional abuse can all cause a child to retreat to whatever leads to pleasure or stops the abuse. All forms of addictions have been linked to childhood abuse. Some women who were sexually abused in childhood have built up a "fortress of fat" where they can be insulated and protected from contact with others. Some children and adolescents who are abused find that, if they become physically unattractive, sexual abuse will cease.

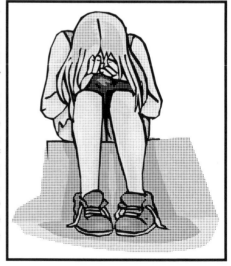

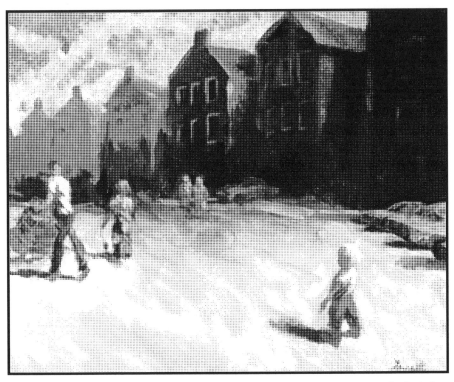

statement, but it just doesn't work by itself nor is it in any way helpful to the patient. Few doctors recognize the ongoing suffering in their over-weight patients. Unfortunately, if health professionals did recognize the suffering of the overweight, most wouldn't know how to handle it anyway.

Childhood Abuse Issues

There is no doubt that many children are abused sexually, physically, and emotionally. Population estimates (more like guessti-mates) of the extent of childhood *sexual* abuse vary widely, but the mid-point estimates are that about 33% of females and 14% of males experi-ence some sexual abuse before age 18.[34] Many, many treatment profes-sionals believe that victims of childhood sexual abuse are at high risk for the development of eating disorders later in adult life. Some cases of obesity are, no doubt, related to childhood sexual abuse. Psychologist Paul D'Encarnacao (now deceased) spent decades developing his "Octopus Theory of Addictions."[35] This theory proposes that childhood abuse, especially sexual abuse, is the primary *cause* of later-life addictions. The octopus' head symbolizes the original cause (the childhood abuse) while the many "arms" of the octopus are the many possible addictions. Addictions that can develop because of childhood abuse are eating disorders, drug & alcohol addictions, codependency, gambling, workaholism, sex addictions, and more. Writers like John Bradshaw, Jane Middleton-Moz, and Sharon Wegscheider-Cruse have proposed various forms of "inner child" therapy approaches to work with victims.

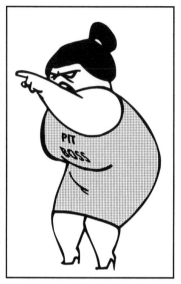

Building A Fortress Of Fat

There is valid evidence that adult survivors of childhood sexual abuse suffer from many of the same emotional issues as obese adolescents and adults. Low self-esteem, shame, guilt, anxiety, depression, poor body image, distorted self-perceptions, and suspicion are all found in both the obese and the sexually abused.[35] One explanation has been that some obese adults (especially females) literally put on fat to create a physical protective barrier between themselves and others. In some ways, it is like the abused child is trying to hide inside a *fortress of fat*. Another related idea is that obese people who were sexually abused are trying to unconsciously make themselves as sexually unattractive as possible. All of these speculations are controversial, although, it is known that some obese adults were sexually abused as children. In such cases, treatment and management of obesity should probably address this issue.

While childhood sexual abuse has gotten the majority of the publicity, other forms of childhood abuse are even more rampant. Physical abuse, emotional abuse, and neglect in childhood are more common than sexual abuse.[36] In addition, reported levels of childhood abuse are steadily increasing[36] — in some ways paralleling the increase in the percentage of overweight people in American society. For example, levels of both child abuse and obesity increase as socioeconomic level decreases. Research indicates that abuse of children and adolescents leads to increased psychiatric problems — including eating disorders.[37] Some researchers speculate that early life abuse can lead to permanent changes in brain chemistry including serotonin[38], a neurotransmitter directly implicated in obesity and overeating.

Few studies have directly addressed the relationship between childhood abuse and obesity. One significant study[53] looked at 100 adults entering a "calorie restriction" program and compared them to a matched group of 100 never-obese adults. Most (79%) of the study's subjects were women who were an average of 65 pounds overweight. The study showed that nearly half (48%) of the obese people suffered the death of a parent during their first 12 years of life as compared to only 23% in the always-slender matched control group. In addition, 40% of the obese group had an alcoholic parent as compared to only 17% in the controls. Childhood sexual abuse was found in 25% of the obese group as compared to only 6% in the controls. Finally, childhood physical and emotional abuse was found in 29% of the obese patients and only 14% in the controls.

It is very probable that obesity and childhood abuse are related issues with some people. Perhaps 25% to 35% of all obese people were abused in childhood, and it is likely that the childhood abuse had a significant impact on their subsequent weight gain, self-concept, and self-esteem. Not *all* overweight people were abused in childhood — but *some* were. An underlying early-life family environment issue (a fundamental family dysfunction) is obviously present in some obese people. When combined with a genetic predisposition to obesity, treatment becomes very complicated.

Codependence & Family Issues

Codependence is a controversial concept in psychology and counseling.[40] Virtually every book on codependence lists eating disorders and overeating as typical codependent behaviors. Most codependency books define codependence as the result of living in an addictive family or an addictive relationship. "Codependency results from the process of relationships. ... **It is an unhealthy pattern of behaviors that develops because of a relationship.**"[40]

Codependent people usually have problems with intimacy (emotional closeness to others). Anne Wilson Schaef,[41] believes this is because the codependent person has a poor idea of **self**. Codependents want to please others, be "good," and live up to the perceived expectations of others. Codependents believe that they should be able to solve other's problems — and their own. When they don't live up to these expectations (no one can), they internalize it and suffer in their self-esteem. The external source of self-esteem in codependents is rooted in overconcern with other's feelings rather than a firm sense of self-image.

Codependent people ultimately want to "possess" other people — because they have no real sense of who they themselves really are. A result of all this is the distortion and denial of feelings in the codependent person. Underlying anger, resentment, low self-esteem, depression, and guilt emerge in devious and distorted ways that confuse others and the codependent person. One way that these feelings are handled is by overeating. Feelings can be numbed by massive food intake. This is a fact. We know that eating some foods causes chemical changes in the brain that lead to "satiation" and a feeling of "fullness." Deep feelings about oneself can be simply crowded out — numbed — by overeating.

The issue of *self* is deeply connected to codependence. Many people define their self as their appearance. Other people define their self in relation to others. Both are styles typical of codependence. The codependent person usually has no sense of purpose in his or her life — other than the connection to a few other people and concern for physical appearance. For example, we encounter female patients who say, "My husband tells me I'm fat and that's why he rejects me sexually." Wayne Dyer[42] states, "Most eating disorders are, initially, efforts to meet a standard of appearance that someone believes will bring happiness. ...that their true essence is located in the value of their appearance to others." Melody Beattie[43] says bluntly, "We don't like the way we look. We can't stand our bodies. We think we're stupid, incompetent, untalented, and, in many cases, unlovable. ... We think we're inferior to and different from the rest of the world — not unique, but oddly and inappropriately different."

Before delving deeper into codependence, consider a few simple examples. Many people eat when they are depressed, angry, disappointed, bored, or stressed. What is important to understand is that depression, anger, disappointment, boredom, or stress are almost always somehow related to other people. Whether it is the disappointment of a lost love, an angry boss, a stressful relationship, or a longing for love, someone else is nearly always involved. The codependent person views *someone else* as the solution to her dilemma. When efforts to resolve the problem fail, the codependent person "stuffs" the emerging feelings in many ways — one of these ways being to stuff themselves!

Another characteristic of codependent people is gullibility.[41] Schaef states that codependent people will believe almost anything if it fits what they *want* to believe. This could be one reason why so many overweight people will buy one "miracle" weight-loss product and gadget after another despite knowing that it won't really work. Lots of people buy the useless products advertised on expensive full-page ads promising, "No Exercise, Eat Anything You Want, And Lose Weight!" Such people *want* to believe they can eat all they want, and by just taking a few expensive pills with each meal, the weight will simply melt off.

As stated earlier, coming to terms with one's self is an important component to overcoming codependence. **You are more than a body. You are more than what you eat. You are more than your appearance.** But you may have struggled and suffered with weight for so long, that you can't see anything else in your life. Think for a moment about who you'd be if you were slim. What would change in you? People would probably respond to you in different ways and you'd probably be healthier, but how else would you change? The truth is, you'd still be you. If all you can think about as you read this is that you'd look better and people would treat you better, you may have a problem with codependence.

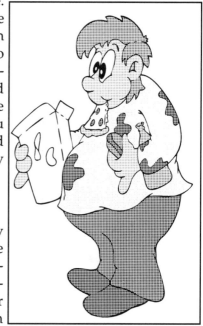

Eating Addiction

Overeating and obesity clearly mimic other addictive behaviors. The yo-yo dieter who cycles between periods of forced starvation and binge eating is, in many ways, like the addict or alcoholic who regularly cycles between relapse and recovery. Many researchers have addressed the compulsive nature of all addictions and how specific addictive behaviors develop in particular people. The fact that brain chemistry is intimately involved with all addictive behaviors is apparent. "Most addictionologists — even those who disagree about other matters of causation and treatment — agree that low self-regard is a crucial factor in all forms of addiction. The chronic absence of good feelings about oneself provokes a dependence on mood-changing activity. Manifest or masked, feelings of low self-worth are basic to most dysfunctional life-styles. One way of coping with disquieting factors is to immerse oneself in an activity that is incompatible with serious self-evaluation."[44] What this means to a person who has tried to lose weight repeatedly is probably not going to be pleasant. You have to confront yourself to save yourself. You can't do it by trying to control yourself. For example, during the drastic diets that you have tried, what did you think about? Chances are you were obsessed with food. It was all you could think about. What the obsession with food does is keep you from confronting deep-seated issues. Few dieters actually come to terms with their self-image, self-worth, or life purpose — they are either too busy eating (and feeling bad about it) or dieting (and being obsessed with food). Either way, food is the focus.

When a baby cries, it is cuddled, changed, and fed. Just as an infant's discomfort is relieved by food and touch, many adults seek solace in food and touch. When touch isn't present, food can be all that's left. The soothing influence of food is sometimes referred to as "a substitute for the thumb" or the chemistry of contentment. Some foods release the pain relieving and soothing brain chemicals endorphin and serotonin.[44]

Addictions come in many variations, but all share in common a repeating pattern of behavior designed to change mood and feelings in a way that is ultimately harmful. *The Many Branches of Addiction* illustrated on the next page depicts how addictions develop.

Overeating In Response To Environment & Emotion

For some people, sitting in front of the television provokes eating behavior. This can be such an ingrained habit that the person doing it is

THE MANY BRANCHES OF ADDICTION

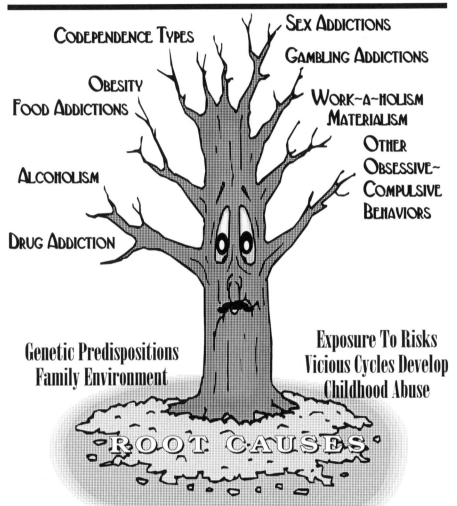

CODEPENDENCE TYPES

SEX ADDICTIONS

GAMBLING ADDICTIONS

OBESITY
FOOD ADDICTIONS

WORK~A~HOLISM
MATERIALISM

OTHER
OBSESSIVE~
COMPULSIVE
BEHAVIORS

ALCOHOLISM

DRUG ADDICTION

Genetic Predispositions
Family Environment

Exposure To Risks
Vicious Cycles Develop
Childhood Abuse

ROOT CAUSES

Addiction is a controversial term. In its purest definition, addiction is a form of *enslavement*. A frequently used definition is that *addiction is rotating one's life around something ultimately harmful*. From that simple perspective, lots of behaviors are addictions — they can be represented by many branches of a single tree. The root causes of them are similar. Genetics, environment, early family life, exposure to certain risk-producing events, the development of self-reinforcing prophecies (vicious cycles), and all forms of childhood abuse contribute to the development of addictions. Which specific branch the addiction takes is probably determined by several factors. Perhaps biological predispositions and childhood environment are the most important determining factors.

totally unaware of it. Others eat when they are bored, nervous, tired, angry, or experiencing any of a host of other emotions. Many researchers believe that food can sometimes be a form of self-medication in that stuffing oneself can lead to a release of brain chemicals that are experienced pleasantly.[44] With other people, it may simply induce the development of bad habits.

Habits are hard to break — especially bad habits. Father Bill Stelling has said that he wishes bad habits were as easy to break as good habits. He made this statement after having 5 heart bypasses performed. He explained that before his bypass surgery he owned a treadmill on which he "religiously" walked several miles everyday for over a year. Then one day he didn't walk for some reason or another. Without consciously realizing it, his good habit was broken and he quit walking altogether. Eventually, after being confronted by the daily sight of the unused treadmill — and the guilt he experienced — he finally sold it. (He now has another one.) The same thing occurs when a person goes off a diet and exercise plan. Diet books and scales are avoided and put out of sight until all of the weight has returned.

Eating in response to boredom, stress, anxiety, or rejection is a habit that obviously leads to some kind of relief. Quitting an exercise program can also be a relief to some people. How a person consistently copes with stress and boredom is a habit — and it could be a good one or a dysfunctional one. And, that is your choice.

All of the prior issues addressed in this chapter relate to the habits a person develops in his or her attempt to cope with day-to-day life. Personality style consists of what you usually do in response to particular events. There are many ways a person can handle stress and tension in life. Some ways are better than others.

Overweight people often cope with stress in dysfunctional ways. Of course, these behaviors were learned early in life in response to a lot of factors. It should not be forgotten that one of these factors is a genetic predisposition. But, changing these dysfunctional coping behaviors requires that they be identified and acknowledged. A few clarifying statements can show the importance of psychological issues to obesity treatment:

1. Psychological factors are definitely related to obesity, over-eating, and other eating disorders. (Treatment with appropriate medications [such as antidepressants] can help with some problems. Individual counseling and group support are usually necessary interventions to assist with other factors.)

2. Chronic, low grade suffering is present in the vast majority of the obese. (Subclinical depression, anxiety, fear, and other negative emotions are present in the obese and overweight with low self-esteem, poor-self concepts, and destructive beliefs. Shame, guilt, feelings of inadequacy, and subtle discrimination take a constant toll on the obese. Treatment approaches must somehow address these issues.)

3. Because of the chronic suffering and discrimination experience by the obese from an early age, personality coping styles are developed that worsen the problem. (Codependency, a distorted sense of self, and the "stuffing" or numbing of feelings with food are examples of vicious, self-reinforcing cycles that develop. These behavioral patterns must be addressed.)

4. Some obese and overweight people, who were abused as children, have unconsciously created a "fortress of fat" designed to keep others at a distance. For many of these people, food may be their only solace in life. (This deep-seated issue must be addressed in professional counseling.)

5. Overeating and obesity clearly mimic other addictive behaviors and should be treated just as any other addictions. (The fact that brain chemistry is intimately involved with all addictive behaviors is not scientifically disputed.)

6. Coping with obesity involves one of two choices. (One choice is to accept the condition, quit worrying about it, and get on with leading a balanced life. The other choice is to take full responsibility for weight and do what is necessary to become healthy. A very interesting fact about these two choices involves dealing with the psychological issues. Either way, underlying shame, guilt, and feelings about oneself have to be addressed.)

Chapter References & Notes

[1] David G. Myers (1992) *Psychology*. New York: Worth Pubs.

[2] Ellen Berschied (1981) An overview of the psychological effects of physical attractiveness and some comments upon the psychological effects of knowledge of the effects of physical attractiveness. In: *Psychological Aspects of Facial Form*. Ann Arbor, MI: University of Michigan.

[3] S. L. Gortmaker, Must, A., Perrin, J. M., Sobol, A. M., & Dietz, W. H. (1993) Social and economic consequences of overweight in adolescence and young adulthood. *New England Journal of Medicine*, 329, 1008-1011.

[4] E. Pamuk, et. al. (1998) *Socioeconomic status and Health Chartbook. Health — United States, 1998*. Hyattsville, MD: National Center for Health Statistics.

[5] M. A. Friedman, & K. D. Brownell (1995) Psychological correlates of obesity: Moving to the next research generation. *Psychological Bulletin*, 117, 3-20. When we say that the "trend indicates..." it means that more often than not the effect is found. For example, while many obese children have very poor self-image, low self-concept, and low self-esteem, other obese children have high or normal levels of these factors. In general, obese children have negative self-evaluations, but it cannot be said that the vast majority of them do. There are many interesting exceptions to these findings that puzzle researchers.

[6] N. Allon (1982) The stigma of overweight in everyday life. In: B. Wolman (Ed.) *Psychological Aspects of Obesity*. New York: Van Nostrand Reinhold. Larkin, J. E., & Pines, H. A. (1979) No fat persons need apply. *Sociology of Work and Occupations*, 6, 312-327.

[7] Karris, L. (1977) Prejudice against obese renters. *Journal of Social Psychology*, 101, 159-160.

[8] Canning, H., & Mayer, J. (1966) Obesity — its possible effects on college admissions. *New England Journal of Medicine*, 275, 1172-1174.

[9] Kelly D. Brownell & Thomas A. Wadden (1991) The heterogenity of obesity: Fitting treatments to individuals. *Behavior Therapy*, 22, 153-177.

[10] C. G. Fairburn, H. A. Doll, S. L. Welch, P. J. Hay, B. A. Davies, & M. E. O'Connor (1998) Risk factors for binge eating disorder. *Archives of General Psychiatry*, 55, 425-433.

[11] L. R. Lilenfeld, & W. H. Kaye (1996) The link between alcoholism and eating disorders. *Alcohol Health & Research World*, 20, 94-99.

[12] Istvan, J., Zavela, K., & Weidner, G. (1992) Body weight and psychological distress in NHANES I. *International Journal of Obesity*, 16, 999-1003.

[13] Holland, J., Masling, J., & Copley, D. (1970) Mental illness in lower class, normal, obese and hyperobese women. *Psychosomatic Medicine*, 32, 351-357.

[14] Leckie, E. V., & Withers, R. F. (1967) Obesity and depression. *Journal of Psychosomatic Research*, 11, 107-115.

[15] Scott, R. L., & Baroffio, J. R. (1986) An MMPI analysis of similarities and differences in three classifications of eating disorder. *Journal of Clinical Psychology*, 42, 708-713.

[16] Hafner, R. J., Watts, J. M., & Rogers, J. (1987) Psychological status of morbidly obese women before gastric restriction surgery. *Journal of Psychosomatic Research*, 31, 606-612.

[17] Black, D. W., Goldstein, R. B. & Mason, E. E. (1992) Prevalence of mental disorder in 88 morbidly obese bariatric clinic patients. *American Journal of Psychiatry*, 149, 227-234.

[18] Moses, N., Banlivy, M. M., & Lifshitz, F. (1989) Fear of obesity among adolescent girls. *Pediatrics*, 83, 393-398.

[19] Brownell, K. D. (1991) Dieting and the search for the perfect body: Where physiology and culture collide. *Behavior Therapy*, 22, 1-12.

[20] Rodin, J. (1992) *Body Traps*. New York: Morrow.

[21] Wadden, T. A., & Stunkard, A. J. (1985) Social and psychological consequences of obesity. *Annals of Internal Medicine*, 103, 1062-1067.

[22] Cash, T. F. (1993) Body-image attitudes among obese enrollees in a commercial weight-loss program. *Perceptual and Motor Skills*, 77, 1099-1103.

[23] Wadden, T. A., Foster, G. D., Stunkard, A. J., & Linowitz, J. R. (1989) Dissatisfaction with weight and figure in obese girls: Discontent but not depression. *International Journal of Obesity*, 13, 89-97.

[24] Cash, T. F., Counts, B., & Huffine, C. E. (1990) Current and vestigial effects of overweight among women: Fear of fat, attitudinal body image, and eating behaviors. *Journal of Psychopathology and Behavioral Assessment*, 12, 157-167.

[25] Cash, T. F., & Green, G. K. (1986) Body weight and body image among college women: Perception, cognition, and affect. *Journal of Personality Assessment*, 50, 290-301.

[26] Young, M., & Reeve, T. G. (1980) Discriminant analysis of personality and body-image factors of females differing in percent body fat. *Perceptual and Motor Skills*, 50, 547-552.

[27] Brodie, D. A., & Slade, P. D. (1988) The relationship between body-image and body-fat in adult women. *Psychological Medicine*, 18, 623-631.

[28] Faubel, M. (1989) Body image and depression in women with early and late onset obesity. *Journal of Psychology*, 123, 385-395.

[29] Mendelson, B. K., & White, D. R. (1982) Relation between body-esteem and self-esteem of obese and normal children. *Perceptual and Motor Skills*, 54, 899-905.

[30] Klesges, R. C., Haddock, C. K., Stein, R. J., Klesges, L. M., Eck, L. H., & Hanson, C. L. (1992) Relationship between psychosocial functioning and body-fat in preschool children: A longitudinal investigation. *Journal of Consulting and Clinical Psychology*, 60, 793-796.

[31] Hill, A. J., & Silver, E. K. (1995) Fat, friendless and unhealthy: 9-year old children's perception of body shape stereotypes. *International Journal of Obesity*, 19, 423-430.

[32] Little, G. L., & Robinson, K. D. (1997) *Understanding and treating Antisocial Personality Disorder: criminals, chemical batters, and batters.* Memphis: Eagle Wing Books. Some of the most interesting findings about self-esteem and self-concept comes from research on criminal and drug abusers. Criminals have much higher than average self-esteem but negative self-concept.

[33] Nir, Z, & Neumann, L. (1991) Self-esteem, internal-external locus of control, and their relationship to weight reduction. *Journal of Clinical Psychology*, 47, 568-575.

[34] D'Encarnacao, P. S., D'Encarnacao, P. W., & Little, G. L. (1990) Treating sexual dysfunction as a function of childhood. Sexual Abuse: ACCERT. In F. J. Bianco & R. H. Serrano (Eds.) *Sexology: An Independent Field.* Amsterdam: Elsevier Science Pub.

[35] D'Encarnacao, P. D. (1995) *Healing Formula For Your Inner Child.* Memphis: Metamorphosis Press. This 542 page book details the ACCERT method which the author developed with his psychiatrist wife for over 25 years. Dr. D'Encarnacao died in 1997 leaving behind masses of manuscripts and data related to sexual abuse problems. *The Healing Formula* book is extremely difficult to obtain today, but the publisher of this book has attempted to obtain some copies. Write for information. Many studies have shown elevated levels of depression, anxiety, suspiciousness, along with poor self-esteem and other self-evaluations in both the obese and adult victims of childhood sexual abuse.

[36] NCCAN (1988) Study Findings: Study of National Incidence and Prevalence of Child Abuse and Neglect.

[37] S. J. Kaplan, et. al. (1998) Adolescent physical abuse: Risk for adolescent psychiatric disorders. *American Journal of Psychiatry,* 155, 954-959.

[38] B. L. Weiler & C. S. Widom (1996) Psychopathy and violent behaviour in abused and neglected young adults. *Criminal Behaviour and Mental Health,* 6, 253-271.

[39] V. J. Felitti (1993) Childhood sexual abuse, depression, and family dysfunction in adult obese patients. *Southern Medical Journal,* 86, 732-736.

[40] G. L. Little & K. D. Robinson (1998) *Untangling Relationships: Coping With Codependent Relationships Using The MRT® Model.* Memphis: Eagle Wing Books, Inc.

[41] A. W. Schaef (1986) *Co-dependence: Misunderstood — Mistreated.* New York: Harper-Collins.

[42] Wayne W. Dyer (1995) *Your Sacred Self.* New York: Harper Collins.

[43] Melody Beattie (1987) *Codependent No More.* Minneapolis: Hazelden.

[44] Milkman, H. B., & Sunderwirth, S. G. (1987) *Craving For Ecstasy: The Consciousness & Chemistry of Escape.* Lexington, MA: Lexington Books.

Chapter 11
COPING WITH PSYCHOLOGICAL & SOCIAL FACTORS

Gluttony is an emotional escape, a sign something is eating us.
Peter De Vries — *Comfort Me With Apples*

Eat to live, and not live to eat.
Benjamin Franklin — *Poor Richard's Almanac*

Summary — The ongoing suffering observed in obese people actually helps to maintain avoidance of the problem. Many obese people use food in an attempt to "medicate" uncomfortable feelings. Subsequently, the constant, low-level suffering accompanying obesity becomes their "normal" mood state. When the obese person makes an attempt to change behaviors in ways that could improve the situation, she often becomes "socially exposed" causing uncomfortable feelings to emerge. For example, an obese female attending an aerobics or exercise class the first times will, most likely, feel very self-conscious. She may experience feelings of shame, guilt, or even anger as a result of the increased visibility of her "problem." These emotional reactions will likely lead her to quit the class and return to her prior habits. Food will then provide some comfort to her and the low-level suffering that remains will seem preferable to the extreme anxiety state precipitated by her exposure. This "vicious cycle" must be addressed by exploring the individual's priorities.

Various psychological issues are related to obesity. Self-esteem, guilt, shame, feelings of inadequacy, and the effects of discrimination all should be addressed. However, uncovering these feelings is only the starting point. Goals must be set and action must be taken. A structured counseling program, preferably conducted in ongoing groups, is the most effective means for exploring issues common to obese patients, providing adequate information and coping tools, and forming realistic plans of action. Clients must learn to self-monitor behaviors and feelings related to eating and activity level. A daily journal is recommended as the best method for teaching self-monitoring skills. Another counseling component is building an awareness of how environmental factors can stimulate eating behavior and then teaching coping skills and strategies that lessen their impact. Learning effective stress management techniques is also essential. Client excuses and rationalizations, self-esteem issues, and priorities can be confronted and altered appropriately in structured groups operated as part of a comprehensive obesity treatment program.

Numerous self-help and support groups are available for obese people. Each of these groups has a unique philosophy and orientation. On one extreme are self-help groups that advocate acceptance of fatness and obesity. On the other extreme are self-help groups that provide support for patients awaiting gastric surgery for obesity. Other groups lie somewhere between these extremes. Deciding whether you will accept the condition of obesity (and opt for "health"), or battle obesity, will determine which of these groups best supports your needs.

Some obese people need deeper psychological counseling or psychotherapy. When childhood sexual abuse, severe depression, or deep emotional issues are related to obesity, extended therapy is advised. Finally, some obese people show all of the characteristic behaviors of addiction. In this case, support groups designed for treating addictive behaviors are ideal treatment components. A focus on preparing and practicing coping strategies for situations where a "high relapse risk" is present is very appropriate.

• • •

Perhaps the most painful aspect of obesity is rooted in the realm of deep-seated feelings and emotions that form over a lifetime of struggle with weight. As related in the prior chapter, research has shown that many obese people continually suffer at a "subclinical" level. That is, their feelings of depression and anxiety rarely get to the level where they could be diagnosed as pathological. We suspect that this subclinical "chronic suffering" endured by the obese becomes the typical, expected psychological state day in and day out. It becomes their "normal" condition. As such, it represents a psychological accommodation to obesity. At the same time, many people medicate this emotional state with food. **People learn to love themselves with food** and change their mood by eating. Food and eating can be substituted for unmet needs and even serve as a way to medicate or bury deeper problems.

Some long-term psychological adaptations are especially resistant to change. That is, people get so accustomed to feeling or acting in a certain way that changing can seem threatening — if not impossible. For example, a female who has lived her entire life as if she was unattractive might have problems adapting to marked improvements in appearance from weight loss, fitness, and cosmetic changes. This woman might feel increased (and quite different) social pressure because of her new found attractiveness. Even deeper psychological issues are present in people who have feelings of failure or were abused. They often use eating and weight as a coping mechanism. For them, continuing to eat to cover the problem often appears to be less painful than confronting the underlying issues.

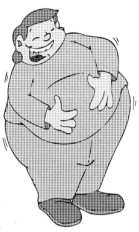

The Vicious Cycle Of Suffering

Because it is usually "low grade" in severity, the chronic emotional anguish of the obese person gradually becomes so ingrained into the personality style that it is accepted as a permanent reality. When the individual attempts to lose weight or begins to exercise, this part of her behavior becomes exposed to a powerful social influence and various feelings (e.g., shame, guilt, failure) rapidly emerge. For example, lots of overweight people are extremely self-conscious (and embarrassed) in social and public situations. Behaviors that bring attention to their attempts to control the "problem" (such as going to an aerobics class) frequently result in a great deal of negative emotion and discomfort. The obese person quickly realizes that she had much less negative emotion when she stayed home. Since going to the aerobics class is so socially uncomfortable, she may decide to quit.

This example depicts how "vicious cycles" operate. A vicious cycle is a self-perpetuating, self-reinforcing pattern of behaviors and feelings. Many obese people make adjustments in behavior designed to minimize exposure to situations that create too much emotional discomfort. These adjustments could include social isolation, avoidance, self-degradation (joking or making fun of the problem), or even depression. When the person does get into situations that stimulate a lot of negative emotion, she will tend to withdraw. This produces a quick lessening of negative feelings and increases the chances that she will avoid similar situations in the future. That is, the constant, "low-grade" suffering that accompanies obesity is definitely more comfortable and tolerable to the person than is the more acute emotional crisis that comes with a socially exposed attempt to work on it.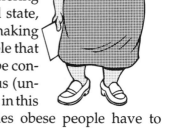

Thus, the low grade psychological suffering of obesity becomes the preferable emotional state, although the individual is seldom aware of making this choice. Social exposure is so uncomfortable that it is powerfully avoided. The avoidance can be conscious — but is more likely at an unconscious (unaware) level. The unconscious process at work in this vicious cycle is one of the greatest obstacles obese people have to overcome in order to make a genuine effort at managing weight.

The pervasiveness and influence of this vicious cycle in the obese person's personality is far greater than many professionals would assume. Most obese patients avoid frequent visits to an obesity specialist's office or even their own family doctor. They will avoid going to specialized groups designed to teach coping skills. They avoid discussing deeper emotions accompanying obesity. They avoid exercise if anybody can see them. It is very likely that the vast majority of obese patients who discontinue treatment efforts do so because they believe there is more acute discomfort experienced in trying to deal with the problem than there is in ignoring it.

You Must Work With The Psychological Piece Of The Obesity Puzzle

Psychological factors interact with underlying biological predispositions, childhood environment, and culture. Depression, anxiety, fear, and other negative emotions are found in the obese and overfat. Low self-esteem, poor self-concepts, and destructive beliefs plague the obese. Shame, guilt, feelings of inadequacy, and subtle discrimination render a constant toll by causing ongoing suffering. Many obese people respond to the suffering by overeating. Understanding all this is one thing, but acting on the problem is another story.

Coping With The Obesity Puzzle: Medication and Counseling Can Be Necessary To Treat Underlying Psychological Factors

Psychological factors that contribute to obesity can be greatly aided with medications and counseling. These include a wide range of possible problems including:

Ineffective Stress Coping
Depression and Anxiety
Lack of Support
Low Self-Esteem
Shame & Guilt
Feelings of Inadequacy
Codependency
Vicious Cycles
Addictive Behaviors

If the psychological puzzle piece is adequately addressed, an individual's mood can be significantly improved and motivation can be increased. Factors leading to overeating can be identified and coping plans formed.

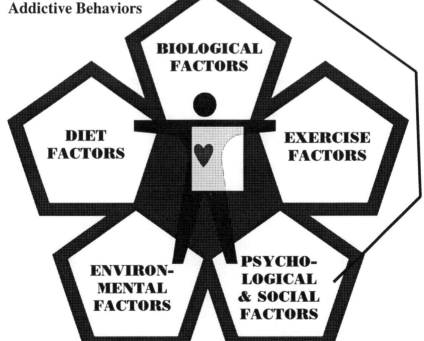

BIOLOGICAL FACTORS

DIET FACTORS

EXERCISE FACTORS

ENVIRON-MENTAL FACTORS

PSYCHO-LOGICAL & SOCIAL FACTORS

When Sigmund Freud first discovered that childhood trauma could cause serious psychological problems in adulthood, there was a great deal of excitement in the emerging field of psychology. Freud devised therapy methods that appeared to uncover the root causes of patients' problems. With the insight that came with this understanding, it was believed that the symptoms and problems would disappear. Patients did, in fact, tend to improve somewhat with their new understanding. But the improvement was short-lived and either the initial psychological problem or a new one appeared. The message in this *is* simple. Understanding isn't enough. It is a start, but some action has to be taken.

Let's make a simple comparison. Imagine that you have a flat tire while driving your car. You probably completely understand the problem a flat tire creates, but **understanding it doesn't change it.** There is some work involved. It usually simplifies things if you have the right tools. The job is made easier if you have someone else with you who has done it before. This is exactly how confronting psychological issues contributing to obesity is done. You have to recognize the problems that obesity causes and understand how your specific issues are tied into the problem. You will probably have to explore some significant events from your past and these could elicit some temporarily unpleasant feelings. Then you have to make specific plans to make changes in behaviors, attitudes, beliefs, and even feelings. The tools employed can be groups, workbooks, and individual counseling. It also helps to have a competent professional to assist in the process. Having social support is a critical element in coping with psychological factors.

Some Form Of Counseling Is Necessary

One of the first tasks obesity treatment programs must accomplish is to convince patients that a form of life-style counseling is necessary for success. A structured counseling component, consisting of weekly group meetings, is the preferred format. The focus of these groups is on evaluation and modification of eating habits, habits of inactivity, and emotional responses to eating.[1] The *LEARN* manual[1] is often recommended as a program guide, although we have developed our own structured workbook to accomplish this purpose. The *SmartLoss*

MRT Group Workbook[2] is based on a systematic approach to personality change over 12 sessions and has a set of supplemental tapes. Other usable program approaches are also available.

The essential counseling components teach self-monitoring, stimulus control, stress management, and address self-esteem/self-concept. In **self-monitoring**, patients keep a daily diary or journal of eating, activity, and feelings. This allows the patient to become aware of how eating, activity level, stress, and mood relate to each other. Problems are more easily identified with a journal and it can be a very useful tool to monitor patient success.

Stimulus control refers to becoming aware of how specific environmental factors can stimulate eating. For example, the sight or odor of certain foods, restaurants, specific stressful situations, or holidays may stimulate overeating. As patients become aware of these "dangerous" cues, they can learn avoidance and coping techniques.

Stress management teaches a set of skills designed to reduce stress and thereby reduce emotional eating and loss of control. Few obese people are even aware of the stress they endure or how their gut level responses are counterproductive. Stress management can be effectively learned in groups or individually with specialized tapes.

Self-esteem & self-concept counseling focuses on beliefs and attitudes related to how a person thinks about obesity and associated feelings. Structured groups in which all the participants are struggling with the same issues are an ideal format for exploring self-esteem, self-concept, and self-worth. Identification of positive aspects about self, making affirmations, and the use of visual imagery are all effective techniques.[1]

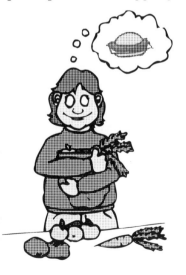

Cognitive-behavioral approaches are preferred for the group counseling component.[1] Cognitive-behavioral groups explore how beliefs, attitudes, and behaviors can be modified to produce beneficial changes. Deeper issues, perhaps related to abuse or emotional conflicts, are best handled in individual psychological counseling sessions.

What Are Your Real Priorities?

The long-term psychological adaptation that occurs in response to obesity actually makes it very difficult for people to become motivated to address the problem in a comprehensive manner. We have noticed this when obesity patients treated with medication are encouraged to enter supportive counseling groups. What happens is that many patients are quite willing to comply with medication recommendations and say that they will "try" to exercise and diet, but they don't believe they have the time for a weekly group. A month later they come in for an appointment stating that they didn't have time to exercise and didn't diet. When encouraged again to enter behavioral counseling, they still resist. In short, lots of obese patients want to rid themselves of their excess fat, but only on their own terms. Unfortunately, these terms usually include a refusal to confront the deeper issues intimately entwined with obesity, as well as avoiding any discomfort.

All of our new patients are asked to rate whether they agree or disagree with this statement:

> *I would do almost anything that was legal, moral, and not physically dangerous to lose weight.*

What do you think our patients say in response to this statement? Almost all of them strongly agree with it. Yet their behavior shows that this isn't true. "I don't have time for a weekly group, I don't have time for exercise, and it's too hard to plan meals," are the excuses from these artful dodgers. In view of this, what is the person's true priority? What are the most important goals to him or her? It doesn't appear to include coping with obesity.

If you are truly serious about managing obesity and lowering body fat permanently, **it has to be made a top priority**. Fulfilling a top priority in life — any top priority — requires the ability to tolerate some discomfort. You may have to tolerate the stares and smiles of others when you are walking. You may have to expose some of the feelings you have. You have to rearrange how you spend your time. This means that you must make time for a group that might last a little over an hour or for a brief one-on-one session occasionally. You must find 15 to 30 minutes a day for some form of physical activity. You must take the few hours a week required to plan meals. And yes, it might cost you some money in the beginning, perhaps as much as $100-$200 a month give or take a little. But if you can conquer obesity, you will save far more money in the long-run. This really isn't much of a sacrifice for a top priority, is it? Think of it like this. A week has 168 hours in it. Can you find 8 hours during each week when you can focus on managing a serious physical problem? If you can't, your future is probably decided.

The First Steps To Freedom From Obesity's Psychological Traps

1. The first thing you have to do is truly understand and accept that obesity is a disease. You probably never made a conscious decision to be overweight or obese — it has just happened. *You can choose to accept the condition or you can choose to really do something about it.* There are support groups available for people who make either choice and we highly recommend that you use them. The choice here is completely yours.

2. If you have been through several cycles of dieting with weight loss followed by relapse with weight regain, *you probably feel some shame and guilt.* A part of you blames your lack of will-power for the condition.

Changing Anything Is Usually Uncomfortable

Making any type of major life change usually involves some uncomfortable emotions. It's probably human nature for us to avoid discomfort, but this avoidance comes at a real cost. People lose job opportunities because of embarrassment and avoidance. People quit educational programs because of avoidance and embarrassment. We've know adults who refused to go classes that could teach them how to read because they were embarrassed that people would know they couldn't read. It's a vicious cycle: "Because I can't read, I won't go to a class that will teach me to read." The same cycle is present in some obese people: "Because I'm 'fat' and embarrassed about it, I can't go walking."

You believe that it's your own fault. Once again, you've got to understand and accept that obesity is a disease. It's a chronic, relapsing condition that **you can never cure**. You may never get to the point where you can manage it on your own. It may take professional help from several different levels and you might need medication indefinitely. **It makes good sense to actively seek out all the help you can get.** Once again, you have several choices ranging from learning to accept and live with obesity to entering various treatments and support groups that attempt to help. Remember that, if you choose to battle obesity, you will have to tolerate some increased discomfort. The temptation to run from emotional pain will be great, but avoiding it by running will only worsen the condition.

3. Today we know that many diseases come from exposure to certain environmental factors interacting with underlying biological and hereditary predispositions. For example, lots of skin cancers come from sun exposure interacting with cancer producing genes. (You make the decision to get a tan.) The truth is that your behavior does play a role in the development of some diseases — including obesity. **You must accept that your hereditary predispositions probably are not suited to living in a world of food abundance and inactivity.** This means that you either accept your genetic fate in the environment present in the world today or modify your life-style. The nature of obesity is that there is no apparent middle ground. You must choose one way or the other.

Available Help For These First Steps

You have already taken action in fulfilling some aspects of the first steps in escaping obesity. By obtaining and reading this book you are hopefully gaining an understanding of obesity as a disease and how various factors influence it. Next, you must seek help. Some weight loss and obesity programs offer psychological and social support. You may find some of these support groups very helpful.[3] However, we recommend that you enter a group program that supports medical treatment rather than discouraging it. Keep in mind that the biological factors underlying obesity are often so powerful that few people can actually lose weight and maintain it without some ongoing medical assistance. But also remember that medical assistance is rarely sufficient in and of itself.

The best support groups (or programs) for obesity are comprehensive. They offer education about obesity, information on nutrition and making realistic eating plans, have workable suggestions and options for physical activity, and offer suggestions for dealing with various environmental factors. In addition, group counseling for shame, guilt, self-esteem issues, and other low level stress issues are also provided in a caring, non-shaming group setting. The support group is typically composed of people who share a common struggle. Finally, the best programs have professional resources available for people with deeper psychological issues.

Support Groups That Promote Acceptance Of Obesity

As we have stated many times, you can treat obesity or you can accept it as a part of your life. A strong movement has been underway in the United States since the early 1970s to promote the acceptance of obesity. The "Fat Underground" is often credited with starting this movement. Lynn McAfee, a medical researcher who had struggled with weight since childhood, reviewed outcome literature on diets and was astonished to find that virtually all diets had massive failure rates. McAfee and a group of friends began issuing articles and brochures on the failure and perils of dieting and how society's reaction to obese people was the main issue. Many of these women viewed the male-dominated medical community as the prime culprit in promoting thinness. Many feminists embraced this idea and the publication of the *Fat Manifesto* was their visible beginning. This event coincided with the death of singer Mama Cass Elliott of the *Mamas and Papas* in 1974. The Fat Underground planned and carried out "raids" against Weight Watchers and at diet/obesity conferences. Many of their members eventually entered NAAFA (see next page).

For *some* individuals, embracing and accepting obesity is perhaps the best course of action. When we say this, we are not saying that they should give up trying to be healthy. We are saying that they should reevaluate why they are trying to lose weight and become thin. This may be especially true for people who have a powerful genetic component.

National Association to Advance Fat Acceptance (NAAFA)

NAAFA is a social support group begun in 1969 that actively embraces fatness and obesity. NAAFA works to promote civil rights for the obese by suggesting and supporting laws and regulations against discrimination. NAAFA accepts that obesity is the result of genetic factors, not personal failure. The organization has almost 5,000 members and is headquartered in Sacramento, CA. Its meetings are described as lighthearted and fun. There are no shaming or guilt-producing activities. To the contrary, NAAFA extols the beauty of fatness and even holds well-publicized fashion shows. NAAFA's web address is: www.naafa.org

Association for the Health Enrichment of Large People (AHELP)

AHELP is a nonprofit organization of diverse professionals who serve obese or "fat" clients. Its main focus is on improving the health of clients rather than fatness or obesity. The organization maintains a referral list of providers in the United States who adhere to their philosophy of improving health rather than just losing weight. Its web site address is www.usit.com/ahelp

Social Support For Fat Acceptance

This is a primarily internet based support resource for fat acceptance. An internet search listing "Fat Acceptance" or "Big Folks" will produce thousands of web pages devoted to various products, support groups, and services for the obese. These include clothing, food, group activities, chat rooms, and sexual preferences. If you are easily embarrassed or offended by various sexual connotations — often quite overt — use some caution in accessing these sites.

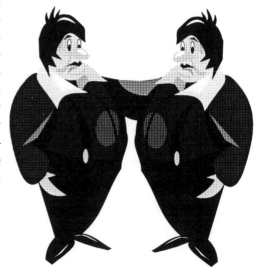

National Organization for Lesbians Of SizE (NOLOSE)

As stated in the NOLOSE description, "Fat Lesbians" probably experience some of the most painful and isolating experiences in society. The organization serves as a support group and resource for lesbians who are overweight or large. NOLOSE is a membership organization that states it will soon close its web site to nonmembers. The web address is www.nolose.org

Radiance Magazine

Radiance: The Magazine For Large Women is a quarterly magazine devoted to worldwide acceptance of women of size. It is a full color, high class magazine. It bills itself as "one of the leading sources of support, information and inspiration in the worldwide Size Acceptance Movement." It certainly appears to fulfill its stated role well. This magazine is highly recommended to all overweight women (many articles should interest men) as it mounts strong attacks against societal discrimination and prejudice against large women. This resource stands as a counterbalance to the super slim models depicted in other women's magazines and

Right: Fall 1998
cover of
Radiance
with
Camryn Manheim.

Reprinted by permission.

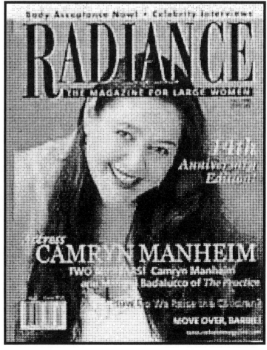

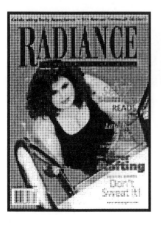

strongly questions the appropriateness of society's pressure on females to be slim. Radiance began in 1984 and has a strong internet presence: www.radiancemagazine.com

Their web page counter in mid-September 1999, showed that nearly 250,000 people visited their site. A four issue subscription in the U.S. costs $20. Address: P. O. Box 30246, Oakland, CA 94604. Their phone number is 510-482-0680.

Support Groups For Losing Weight

The lines that distinguish support groups from commercial diet programs are slowly blurring. Commercial programs have come to recognize that some form of social support is an essential component in weight loss and weight maintenance. Commercial diet programs are reviewed in **Appendix B**. Below are the major social support groups designed to help people who are actively trying to lose weight. (Several of these are also reviewed in **Appendix B**.)

Overeaters Anonymous (OA)

OA was started in 1960 by a Los Angeles housewife who modeled it on the principles of Alcoholics Anonymous (AA). The nonprofit group today has over 10,000 "groups" meeting routinely in virtually every city and almost every town in the United States. OA views obesity and overeating as an addiction and stresses a form of "abstinence" from some foods and eating situations. The program focuses on reliance on a higher power (spirituality) and addresses physical and emotional aspects of overeating. The program definitely is affordable (donations are accepted) and is available everywhere. Many people find the personal support from others in the same situation very helpful.

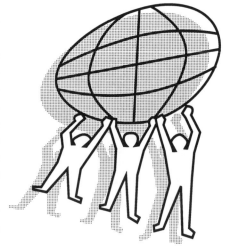

OA groups each tend to develop a personality of their own

based on the unique mix and blend of the people who attend. OA does not endorse any diet plans, but members will commonly suggest one diet over another. If a 12-step spiritual approach appeals to you and you see an addictive component in your eating, OA may be ideal. It's important to not judge OA by any particular meeting or group. It is a good idea to "shop around" and attend several different OA meetings until you find one that seems to have an environment and mix of people that feels right to you. OA is listed in every phone book under weight or social support agencies. You can get information about the group closest to you by calling 505-891-2664. The OA web site is www.overeatersanonymous.org

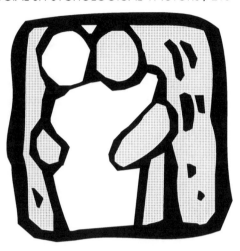

Take Off Pounds Sensibly (TOPS)

TOPS is a nonprofit organization that provides social support in weekly groups. The program requires that members make weight and diet goals. The first group visit is free, but there is an annual membership fee and chapters have a locally set due's structure. TOPS meetings are fun and usually upbeat. Contests and awards are frequently given for weight loss. Call 800-932-8677 to find the nearest group. TOPS web address is: www.tops.org

Association For Morbid Obesity Support

This an online support group devoted to reducing "the suffering and isolation" of people with morbid obesity. Most of the people in the group are either awaiting obesity surgery or have recently had the surgery. It contains a search option that allows you to find a local bariatric surgeon (these are physicians specializing in stomach surgery.) (**Appendix A** reviews surgery options for obesity.) The web site has chat groups, individual stories, and a gallery of member pictures. In August 1999, the site had 1,866 members. The address is: www.obesityhelp.com

Taking More Steps To Free Yourself From Psychological Traps

Whether you decide to lose weight or not, you will find yourself happier and more worry free by confronting deeper issues. Shame and guilt take considerable time to overcome. Continuing in ongoing support groups can greatly aid this effort. However, there are deeper issues that often emerge in obese patients.

Depression, anxiety, and obsessive compulsive behavior are frequent companions to many obese people. Depression, anxiety, and obsessive compulsive behavior all have a biological basis and modern antidepressants can sometimes work wonders. Chapter 9 reviewed several of the SSRI medications that can be helpful for depression and obsessive-compulsive behavior. Since serotonin is so involved with both depression and overeating, it is not surprising that many people lose weight when they begin taking drugs that increase serotonin.

For some obese people, obesity has its roots in childhood abuse or other emotional factors such as codependency. Extended counseling or psychotherapy may be necessary to uncover and treat these issues. One study[4,] for example, evaluated the weight loss of 84 obese patients after an average of 42 months of psychotherapy. Results showed that almost half of the patients lost over 20 pounds despite the fact that the focus of the therapy was not on weight or obesity! Psychologists, licensed counselors, music therapists trained in the Bonny Method[5], and other psychotherapists may be quite helpful; however, it is wise to check out credentials and techniques, There is a wide variation in skills, ability, and training among these professionals.

Binge Eating Disorders

Adapted from *Binge Eating Disorders* (1993, 1998),
National Institute of Diabetes and Digestive and Kidney Diseases

Many obese people have symptoms of binge eating disorder. It is a newly recognized condition that probably affects millions of Americans. People with binge eating disorder frequently eat large amounts of food while feeling a loss of control over their eating. This disorder is different from binge-purge syndrome (bulimia nervosa) because people with binge eating disorder usually do not purge afterward by vomiting or using laxatives. Binge eating disorder usually requires professional help and medication.

How Common Is Binge Eating Disorder?

Although it has only recently been recognized as a distinct condition, binge eating disorder is probably the most common eating disorder. Most people with binge eating disorder are obese, but normal-weight people also can be affected. Binge eating disorder probably affects 2% of all adults, or about 1 million to 2 million Americans. Among mildly obese people in self-help or commercial weight loss programs, 10% to 15% have binge eating disorder. The disorder is even more common in those with severe obesity. Binge eating disorder is slightly more common in women, with three women affected for every two men. The disorder affects blacks as often as whites; its frequency in other ethnic groups is not yet known. Obese people with binge eating disorder often became overweight at a younger age than those without the disorder. They also may have more frequent episodes of losing and regaining weight (yo-yo dieting).

Binge Eating Disorder Symptoms

Most of us overeat from time to time, and many people feel they frequently eat more than they should. Eating large amounts of food, however, does not mean that a person has binge eating disorder. Most people with serious binge eating problems have:

- Frequent episodes of eating what others would consider an abnormally large amount of food.
- Frequent feelings of being unable to control what or how much is being eaten.
- Several of these behaviors or feelings:
  1. **Eating much more rapidly than usual.**
  2. **Eating until uncomfortably full.**
  3. **Eating large amounts of food, even when not physically hungry.**
  4. **Eating alone out of embarrassment at the quantity of food being eaten.**
  5. **Feelings of disgust, depression, or guilt after overeating.**

What Causes Binge Eating Disorder?

The causes of binge eating disorder are still unknown. Up to half of all people with binge eating disorder have a history of depression. Whether depression is a cause or effect of binge eating disorder is unclear. It may be unrelated. Many people report that anger, sadness, boredom, anxiety or other negative emotions can trigger a binge episode. Impulsive behavior and certain other psychological problems may be more common in people with binge eating disorder. Dieting's effect on binge eating disorder is also unclear. While findings vary, research suggests that about half of all people with binge eating disorder had binge episodes before they started to diet. Still, strict dieting may worsen binge eating in some people, especially adolescents. Recent research has centered on low serotonin levels as a possible cause of the disorder. Prozac and several other SSRI antidepressants can be very helpful and are often prescribed.

Should People With Binge Eating Disorder Try to Diet?

People with binge eating disorder who are not overweight or are only mildly obese should probably avoid dieting, since strict dieting may worsen binge eating. However, many people with binge eating disorder are severely obese and have medical problems related to weight. For these people, losing weight and keeping it off are important treatment

Night Binge Eating

Many obese people find that they are able to control eating throughout the day, but at night they seem to lose control. Night-eating syndrome was first described in 1955, but little research was conducted on it until recent times. A 1999 study[5] evaluated 12 obese people with night-eating syndrome. The patients were observed for a week in their homes and then for a 24-hour period in a hospital. Twenty-one normal eaters served as a control comparison group.

The night-eaters consumed 56% of their daily caloric intake at night compared to 15% in the controls. Night-eaters awakened nearly four times each night and ate during half of these awakening periods. Controls awakened an average of less than once per night with no night eating behavior. Low levels of melatonin and leptin were found in the night-eaters.

Melatonin is produced from serotonin and is associated with sleep and our normal pattern of sleep. It is not known whether taking melatonin supplements at bedtime will help with the syndrome. However, restraint in eating during the day is one factor associated with night eating.

goals. Most people with binge eating disorder, whether or not they want to lose weight, may benefit from treatment that addresses this eating behavior.

Treatment Options For Binge Eating Disorder

Several studies have found that people with binge eating disorder may find it harder than other people to stay in weight loss treatment. Binge eaters also may be more likely to regain weight quickly. For these reasons, people with the disorder may require treatment that focuses on their binge eating before they try to lose weight. Even those who are not overweight are frequently distressed by their binge eating and may benefit from treatment. Several approaches are being used to treat binge eating disorder. Cognitive-behavioral therapy teaches patients techniques to monitor and change eating habits as well as to change the way they respond to difficult situations. Interpersonal psychotherapy helps people examine relationships and to make changes in problem areas. Treatment with medications such as SSRI antidepressants (Celexa or Prozac) may be helpful for some individuals. Self-help groups may also be a source of support. Researchers are still trying to determine which method or combination of methods is the most effective in controlling binge eating disorder. The type of treatment that is best for an individual is a matter for discussion between the patient and his or her health care provider. Most people who have the disorder have tried unsuccessfully to control it on their own.

Addiction Issues

Addiction is a complicating issue in obesity treatment and, many, if not most, obese patients show addictive eating patterns. As related in the prior chapter, addictions can take many forms with the root causes being genetic predispositions, childhood abuse, childhood environment, and other factors. Addiction treatment can be in-patient or out-patient, with the severity of the addiction often determining the most appropriate treatment.

A host of issues are addressed by addiction treatment programs. These range from exploration of childhood to the people, places, and things in the addict's current life. Spirituality is often a core issue.

One important consideration in treating obesity is the cultural or ethnic identity of the individual.[7] Different cultures tend to have different views of ideal body size, vastly differing eating habits and food preferences, and spiritual beliefs. These differences have to be respected.

In general, the addictive aspects of obesity can be addressed by some self-help programs (OA) or through the systematic group counseling component of obesity treatment. Some obese patients will need more intense counseling.

One of the most important concepts developed in addiction treatment as it applies to obesity, is **relapse prevention**. A "return to old habits" is the most cited reason explaining why people who lose weight tend to regain it. Relapse prevention strategies begin by identifying specific environmental cues, people, and mood states that can make patients susceptible to "slips" and lapses back to prior eating habits. Patients then are assisted in developing coping strategies for each of these "high risk" situations.

In sum, addiction treatment for obesity explores some of the causal factors of the disorder and gives the patient tools for changing behavior and emotions. Specific people, places, things, and emotional states that create high risk relapse situations are uncovered for each individual. Finally, specific coping strategies and plans are formulated for preventing relapse.

Chapter References & Notes

[1] American Association of Clinical Endocrinologists and The American College of Endocrinology. (1998) *AACE/ACE Position statement on the prevention, diagnosis and treatment of obesity.*

[2] Little, G. L., Robinson, K. D., & Milnor, J. P. (2000) *SmartLoss MRT Group Workbook for Fitness & Weight-Related Issues.* Memphis, TN: Eagle Wing Books.

[3] Weinew, S. (1998) The addiction of overeating: self-help groups as treatment models. *Journal of Clinical Psychology,* 54, 163-167.

[4] Rand, C, & Stunkard, A. J. (1978) Obesity and psychoanalysis. *American Journal of Psychiatry,* 135, 547-551.

[5] Bonny, Helen (1989) Sound as symbol: guided imagery and music in clinical practice. *Music Therapy Perspectives,* 6, 7-10. Bonny Method practitioners (called Fellows) are listed in an international registry available through the Association for Music & Imagery (contact: James Rankin), P.O. Box 4286, Blaine, WA 98231-4286.

[6] Birketvedt, G. S., et. al. (1999) Behavioral and neuroendocrine characteristics of the night-eating syndrome. *Journal of the American Medical Association,* 282, 657-663.

[7] Davis, N. L., Clance. P. R., & Gailis, A. T. (1999) Treatment approaches for obese and overweight African American women: a consideration of cultural dimensions. *Psychotherapy,* 36, 27-35.

Chapter 12
ENVIRONMENTAL COMPONENTS OF OBESITY: LIFE-STYLE ISSUES

Mechanization limits the necessity of physical activity required to function in society. Many people are entrenched in sedentary daily routines consisting of sitting at work, sitting in traffic, and sitting in front of a television or a computer monitor for most of their waking hours.
National Heart, Lung, and Blood Institute —1998

Summary — Today, more than half of Americans are overweight and 23% are obese. Since 1960, the rate of obesity has doubled. Much of the modern world is experiencing the same epidemic of obesity. Germany, Britain, Canada, and other countries all face escalating rates of obesity. The simple reason for this is that we retain genetics designed for periods of starvation. At the same time, we live in a world where food is abundant and the required amount of physical activity is greatly decreased. Our overall life-style has changed rapidly adapting itself to massive technological advances. Television viewing time has dramatically increased and computer games have replaced participation in physical activities. A quarter of American adults are completely inactive and another 42% are seldom active. Almost half of American teenagers are sedentary.

The work world has gradually replaced labor-intensive jobs with sedentary office jobs. Corresponding to reduced activity levels at work are lowered energy requirements in other day-to-day tasks. Modern conveniences of all types have reduced our overall physical activity level. From electric car windows to leaf blowers, chores that once took time and effort have been reduced to button pushing. Shopping has become easier and less energy consuming with catalogs, computers, and other shop-at-home services.

These small changes in our overall activity level lead to big changes in weight. The elimination of a daily activity equivalent of a 10-minute walk results in a five pound weight gain over the course of a year. Over a decade it's a gain of 50 pounds! At the same time our activity level has increased, food intake has also changed. Americans are eating in restaurants in ever-increasing numbers. Fast food and restaurant dining account for 44% of all food purchases in the United States. We are enticed to eat fat and calorie-laden meals at restaurants, and we often have no idea of the actual calorie content in these meals.

Americans as a whole fail to exercise adequately in order to make up for decreased daily activity level and increased food intake. Exercise is often viewed as a boring chore. In addition, our reduced activity level leads to increased stress and anxiety. In turn, stress produced in our technological, fast-paced environment, leads to both inactivity and overeating. Few people struggling with obesity confront either their stress-coping strategies or their life-style.

• • •

More than half of American adults are overweight (97 million), approximately 23% (40 million) are obese, and the rate of obesity in America is still increasing.[1] While the rate of obesity in this country has almost doubled since 1960, most of the increase has occurred over the past 10 years. "The increase in overweight and obesity appears to have occurred among U.S. adults across all ages, genders, and racial/ethnic groups."[2] Even immigrants who establish residency in the United States experience a rapid increase in obesity level. This would seem to indicate that our environment and life-style somehow promote obesity.

Most industrialized countries are experiencing an epidemic of obesity similar to the United States. Over the past 10 years, the rate of obesity in the United Kingdom has doubled.[1] Half of Germans are overweight and 20% are obese.[3] Half of Bulgaria's population are over-weight or obese and nearly two-thirds of Czechs are overweight or obese.[4] In Canada, the rate of obesity in children has increased by 50%. The Ottawa Heart Insti-

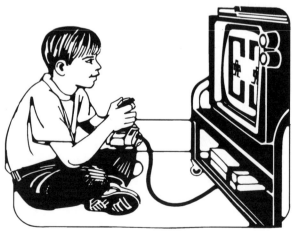

tute found that Canadian children expend 4 times less energy today than did children in the 1950s. Watching sports and passively playing computer games have replaced participation in sports and other play activities. In addition to sitting in school 25 hours each week, Canadian children sit in front of the television 25 more hours.[5] There is every reason to believe that American children watch just as much television 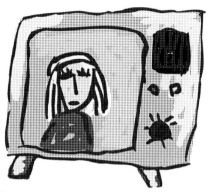 as Canadian children do and that this behavior starts at an early age. It has been reported that American children age 2 months to 5 years currently have a rate of obesity (10.1%) nearly double that observed in the years 1971 to 1974 (5.8%).[6]

Why We Are Fatter:
We Have Quickly Adapted Our Behavior To Modern Conveniences And Food Abundance — But Our Bodies Are Still Programmed For Starvation Survival

The astonishing increase in obesity in the modern world can be explained in a few brief statements. **The obese are genetically programmed to survive in a world with regular periods of starvation. However, we now live in a society of abundance.** Our body is designed to expend a lot of energy to maintain basic survival. Growing and gathering food, building a shelter, making tools, clothing, implements, and trade goods took up almost all of the waking hours and energy of people in the not-too-distant past. Today, inexpensive food is everywhere. All-you-can-eat buffets were unheard of just a few decades ago. People now work an average of only 40 hours a week to ensure a standard of living which exceeds that of ancient royalty. Few people in the modern world grow or gather their own food, make their own clothes, build their own shelter, or even expend energy maintaining their shelter. At the same time, our entertainment and recreation has become more passive while the world of work has altered from primarily physical labor to sedentary high-tech jobs. The availability of transportation has made walking nearly obsolete. Inactive vacation and leisure time have markedly increased, and routine chores like washing clothes and mowing the yard have been reduced to virtually passive activities. In truth, modern "conveniences," designed to make our lives easier and more enjoyable, are playing a large role in making us fat. We are eating more yet we are less active. Our genes, however, are still programmed for possible starvation. Everything we do in our lives — our overall *life-style* — has dramatically changed over the past 100 years in response to the changing societal *environment*. This has been especially true in just the past 50 years. Our survival-ensuring genetics haven't caught up to the changes in our environment.

Christianity, Obesity, & Life-Style Issues

The influence of life-style on obesity is an issue many obese people seem to want to avoid. Occasionally, obese patients come in for weight loss medications and quickly make it a point to tell us that they are Christians. Their point is made in response to our questions about stress-producing "issues" and "problems" they might have which could be contributing factors to their obesity. They will usually say that they have no unresolved issues or problems, because they have "placed them in the Lord's hands." It's plain that they want this part of our interview to be ended quickly. They tell us that they simply need some medication that will take off the excess weight. Some also say that being overweight or fat sets a poor example for other Christians and they want to better serve their religion.

As Christians, we have given a lot of thought to this line of reasoning. We do believe that placing problems in God's hands, the Lord's hands, or even a "higher power" (as 12-steppers do) is appropriate and beneficial. But is that all there is to it? If it was, wouldn't these patients lose weight or at least be at peace with the condition of obesity?

An important fact is often missed among people who reason that their problems are "in God's hands." These people will readily admit that their model for living is Jesus and that they are trying to emulate his way of life. What is missed is that Jesus' way of life consisted of more than his care and concern for others. It was *everything* he did. Other than his brief, triumphant donkey ride into Jerusalem, how did he get around? He **walked**. He obviously walked a lot during his three brief years

Our Changing Environment

Environmental influences that impact obesity levels are usually divided into two major areas: 1) Physical activity and 2) food intake.[1] Both of these areas are functions of an individual's life-style. In many ways, increasing levels of obesity mirror an ever-increasing technological society. For example, surveys show that gasoline consumption and hours spent watching television correlate well with obesity levels.[7]

Physical Activity Changes

"For many people, even when caloric intake is not above the recommended level, the number of calories expended in physical activity is insufficient to offset consumption. Mechanization limits the necessity of physical activity required to function in society. Many people are entrenched in sedentary daily routines consisting of sitting at work, sitting in traffic, and sitting in front of a television or a computer monitor for most of their waking hours."[1]

of ministry. He often fasted, but feasted occasionally. He took long periods of time away from others for reflection to maintain balance. Prior to his ministry, he was probably a carpenter—an honorable, creative, and very physical occupation. We ask these patients if they thought Jesus was fat? The reply, of course, is "no."

In our week-long professional training sessions for counselors in Moral Reconation Therapy (MRT®) we have encountered many ministers who tell us they are stressed out because they have so much important work to do. They go on to say they haven't had a vacation in 5 years or more and they are working 80 hours a week. We like to remind them that Jesus frequently took 40 days and nights away from others despite the fact that problems and troubles were everywhere. It might not have been a vacation, but it prepared him for what he had to face. In addition, walking everywhere allowed him time to think, prepare, organize and make plans, and talk to others. Today, we rush home from a stressed work environment and arrive minutes later at home where we face more stress. Modern transportation takes us in minutes to entertainment, educational activities, stores and restaurants, religious activities, children's events, and on and on the list goes. How much like Jesus' life are all of these things?

There are more examples we could cite, but the point is hopefully made. Life-style has a lot to do with obesity. God and religious beliefs are definitely important, but it is helpful to take a good look at the overall life-style of our spiritual role models.

Fewer and fewer Americans are engaged in simple physical activities in our day-to-day lives.[2] If we want to change a channel on television, all we do is click the remote control. If the volume is too low, we use the remote. We can watch movies 24 hours a day without leaving our living rooms. We can order first run movies over cable television. People who decide to burn the calories to drive their car to a movie theater 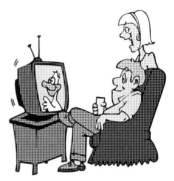 can consume several days of fat in a large tub of popcorn. Almost every food available in theaters is high in fat, calories, and sugar.

When people aren't watching television they are playing "games" on a computer. Jumping, running, kicking, playing golf, football, and baseball seem to be more fun on a computer screen than in reality. Besides, if it's hot outside, we'd rather stay inside in the air conditioning than take a walk or play a game in the reality of the outdoors.

Food is produced in ever-increasing quantities by mechanized, high-tech farming. Gigantic, corporate farming operations are absorbing smaller, family-owned farms decreasing steadily the amount of physical 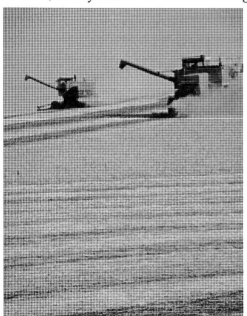 labor required to produce commodities. Soil preparation, planting, weed control, pest control, harvesting, and food processing are all accomplished much more efficiently due to mechanization. It is interesting that few Americans are now involved in the labor-intensive harvesting required in the gathering of some foods (like fruits and some vegetables). We rely on "cheap" labor forces imported from poor neighboring countries. All of these factors result in constant year-round availability of cheap food.

The American work environment continues to undergo drastic change. Some physically active occupations have been replaced by automation. Robots make many of the components in automobiles and even assemble them. Fewer human beings are involved in this once labor intensive occupation. Most other types of manufacturing are also automated. Roofers and carpenters use nail guns; it's faster and easier than using a hammer. Spray painting and power paint rollers have reduced the energy required to complete those chores. Computer communication and videoconferencing eliminate the need to move from a chair in a cubicle or office. We don't have to take the time and energy to roll a piece of paper into a typewriter. This reduces the need to pull open a filing cabinet and place the paper in a file. A single computer disk can store the equivalent of an office full of records. Virtually every job and occupation has undergone changes which have reduced the amount of physical activity required.

Many people today spend 8 hours at work in a chair. More and more jobs are eliminating the need to expend the energy required to get ready for or even go to work. Many companies are delighted to have employees work from home since it saves the company money due to

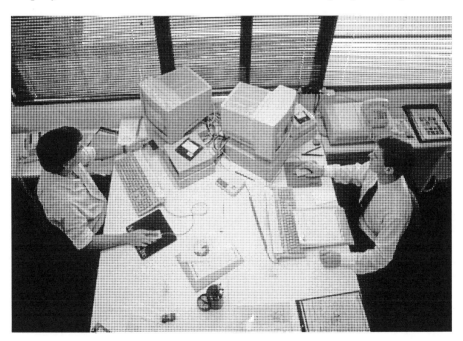

less sick time, less office space, lower utility consumption and equipment use, and fewer conveniences afforded employees. Soon, anyone who actually moves his hands and fingers to type on a keyboard will be considered obsolete or behind the times. Computers with voice recognition word entry are already in use.

All of our habits are changing in response to technological advances. Newspaper subscriber numbers are falling. The once common early morning walk to the front yard to pick up the paper is being replaced by sensationalized, 24-hour "news" available on television or a click to a computer news site. The few calories people were expending while turning the pages of a newspaper or book are being absorbed into fat cells as we read more and more from computer screens or passively watch television.

While in our car we only have to push a button to roll a window down. There's no need to burn a few calories turning a handle. And if we get a flat tire, we'll call a prepaid emergency service. We even have tires today that can't go flat. Few people today service their own cars. This energy consuming task is being done faster, better, and cleaner by services that specialize in "quick" jobs. In addition, computerization of automobiles is making the "yardtree mechanic" a thing of the past.

If we need to use a phone, we don't have to get up and walk to one. We just take our small digital phone out of our pocket. If we need to mail something to someone, we can do it in front of the computer screen. "Snail mail" is dying and so are trips to the post office with short walks from the car to the counter. In recognition of this, the post office has instigated a pick-up service and stamps can be ordered from your computer.

Shopping is taking less energy. Computer (on-line) shopping is now available for virtually everything including automobiles. You can buy a car without leaving your home and have it delivered to your driveway. Even groceries can be delivered to our doorstep from on-line sites. Prescriptions can be ordered over the phone or internet, and they are hand delivered by mail or a messenger service. You can visit with a physician on the internet. Catalog shopping is also a hot business eliminating gift buying trips. Virtually all of our bills can be paid over the phone or on computers. All of our banking can be handled the same way. There's no need to burn the energy required to write checks, put them in envelopes, put the stamps on, and somehow get them to a post office.

For those people who go on shopping trips, finding a good parking space with the smallest amount of walking possible has become a science. Americans will spend 10 minutes or more driving around in a parking lot waiting for a space to open up near the door. When we come out with our cart, few people burn the calories necessary to return the cart or push it to a safe area.

Americans are buying bigger houses with smaller yards. Why? Because yard maintenance is a hassle. Seeing a man cutting a postage stamp-sized lawn on a huge riding mower is a common sight today. Raking the lawn is becoming obsolete. We use leaf blowers or pay someone to do it. Electric hedge clippers, chainsaws, limb clippers, and every conceivable implement that can be pulled behind a yard tractor are used by those souls who insist on having a maintained yard. All of these tools are designed to quickly do chores that were once tiring, dirty jobs.

About 20 years ago, wood-burning fireplaces or stoves were desired amenities in a home. Today gas fireplaces with remote controls are the "hot" item. Bringing in wood from the cold is a hassle and the ash removal is work. Gas is "cleaner" and easier to use.

Preparation of meals used to be time and energy consuming. Just try baking bread or a cake from scratch or make the entire traditional American Thanksgiving meal — you'll know how exhausting it can be. Today we take excellent pre-cooked meals and put them in the microwave or we preorder from a caterer. And when we're done eating, almost all of us put dirty dishes in a machine that does all the work for us. When a machine is made that puts the clean dishes away for us, we'll all buy it and someone will make a bundle of money.

Of course, more and more people are avoiding all of the hassles involved with meals. We can drive to a nearby fast food outlet where we can get everything we need from a handy window. There's no need to even get out of the car. Or we can have a complete meal delivered to our house by making a phone call. For others, a trip to a nice restaurant eliminates all of the food and meal preparation as well as the clean-up.

We Aren't Against Technology And Conveniences

Don't misunderstand what we are saying here. We certainly avail ourselves of all the modern conveniences we can. We enjoy riding mowers, cell phones, restaurants, catalog shopping, computers, coffee makers, dishwashers, microwave meals, remote controls, electric car windows, air conditioning in the summer, and we'd probably get a robot maid if a reliable model was available. We don't like to clean houses, either. We'll also buy the dishwasher that automatically puts away the dishes as soon as it's available. (A tip for the inventor: it'd be nice if it would also put the dirty dishes *in* the washer for us.) We like computers and all of the gadgets and handy devices that seem to be put on the market every day. The real point is that the amount of energy we consume each day is falling. It may not seem like much to you, but over a year, a decade, or a lifetime, it adds up.

What Energy Saving Technology Means To Obesity

Although we haven't addressed diet and nutrition yet, most of you are probably aware that a pound of fat contains 3,500 calories. (We Americans commonly refer to what is actually a *kilo*calorie as a *calorie*.) Calories are burned by the body to keep us alive and allow us to do work by providing energy. Every movement we make burns some extra

Calorie Calculations

We employed several computer-based programs to calculate calories consumed by various activities. The *DINE® Healthy* system allows you to analyze diet, weight, and exercise and plan meals based on individual dietary needs. The program is fairly expensive ($170 or so) and could be used by nutritionists and physicians. It allows for unlimited personalized files and creates several useful charts and graphs to plot individual progress. The program is available from the manufacturer (716-688-2400).

Another system we tested was The *Diet Balancer®*. It was slightly more complicated to use but gives good results and is much less expensive ($40). It performs many of the same functions as the more expensive programs. Multiple files for individuals can be created. It is available from the manufacturer (800-922-2988).

In addition, many computer programs with recipes exist as do many internet sites. The *Home Gourmet®* was exceptionally useful. It has 10,000 recipes as well as full nutritional data on 4,500 food items. It was also cheap ($10). Many computer stores carry it as well as many other recipe programs. Weight Watchers® and other weight-loss oriented organizations have both recipe software and books available at inexpensive prices.

calories because it takes energy for muscles to move. To demonstrate how important small movements can be to weight gain, let's take a few simple hypothetical examples.

A 20 minute walk at a 2 m.p.h. pace (more like a stroll), burns about 100 calories in a person who weighs 175 pounds. If technology has reduced the amount of work this person does by the daily equivalent of a 20 minute stroll, it means that the person will use 100 less calories each day. It doesn't seem like much until you multiply it by the 365 days in a year. Then it's 36,500 calories. Since a pound of fat has 3,500 calories, the yearly equivalent of fat added is over 10 pounds. Over a decade it could add up to 100 pounds!

A 20 minute walk isn't much. Walking to your car parked at the far end of the lot, taking a flight of stairs instead of an escalator or elevator, walking into a restaurant instead of using the drive thru, changing channels at the set instead of using the remote, walking to the convenience store a block away instead of driving, hand washing your car instead of using a service, and countless other small activities would make up the 100 calories.

Every new technological advance reduces calorie burn and increases our fatness. The situation with Americans' overall level of activity has worsened with each new gadget and energy saving device. Today, 25% of all American adults lead totally sedentary, inactive lives.[8] Approximately 67% of American adults are either completely sedentary or seldom active (seldom active is defined as not exercising or walking

The Delicate Balance Of Energy

Over the course of a year, a typical American might consume 1,095,000 calories (based on 3,000 calories a day). A seemingly insignificant reduction in physical activity amounting to a 10 minute daily walk would result in over three pounds of fat gain over a year. If this person continued to do everything exactly the same way, but simply drank an extra soft drink each day (140 calories for 12 ounces), he or she would gain almost 15 pounds of fat over a year. Only 10 extra calories a day, the equivalent of a potato chip and a half, adds a pound of fat in a year. The balance between food intake and weight maintenance is far more delicate than most people understand. The good news is that the reverse is also true. Reduction of daily intake of the equivalent of a soda results in a 15 pound weight loss over a year. Small increases in physical activity level that are consistently performed lead to big changes over time.

at least four, 30-minute periods a week).
Nearly 50% of Americans aged 12-21
years are inactive. In 1991, 42% of high
school students participated in physical education classes, by 1995, only
25% participated.[8] The overall life-style
of Americans has become more inactive and physically passive. In response
to the reduced activity level, we simply don't need as much food.

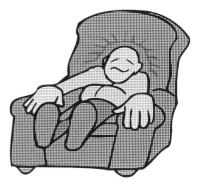

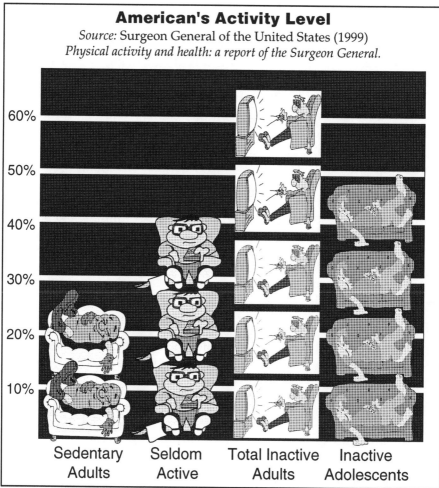

American's Activity Level
Source: Surgeon General of the United States (1999)
Physical activity and health: a report of the Surgeon General.

| Sedentary Adults | Seldom Active | Total Inactive Adults | Inactive Adolescents |

Food Intake Changes

At the same time that our level of activity decreased, our food intake has changed. In 1909, Americans consumed an average of 3,500 calories a day. By 1994, Americans consumed a daily average of 3,800 calories.[9] Over a year, these extra 300 calories each day would amount to 31 pounds. But all of us are a lot "bigger" now than we were in 1909, and it takes extra calories to maintain higher body weight.

American's daily average consumption of fat in 1909 was 123 grams compared to 159 in 1994.[9] Awareness of the risks and hazards of fat consumption to health has increased since 1994, and fat consumption has subsequently decreased. However, many people have increased overall consumption of calories by eating more carbohydrates and sugar. In 1909, sugars and sweeteners supplied 11% of American's calories. In 1994, sugars and sweeteners contributed 18% of American's daily calories.[9] Research has shown that neither fat consumption nor sugar consumption are to blame for obesity level increases. Rather, it appears to be the total increase of calories.[10, 11]

High fat consumption (especially saturated fats) is associated with many of the health risks seen in obesity. Fat also contains more caloric energy, by weight, than do carbohydrates or protein. For these

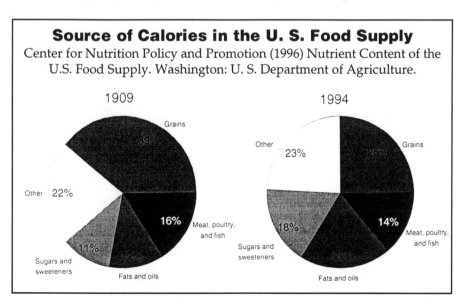

Source of Calories in the U. S. Food Supply

Center for Nutrition Policy and Promotion (1996) Nutrient Content of the U.S. Food Supply. Washington: U. S. Department of Agriculture.

reasons, the U. S. Department of Agriculture's Food Guide Pyramid stresses higher carbohydrate consumption coupled with decreased fat consumption. When this is actually done, many obese people do reduce total calorie intake and reduce weight.[12]

America: Eating Out More

More than 300,000 "fast food" restaurants exist in America. Fast food is "convenient, predictable, and fast. Fast food has become part of the busy American lifestyle."[13] But most fast food is high in calories, fat, and sodium.

A busy office worker might stop at a McDonald's® drive thru for a quick breakfast and then have lunch at a Wendy's®. A simple breakfast at McDonalds® might consist of a coffee, Egg McMuffin®, hash browns, and a cinnamon roll. Lunch at Wendy's® could be a grilled chicken sandwich, "medium" fries (the Biggie®, not the Great Biggie®), and a medium Frostie®. These two meals total 2,030 calories with 80 grams of fat. Too tired and stressed out to cook that evening, a call to a pizza delivery service brings supper. Only three slices of a large cheese pizza and 6 small cheese sticks add another 1,338 calories and 36 grams of fat to the daily total: 3368 calories; 116 grams of fat.

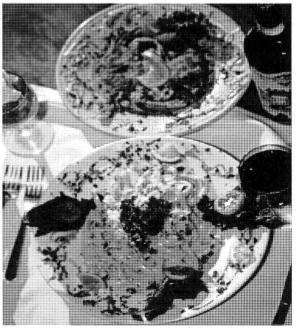

The National Restaurant Association reports that Americans spent $354 billion eating out in over 800,000 restaurants during 1999.[14] They went on to show that 44% of all American food purchases are in restaurants as compared to just 25% in 1950. By 2010 the rate of restaurant food purchase is expected to exceed 53%.

The biggest changes expected by the restaurant industry are in increased high-tech preparation designed to bring restaurant food and service into the consumer's home or office. The implication of this is simple: we are probably going to get even fatter.

Life-Style Issues

Life-style overlaps virtually all of the other pieces of the obesity puzzle. Exercise, diet, personality and psychological issues, and even biological predispositions and medical conditions impact life-style. Life-style exerts a constant, pervasive impact on weight. It is also a life-long issue. That is, **your life-style will influence your weight and health for the rest of your life.** Failure to permanently change life-style is the number one reason why people who lose weight can't seem to maintain that weight loss.

Research by the Calorie Control Council on people who regain weight has indicated several key life-style behaviors as important factors.[15] Failure to exercise is the number one reason people who lose weight regain it. Other factors include snacking, bingeing on favorite foods, emotional eating, and improper eating at restaurants.

Physical Inactivity

American adults and children have gradually become couch potatoes. Two-thirds of us define ourselves as inactive.[8] In 1994, the President's Council on Physical Fitness and Sports polled Americans about their level of activity. Forty percent of us replied that we didn't have time to exercise.

What are we doing with our time? We are going to a stress-filled work environment, driving in stress-filled traffic, attending stress-filled activities, and attempting to manage our lives in a stress-filled, high tech world. We spend our nonwork time paying bills, attending to our children's activities, tinkering with our collection of high-tech material objects, planning some sort of recreation to escape, and trying to relax and reduce stress. Our schedule is too full. Exercise is seen as boring, we're too "emotionally" tired to exercise, or we decide it isn't necessary. Exercise begins to be just another stressful chore to many people trying to cope with other life stressors.

WHY WE FAIL TO MAINTAIN WEIGHT LOSS

The Calorie Control Council's 1998 Consumer Survey evaluated the reasons why Americans are not successful at maintaining desired weights.The key issues in our failures are life-style choices. The figure below shows results from the survey of adult Americans who reported they need to lose weight. The reasons they fail (with the percentage for each) are:

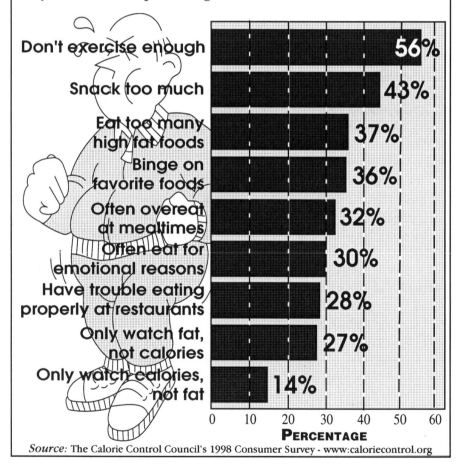

Reason	Percentage
Don't exercise enough	56%
Snack too much	43%
Eat too many high fat foods	37%
Binge on favorite foods	36%
Often overeat at mealtimes	32%
Often eat for emotional reasons	30%
Have trouble eating properly at restaurants	28%
Only watch fat, not calories	27%
Only watch calories, not fat	14%

PERCENTAGE

Source: The Calorie Control Council's 1998 Consumer Survey - www:caloriecontrol.org

Despite our excuses, physical inactivity does relate to our increased fatness. Exercise is necessary in today's world to maintain lean weight and fitness. As we said, Americans are burning less calories in daily life than we were 50 years ago. Whether it's the use of a television remote control, an electric car window, or eliminating the energy required to make a meal by eating out, we are burning less energy. **Thus, without making up the difference through planned exercise periods, we are destined to get fatter.**

As we stated in earlier chapters, our priorities in life determine how much importance we place on things. Exercise is a low priority for many obese and overweight people. We give lip service to "fat loss" and fitness as priorities, but the activities that actually reduce body fat and enhance health are placed at the bottom of our priority list. Something has to give in this situation and, more often than not, it's our waistline.

Family Influences

Our life-style develops over time and is greatly influenced by early family life. The kinds of physical activity each of us will engage in as adults is encouraged in early life. Some parents involve their children in physical activities like sports, bicycle riding, swimming, and swinging. Children will naturally gravitate to a level of activity that is reinforced by parents and peers. Some parents discourage children's participation in physical activity and encourage passive activities such as television. Research shows that obesity in children and adolescents is closely correlated with hours watching television.[16]

Eating habits are also influenced by family life. The tendency to overeat, eat high fat foods, or sugar laden foods develops early. Other influences on eating habits come from the comments of parents regarding wasting food, cleaning plates, or eating to "enjoy" oneself.

While the people reading this book will already have developed a basic life-style, it's important to understand how your actions can and will influence your children. It is a parental responsibility to teach children priorities in life. Encourage them to become involved in physical activity. Teach them healthy eating habits. Change your behavior for your children.

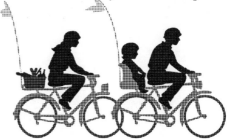

Our Eating Environment

It's impossible to watch commercial television and not get bombarded by food advertisements. Beautifully prepared burgers slowly spin in front of our eyes enticing us to eat. They are perfectly made, succulent, and thick. Of course, they don't look anything like the burger we'll actually get. The ones on television usually aren't food at all, they're a sprayed, plastic goop painted to look like food. Outlets for ice cream, pizza, beer, subs, and elegant dining advertise constantly on television, in newspapers, magazines, and billboards. It's so easy to rush through a drive-thru for lunch or breakfast and it's actually getting cheaper.

Very few people pack a lunch anymore. It just seems too old-fashioned in our hasty, fast world. We rationalize that it takes too much time to get ready and is a hassle to plan and keep fresh. It won't impress co-workers, either. If you are young and trying to further your career, you think packing your lunch might be viewed as cheap or the kind of thing "losers" do. It doesn't matter that, for an obese person who works in an office, it is perhaps one of the healthiest and easiest ways to control exactly what you eat.

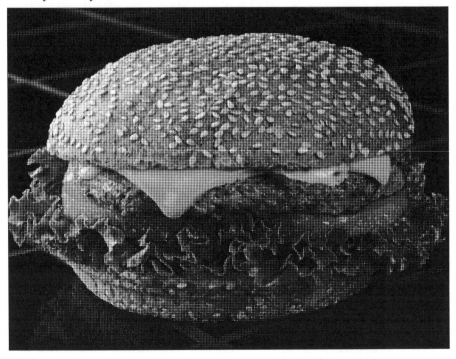

When we go to a restaurant the selections are primarily high-fat and high-calorie. Few restaurants, other than fast food outlets, supply a complete nutritional breakdown of their selections. Some may highlight low-fat selections, but what the consumer doesn't know is that they usually are high calorie. Portions tend to be large — much larger than a "serving" — but the volume we receive and the great taste keep us coming back. Restaurants aren't to be blamed for this; chances are that your grandmother didn't supply you with a nutritional breakdown when she made her wonderful meals. She wanted it to taste good and fill you up. When you've completed your main meal, a covered tray with beautiful, dessert selections is brought by to entice you. It always looks perfect because it's plastic. "You've earned it," our friends encourage, "there's nothing wrong with indulging yourself once in a while."

Our total eating life-style involves impulse buying and impulsive eating. We buy foods in supermarkets based on the package colors and designs. Advertisers know this and so do the companies producing food products. If a product is "good" it won't sell unless it looks right. So advertising and marketing science determines the exact colors and package shapes needed to sell an item. Most of us are too busy to study labels or plan meals. So we grab whatever "looks good" and throw it into the cart. We even buy pet food based on how the package looks to us. Who do you think the beautiful colors, pictures and succulent descriptions on pet food are there for? Marketers know how we make our decisions and how we are influenced.

We aren't laying any blame on advertising, marketing, and packaging. That's not the issue. The issue is obesity and life-style decisions. One important part of solving the obesity puzzle is to take control of the issues that impact obesity and weight. Once again, your priorities enter the picture. If a fast and trouble free meal is your priority, fast foods will play a central role in your life. Impulsive decisions will also be there because, without planning, you will be subject to the influence of carefully chosen marketing ploys.

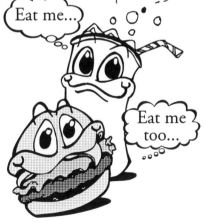

Personality Impacts Life-Style & Stress Coping Strategies

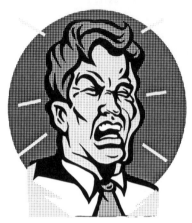

Our personality style has a lot to do with the life-style habits we adopt. Health and fitness are, to some extent, life-style choices. Some people choose to actively engage in healthful activities while others pointedly avoid them. The "couch potato" tends to be a passive style that shuns activity. The reasons for this can be many, but stress can be a factor.

The small annoyances we experience in everyday life tend to produce the most significant stress in our lives.[16] Traffic jams, work hassles, waiting in lines, and trying to meet schedules all produce stress. Sixty percent of Americans report feeling great stress weekly and many overeat in response.

Some people feel a sense of control in their lives while other people see stress as an uncontrollable factor. These perceptions of control tend to determine the vulnerability level individuals have to certain conditions. These conditions include heart disease and obesity.[16]

In a previous chapter we have discussed the idea of *stress defeat syndrome*. Research has consistently shown that stress increases eating behavior in people who are overweight and dieting.[17] People who feel stress is uncontrollable (and who feel defeated by it in the meeting of personal goals) are particularly vulnerable. A related concept is *learned helplessness*. That is, some people come to believe they are helpless to change things in their lives. In response, these people resort to the learned pattern of behaviors that lead to feeling better or to the only behavior that they feel is under their control. This can be any addictive behavior that includes eating.[17]

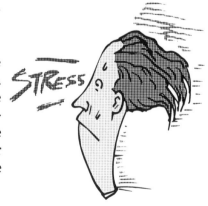

A recent study examining these possibilities found that few overeaters actually understand why they overeat in response to stress.[17] The study showed that some people who overeat do so to mask feelings of failure and negative emotions. Some overeaters believe that dieting efforts are doomed to fail and give in to feelings of helplessness.

Conclusions

1. Obesity has a powerful environmental life-style component that must be adequately addressed by treatment efforts. This component overlaps all other areas of obesity and includes physical activity and dietary habits. Individuals' personal priorities in life have to be explored.

2. Overall physical activity levels must increase in the obese. Small daily increases in activity lead to major long-term changes.

3. Regular periods of sustained activity (walking or exercise) must be planned and completed to make up for environmentally-produced reductions in necessary activity.

4. Eating habits and behaviors have to be analyzed and controlled in the obese. Impulsive eating, fast food and restaurant eating, and food purchases have to become conscious, planned events (not habits).

5. Early-life influences on eating and physical activity must be explored in the obese. These can be difficult to change, however, even small changes can lead to substantial health improvements.

6. The influence of life and environmental stress, perceptions of self-control, and feelings of helplessness are critical factors in weight management in the obese. Obese people need to realize the powerful influence that stress plays in their lives and that their responses are often self-defeating. The stress itself isn't the problem. The problem is in how stress is managed. ("My problem is not *the* problem. My problem is *how I manage* my problem.")

Chapter References & Notes

[1] National Heart, Lung, and Blood Institute (1998) Clinical guidelines on the identification, evaluation, and treatment of overweight and obesity in adults. Washington: NIH (Pub. # 98-4083).

[2] AACE/ACE Obesity Task Force (1998) *Position statement on the prevention, diagnosis and treatment of obesity*. The American Association of Clinical Endocrinologists and the American College of Endocrinology.

[3] Archutt, A. (1998) Fat in spite of hard farm work - tracking down obesity. Research press release. University of Trier; Forschungszentrum fu Psychobiologie und Psychosomatik.

[4] The Milan Initiative (1999) *Obesity Newsletter* (Spring), 7.

[5] Linton, M. (1998) Generation of inactive kids at risk. *Toronto Sun*, February 2, 1998.

[6] American Academy of Pediatrics (1999) More four- and five-year-olds overweight, government study finds. www.pediatrics.org

[7] Gibbs, W. (1996) Gaining on fat. *Scientific American*, (August, 1996).

[8] Surgeon General of the United States (1999) *Physical activity and health: a report of the Surgeon General*. Washington: National Institutes of Health.

[9] Center for Nutrition Policy and Promotion (1996) Nutrient Content of the U.S. Food Supply. Washington: U. S. Department of Agriculture.

[10] Hill, J. O., & Prentice, A. M. (1995) Sugar and body weight regulation. *American Journal of Clinical Nutrition*, 62, 264-273.

[11] Seidell, J. C. (1998) Dietary fat and obesity: an epidemiologic perspective. *American Journal of Clinical Nutrition*, 67, 546-550.

[12] National Institutes of Health. (1998) Clinical guidelines on the identification, evaluation, and treatment of overweight and obesity in adults. www.nih.gov/nhlbi/cardio/obes/prog/guidelns

[13] *Fast Food Finder*. The Minnesota Attorney General. The Minnesota Attorney General's office produced a massive archive of fast food facts and a guidebook to the components of many menus. This has been incorporated into many internet sites as "Fast Food Finder." The Appendix in this book on calorie contents of fast food items was, in part, derived from this source.

[14] National Restaurant Association. Restaurant Industry in the Year 2010: Takeout Sales to Soar. Press release; May 24, 1999. www.restaurant.org

[15] Calorie Control Council National Consumer Survey, 1998. (1999) Trends & Statistics: Why Do We Fail? www.caloriecontrol.org/reasonswhy

[16] Myers, D. (1992) *Psychology*. New York: Worth Publishers.

[17] Polivy, J., & Herman, C. P. (1999) Distress and eating: why do dieters overeat? *International Journal of Eating Disorders*, 26, 153-164.

Chapter 13
COPING WITH
THE ENVIRONMENTAL
& LIFE-STYLE
COMPONENTS OF OBESITY

*Freedom, to me, is being able to avoid what I know I should avoid,
and being able to do what I should do.*
Father Bill Stelling (1998) — *Spiritual Reflections On Everyday Living*

Summary — Your life-style is a global way of describing everything you do in terms of your typical behavior patterns and responses to environment. Life-style overlaps all the other pieces of the obesity puzzle, and by making some carefully planned changes in small areas of behavior, you can significantly enhance fat loss as well as derive substantial health improvements. One of the most important ideas to keep in mind is that small consistent changes in behavior lead to big changes over time.

There are many aspects of our environment and personal circumstances that are out of our control. However, how we interact with our environment and respond to it is a choice we make. There are so many areas in our lives where healthy life-style changes can be made that the task can seem overwhelming. We recommend you start by looking at possibilities listed throughout this book and in this chapter. Then identify a few that seem easy to do and are manageable. After choosing these behavioral changes, make all of the necessary preparations to fulfill the goals you have chosen. We strongly urge people to start a health journal or diary when beginning the change process. The journal should permit you to list daily eating, physical activity, and feelings that emerge. Wearing a pedometer every day is an excellent way of charting daily physical activity levels and measuring how well you are fulfilling your goals. If fat loss is a goal, the journal should have a place where you can routinely chart weight.

For some people, doing anything at home will increase their physical activity level. There are a few simple recommendations that should be easy to implement. First, during commercials, stand up and stretch and stroll through the house. If you hear music you like on the television, stand up and dance. Never eat while watching television. Gum chewing is an alternative. Take a few short walks. Do some yard work or chores for 15 minutes or so every day. If you like reading, browse a library or bookstore regularly. Develop some hobbies like bowling or dancing.

At work, make it a habit to get out of your chair every 15 minutes or so and stretch. Take a few 5 minute strolls during breaks and at lunch. Carry a lunch to work. Eliminate fast food from your life-style. If you must eat it, identify the healthiest food options and always order them. Look at the nutritional analyses of fast foods in the back of this book or get them from the restaurants. Healthy (non fast food) restaurant eating is difficult. Most of their food is calorie and fat dense. In addition, few restaurants have a calorie or fat breakdown of their selections. Try to find a few restaurants that offer truly healthy options. Order foods cooked without fat or oil.

To control binges and hunger, eat more often. Three meals and three snacks should become a daily routine. Be a smart consumer by carefully shopping for low calorie, low fat snacks — learn how to read and understand the nutrition labels on food. Buy all of your food items in grocery stores — not convenience stores.

Understand and accept that a lot of things in life are not under your control. However, you can change your responses to things that happen in your environment by developing a healthy philosophy and a behavioral plan. For example, when stuck in traffic or a checkout line, have something interesting to read. Keep in mind that it only seems like a long time. The unhealthy alternative is to feel frustration, impatience, and anger. These emotions lead many overweight and obese people to overeat.

You can experience real health benefits and a lot of fat loss if you will implement several small life-style changes over the course of a year. Make sure the changes you select are under your control, but keep in mind that you also need to consistently monitor yourself on them. When you become motivated to make another small change, add it to your routine. Just remember, if you truly intend to make health improvements and reduce fat, you have to change something.

• • •

Coping with obesity's environmental and life-style issues doesn't require returning to the stone age or living in a hunter-gatherer society. What it does require is a comprehensive evaluation of how you live your life. Then you must identify those areas where you should make changes — and are willing to change. Finally, you must make a plan of action and then follow through with it.

Regardless of whether you plan to lose body fat or become more accepting of the condition, you can improve your health by making small adjustments in the way you live. Being more active, eating healthy, coping with stress in healthy ways, and taking control of your immediate environment all will produce benefits. If you are seeking to reduce body fat and lower health risks, these changes are critical components of a comprehensive plan.

The next chapters address the exercise and diet pieces of the obesity puzzle in depth. While there is some overlap among all of the components of obesity, life-style can be viewed as a more global way of addressing *everything* you do. Thus, this chapter makes a number of suggestions for establishing small but consistent changes in your day-to-day life. Overweight and overfat people who are the most serious about reducing health risks will want to make more structured, in-depth plans for exercise and eating. However, identifying and changing some of the "small" behavioral patterns that comprise life-style can go a long way toward improving health. Thus, they should be a part of any comprehensive fat reduction strategy.

Make Small Changes And Maintain Consistency

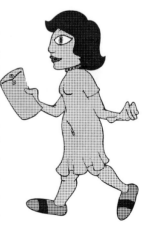

For the vast majority of obese people, it is best to start by making small changes. Hopefully you remember a few examples we gave in the last chapter. If a 175 pound woman increased her activity level by 20 minutes a day (reaching the equivalent of walking or strolling for 20 minutes), it would her reduce body fat by 10 pounds each year. (A 350 pound person doing the same thing would lose 20 pounds each year.) Reducing daily caloric intake by the equivalent of a single cola results in a 15 pound fat loss over a year. Obviously, if you can make a few small

Coping With The Obesity Puzzle:
You Must Exert Some Control
Over Your Environment and Life-Style

If the environmental and life-style puzzle piece is adequately addressed, substantial improvements in health can be attained. Small but consistent changes lead to big changes over time.

Environmental and life-style issues overlap with and affect every other area of the obesity puzzle. You must assess your activity level, eating habits, and identify stress coping behaviors:

Inactivity
Sedentary Leisure
Fast Food Junkie
Sedentary Work
Avoidance Of Small Chores
Impulsive Food Purchases
Feelings of Helplessness
Refusal To
Take Control

BIOLOGICAL FACTORS

DIET FACTORS

EXERCISE FACTORS

ENVIRON-MENTAL FACTORS

PSYCHO-LOGICAL & SOCIAL FACTORS

changes in what you do, and do them consistently over a year, you could lose a substantial amount of fat. The simple message in this has been stated in this book already, but it is so important that it bears repeating:

> Small consistent changes add up to big changes over time.

We've heard a lot of people reject the cola idea by saying they don't like diet drinks. You can develop a taste for them. Chances are that you didn't love the taste of beer, wine, liquor, or a lot of foods the first time you experienced them either. You probably have acquired a taste for some of them now. So, if you don't like diet drinks, try them all until you find one that eventually tastes good. If you want it to happen, it will.

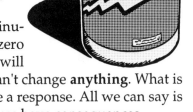

If you can find an excuse for continuing to drink a regular cola when a genuine zero calorie option is available, it is likely you will also find an excuse to explain why you can't change **anything**. What is our response to this? We don't really have a response. All we can say is that you are making a choice and all choices have consequences.

A parallel example is with skin cancer. Everyone has heard the "use sunscreen" warnings. Sun exposure often interacts with several cancer-producing genes. When skin damage (a tan is damage) accumulates over time to a predetermined level, the gene is activated and skin cancer results. It's the interaction between environment and genetics that is the underlying cause. We can't control genetics yet, but we do have some control over our environment and behavior. We make choices and all choices have consequences — some good, some bad.

Using A Health Journal

There are a lot of ways to begin making healthy life-style changes. We recommend that you start by making a list of obvious changes that you could easily fulfill. You may not have thought of all of the possibilities, but this chapter and other parts of this book have a lot of suggestions.

We aren't recommending that you employ *all* of the suggestions we make, just *do something*. As you find ideas that appeal to you, write them down. Once you have created a list of possibilities, choose a few that seem manageable. Then make a schedule of exactly when and where you will do them. Include all of the necessary preparations. For example, if you decide to try the diet drink idea, you will need to dispose of all the sugar-based drinks in your pantry and obtain some diet drinks.

The next thing you should do might seem a bit unusual, but it can really help. You need to begin a health diary or health journal. You can make your own from a notebook and paper, but there are several specially designed journals available in bookstores. Make sure that you use one that has enough space for you to write. Some of these journals are impractical because of their small size. They are printed the size of a paperback book so you can hide it in a pocket or purse. That can be very convenient until you begin writing in it every day. You quickly realize that the writing space is far too cramped.

We recommend you use "two month journals" to chart your planned eating, unplanned eating, physical activity, and feelings that emerge. If weight is a concern, use a journal that includes a weight chart and has a listing of the calorie/fat content of food. Our *SmartLoss 60-Day Health Journal* was specifically designed for all these purposes. It can be obtained from the publisher of this book or any bookstore can easily order it. One reason we recommend 60 day journals is that each 60 days should be perceived as a progressive learning experience. Learn from your successes and failures. At the end of the 60 days, begin another journal with some updated goals and planned changes. Behavioral research shows us that beneficial habits can be learned if we will do them consistently over 60 days or so.[1] Progress, not perfection, is the goal.

If you have professional assistance or a reliable support system for your overall health plan, use the journal to identify specific problems and feelings that seem to be related to stress, inactivity, or unplanned eating. Professionals supporting your weight loss or health effort should appreciate the information and find it helpful. Keep the journal with you every day. Make it a habit to write in at appropriate and consistent times.

Increasing Physical Activity At Home

For a true "couch potato," doing just about anything is an increase in activity. But it's a good idea to have some way to reliably track it. We recommend that everyone who is using a health journal wear a pedometer. This is a small device about the size of a watch that attaches to your belt or waist. A pedometer records the number of steps you take each day.

Aside from planned exercise periods (covered in the next chapter), there are countless things you can do to become more physically active. If you watch a lot of television, put away the remote for a few days. Yes, this means you will have to walk to the television and stand there while you push buttons. At every commercial, get up and stretch and stroll around the house. The typical network television hour includes at least 8 to 10 minutes of commercials. Moving a little during commercials is not much of a sacrifice, but it does increase the activity level of a couch potato.

Another television idea might be best done when you are alone. Every now and then you will hear a song or background music that you like. Instead of tapping your fingers to the music, get up and dance. We know that you've probably heard this before, but you should never eat while watching television. Chew gum if you must, but do not eat. The reason is that television promotes unconscious eating. Many people have essentially been programmed to eat in front of the television and they are seldom completely aware of what they are doing. Better yet, unplug the television.

Taking a few short walks a day is very beneficial. Even 5 minute walks produce health improvements. Plant a small garden and get into the habit of attending to it every day. If you have a yard, do a small amount of work in the yard every day. If you like reading, go to a library and browse. Go to a bookstore and browse. Many bookstores have chairs so customers can sit and read.

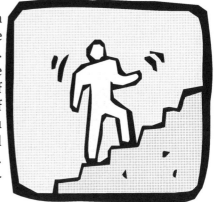

Another possible set of activities includes household chores. Wash your windows — one or two a day. Clean out a closet or cupboard. Do little chores (typically put off as long as possible) bit by bit. If you can bring yourself to do it, wash your own dishes occasionally. Prepare all of your own meals. Set the table for meals. Go window shopping in malls, just avoid the food area.

Try to develop a more *active* family and social life and blend it with leisure. Have healthy, well-planned picnics and cookouts. Go to some social group meetings. Try to go to the movies, a play, or a concert (you have to do *some* walking to get there). Go dancing, go bowling, fish — develop an active hobby or interest. For ideas, look back over your past and identify some activities you really enjoyed. Just be cautious about food and alcohol consumption related to these activities. If you have a lot of free time, you might consider doing volunteer work. For example, you could assist in an exercise/stretching class at a nursing home.

Physical Activity At Work

Chances are that you can find some work time (including breaks and lunch) to increase physical activity. If you have a sedentary job, get out of your chair every 15 minutes and stretch. Some computer programs are available that will remind you to take a brief break as often as you tell it to. Stand up and move while you are talking on the phone. During break periods, take a 5 minute stroll. Walk to lunch if you can. Park further away than you usually do. Take a 5 to 15 minute stroll at lunchtime. If you normally take an elevator, get off one floor below and walk up the last flight of steps. If your job permits it, take a small object (like a book) and do repetitive arm exercises with it from time to time. 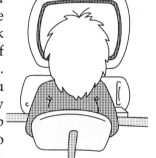 Keep a "stress ball" on your desk, repetitively squeeze it. Do something!

Making Life-Style Eating Changes

Stress, poor planning, and social pressure are the major reasons we consume so much fast food. These three reasons are lumped together by the fast food industry and simply termed "convenience." We feel certain that you know this already, but you should try to eliminate fast food from your diet. You can probably plan and prepare the majority of your meals, and doing this will eliminate a lot of fat and calories from your diet. If you must eat fast food, don't look at the menu and decide what you want. Decide what you will order **before** you get there. **Appendix D** at the back of this book has a listing of the fat and calorie content of the items available at most popular fast food restaurants. Some of them have virtually nothing that a health-conscious, overweight person should eat. Most, however, have a few selections that are healthy. Just don't be swayed by impulse hunger created by smells, pictures, or the little sales pitch always given after you order: "Do you want an apple pie or french fries with that order?" If you can resist the temptations of seeing and smelling food, always walk inside to order. Never "supersize" except maybe with a diet drink.

Eating in most restaurants is a great unknown for dieters. Few restaurants outside the fast food industry have a nutritional analysis of their meals available. Restaurant food is typically very dense in calories and fats. Choose restaurants that serve some obviously healthy foods. Have a plan before you go to a particular restaurant. If you are dining with friends, eat something healthy and low calorie, and plan to eat more when you get home. Better yet, eat before you go to the restaurant. (That *is* a real life-style change.) Stay away from foods with creams, gravies, sauces, or that were cooked in fat. Choose the lowest calorie and lowest fat dressings you can for salads (Remember that some sugars and starches can be more dangerous than fat.). Smart people carry their own dressings and sweeteners with them in small packages. Try to order lean meats either grilled or baked. Tell the waiter you want things cooked without oil or fat. If you order a baked potato, have it delivered to you plain. A delicious trick is to put steak sauce in it rather than butter or sour cream.

Certain snacks and drinks should simply be eliminated and healthy substitutes made. Some mixed fruit drinks, advertised as health drinks, have nearly 1,000 calories. All alcohol contains empty calories. (Alcohol has calories with no nutritional value.) If you must drink, do it moderately (no more than 2 drinks a day) and try to choose the lowest calorie form of drinks.

The chapter on diet goes into greater detail on this, but most of the "low" or "no fat" products and snacks have a lot of calories because of high sugar content. Calories do count. You can add body fat even if you eat no fat at all. Diabetics have to make major adjustments in snacks, fruits, and all other eating areas. If you are obese and age 40 or over, you have a risk of developing diabetes. Eating healthy now can delay or prevent the onset of diabetes. Some snacks are both low fat and low calorie and are available in grocery stores and in food warehouses. They typically don't taste as good as the regular version, but they are healthier and you can acquire a taste for them. Take some time in a grocery store and search carefully for these items.

Try to eliminate convenience store shopping from your life. **Never shop for food when you are hungry.** Buy food in grocery stores. You have to walk more in a grocery store and you have a wider selection of healthy food. Become accustomed to using a shopping list so you can eliminate impulse buying and fulfill your food plans. Be a smart consumer. Choose foods by reading the nutritional labels. These will be fully explained in a later chapter. Look for foods with low calories, low fat, low sugar, and high fiber. Learn to appreciate fresh fruits and vegetables.

You should try to *eat 6 times a day*. A common pattern among dieters is to go most of the day without eating and then overeating in the evening. You do not want to be hungry, so you should plan to eat more often. Never skip breakfast, but make it healthy and filling. One of us routinely makes for breakfast a very filling scrambled egg sandwich with 160 calories and virtually no fat. The 2 slices of bread have 100 calories (50 each). Most large grocery stores will have some selections of bread where each slice is 50 calories or less. The 2 eggs come in a frozen package with 0 cholesterol and 0 fat (60 calories). After a minute in the microwave, the eggs are scrambled in 0 fat oil spray. A diet soda goes with the meal. Of course, not all of us eat this breakfast. Fiber One® or All-Bran® are excellent breakfast cereal options.

In midmorning you should have a snack that you carry with you. If you go to work, carry a lunch several days each week. If a microwave is available, a wide range of soups and low fat, low calorie meals are ideal.

You will also find that doing this will save you a great deal of money over a year. In the afternoon, you have another snack. In the evening, a planned formal meal around a table is best. An evening snack is the sixth meal.

Life-Style And Stress

The prior two chapters reviewed psychological issues associated with obesity. Stress factors are an important component in determining your life-style as well as eating and activity patterns. For example, too many of us come home from work so mentally exhausted that all we do is collapse on the couch and watch television. There are numerous stress inducing interactions we have with our environment. For example, traffic congestion often causes rising blood pressure, worry, and anger. You might decide to leave earlier or later to avoid the high traffic times, but you will still find yourself occasionally stuck in traffic. So, what do you do?

In his first book, *Simply Spiritual*[2], Father Bill Stelling addressed his own frustrations and anger about traffic:

"According to me, I have two faults of impatience: Being stalled in traffic; and moving in traffic. According to many others, there is no way to keep track of the faults I have of impatience. For me, where impatience is, anger is seldom far behind.

Sometime ago I found myself stalled in a traffic jam. I'm not one of those people who lays on the horn. I just sit and fume. Quite by chance the voice on the radio announced the time and I glanced at the clock on my dashboard to see if it was right. It was that glance that led me to a startling discovery. I noted when traffic began moving again that less than three minutes had elapsed. Most of my time in the car is spent alone, so there is no one to pass the time with. Perhaps that is unfortunate. Since I made the discovery of the three minutes, I try to remember to have the *Reader's Digest* or a book of jokes or puzzles in the car with me. I find this helpful whenever I am waiting in line at the checkout counter, at the bank, and other places, too. ... When I get impatient, it means that I am refusing to endure, to accept reality. As the saying goes. I'm refusing to accept life on life's terms."

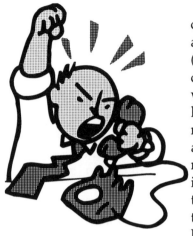

What is meant by "refusing to accept life on life's terms?" If you can take an objective look at your environment (and your genetic predispositions), you can understand it. You came into this world at a time when incredible technological advances are being made. Conveniences that reduce our physical work are everywhere. Travel is quick, convenient, and usually comfortable. Contrarily, we have numerous responsibilities that are imposed upon us that require us to rush from one obligation to another. But accidents happen. Traffic jams happen. Sometimes we get stuck in the back of a line. When you respond to these inevitable delays with impatience and anger, you are refusing to accept life on life's terms. In short, you believe that life's realities should accommodate to you.

Another component of "life's terms" is our incredible food abundance. We came into a part of the world at a time when food was plentiful. Going to a food buffet with others is probably inevitable for all of us even when we are dieting. Some dieters get temporarily frustrated and angered by the situation, but then they often decide to go ahead and binge.

The final piece of "life's terms" is your genetic inheritance. You probably were born with a set of thrifty genes programmed to ensure your survival in times of starvation. But the world you encounter has an abundance of food and doesn't demand a lot of physical activity. Unless you accommodate your behavior to the situation — you are destined to get fat.

Anger and frustration lead many of us to automatically eat. It is *how we respond* to these situations that determines the impact they will have on us. You do have a right to become angry and frustrated at work, in traffic, and in social situations. You have the right to overeat when you go to a restaurant. But as Father Bill wrote in his 1998 book, *Spiritual Reflections On Everyday Living*[3], "Just because I have a right to do a thing, doesn't mean it's the right thing to do." He adds, "Freedom, to me, is being able to avoid what I know I should avoid, and being able to do what I should do."

Since stress, inconvenience, work frustrations, social life conflicts, and lots of other uncontrollable events are inevitable, what's the best course of action. First, as Father Bill related, have a plan of action that enables you to dissipate the stress in a healthy way. Music, relaxation techniques, becoming philosophical, reading, taking medication, and taking walks can all be a part of a plan of action. In addition, by making slight adjustments in your schedule (a part of your life-style), you can reduce the probability of some stressful events. You perhaps know someone who always seemed to be 5 or 10 minutes late for work? The person always had some sort of excuse for it. The real problem was the person left for work 10 minutes too late. The solution was obvious.

Control Issues

Perhaps the most critical issue in planning possible life-style changes is deciding what you can control and what you can't control. You can learn to control and change your emotional responses to frustrations. You can regularly look at your successes in life rather than dwelling on your failures. You can become more active in your environment. You can change food and eating patterns. You can go to support group. You may choose to not exert some control over these situations, but you should understand that you have made a choice to give up control. People who feel a lack of control over their lives tend to have higher rates of obesity and heart disease.[4] People who feel that they will never gain control over stressful situations are especially prone to weight gain and binge eating.[5]

One of the most useful tools we have ever used to assist others (as well as ourselves) in handling control issues is the *Serenity Prayer*. It is widely associated with (AA) 12-Step programs, but its originator is believed to be the Protestant theologian, Reinhold Niebuhr. Even if you don't believe in God, there is a wonderful philosophy embedded in it. The prayer is:

God, grant me the serenity to accept the things
I cannot change, the courage to change the things I can,
and the wisdom to know the difference.

In applying the prayer to obesity, fitness, and life-style, several observations are apparent. Some things about yourself and the world are not under your control — they cannot be changed. You have to come to accept these and become okay with it — that's serenity. For example, you may have major responsibilities that get in the way of walking an hour a day. If that's the reality, come to accept it. You may also have a genetic predisposition to have wide hips and large thighs.

At the same time, the prayer tells us to take charge of the things we are able to control — have the courage to change the things we can. Maybe you can't walk an hour a day, but can you find several 15 minute periods when you can walk? Maybe you'll always have large thighs, but there are a lot of things you can do to reduce and tone them.

The final aspect of the prayer asks for the wisdom to know the difference between things we have the ability to control and things we don't. Wisdom can come from gaining knowledge, doing self-exploration, and seeking help. Ask yourself this simple question: Are you doing *everything* you can to control obesity and become fit? If you can answer "yes," then there is no reason for you to worry. If your answer is "no," you have two choices. You can just accept the condition and quit worrying. Or you can take charge by changing the things you can. It's simple, but it can really help you if you apply it to your life-style and behavior.

Chapter References & Notes

[1] Pettit, J. (1999) Can food become an addiction? Substituting a positive addiction as a treatment approach. *Addictive Behaviors Treatment Review*, 1 (2), 3.

[2] Stelling, B. (1992) *Simply Spiritual*. Memphis: Eagle Wing Books, Inc.

[3] Stelling, B. (1998) *Spiritual Reflections on Everyday Living*. Memphis: Eagle Wing Books, Inc.

[4] Myers, D. (1992) *Psychology*. New York: Worth Publishers.

[5] Polivy, J., & Herman, C. P. (1999) Distress and eating: why do dieters overeat? *International Journal of Eating Disorders*, 26, 153-164.

Chapter 14
EXERCISE & METABOLISM:
THE FOURTH PUZZLE PIECE

Overall, exercise is of marginal benefit in the treatment of obesity.
J. S. Flier & D. W. Foster (1998) — *Williams Textbook of Endocrinology*[1]

Exercise during and after dieting is one of the few predictors
of successful long-term weight loss.
D. G. Myers (1992) — *Psychology*[2]

Summary — Consistent moderate exercise results in health improvements in heart disease, blood pressure, diabetes, osteoporosis, and numerous other conditions. Establishing an exercise routine lasting 30 minutes 5 or 6 days a week leads to reduced stress, increased energy, better sleep, less depression, and reduced body fat. Despite all of the benefits derived from only 3 hours of exercise a week, less than a third of Americans maintain that level of activity.

Exercise is a major component in the treatment of obesity and in the maintenance of weight loss. When weight loss is accomplished by dieting alone, a substantial amount of muscle tissue is lost with fat. This occurs because the pancreatic hormone glucagon is released during restrictive dieting. Glucagon not only signals fat cells to release free fatty acids for consumption as energy, it also produces a break down of muscle fibers in order to produce amino acids that are converted into glucose. Due to the loss of muscle tissue during restrictive diets, the Basal Metabolic Rate subsequently declines. Muscle tissue burns a lot more calories, pound for pound, than does fat. This means that the individual who lost the weight has to continue to restrict caloric intake after the diet because of less muscle.

Exercise is the only sure way to maintain muscle mass during periods of fat loss. Increased muscle mass facilitates additional fat loss by raising basal metabolic rate. In addition, the increased physical activity from exercise consumes calories helping with fat loss.

Two types of exercise are necessary. Aerobic exercise should be established with the eventual goal of having 30 minutes of sustained exercise a day at least 5 or 6 days per week. The daily 30 minutes can be broken into several short time periods if necessary. Walking, jogging, dancing, aerobic exercise, cycling, and swimming are examples of aerobic exercise. Anaerobic exercise, especially resistance training, is the second form of necessary exercise. Anaerobic exercise builds and strengthens muscles. Light weight lifting is the preferred method of anaerobic exercise.

Starting an exercise routine requires planning and goals. You should try to make it as pleasant as possible by listening to music, walking with friends, or using videotapes. Walking is the method the vast majority of people use for their frequent exercise. Walking in malls or using a treadmill can be very helpful. Joining a fitness center or health club is an option, but not necessary. However, having social support for your exercise is very helpful. If you have been inactive, you should begin by making small increases in exercise. Chances are that it will seem to be unpleasant at first, but keep in mind that, with continued effort, it can become enjoyable.

Strength building through weight lifting requires minimal equipment and only a small amount of time. A few sets of different weight dumbbells can be used. The first three weeks of weight lifting requires one or two days a week of less than 30 minutes. During this time you work through a series of repetitive exercises working different muscle groups. After the first three weeks, the weight should be slightly increased and the number of repetitions increased. You should also increase the number of days you lift weights to three each week. This strength and muscle building phase lasts four to 20 weeks until you reach your desired level. Maintenance of muscle mass and strength is much easier than building them. All that is required is working out two times each week without increasing the weight.

Establishing an exercise plan is essential to changing your health and activity level. Goals should be written down and your progress recorded. We recommend using a health journal.

• • •

The health benefits of exercise have been well publicized by governmental agencies, schools, organizations, and the media. Tens of thousands of scientific studies have been carried out and published documenting the effects of exercise. All it takes is 30 minutes of sustained exercise 5 or 6 days a week to derive many health improvements.

Mainstream college and medical textbooks as well as all of the previously mentioned information sources take a consistent stand on regular exercise:[3, 4]

- Exercise reduces the risk of cardiovascular heart disease
- Exercise can lower blood pressure and some cancer risks
- Exercise can help type 2 diabetics manage symptoms
- Exercise reduces the risk of developing diabetes
- Exercise reduces the risk of osteoporosis
- Exercise delays many health problems of aging
- Exercise increases endurance and strength
- Exercise promotes total body flexibility
- Exercise can improve mood and sleep quality
- Exercise reduces stress
- Exercise enhances thinking ability
- Exercise reduces body fat percentage

With all of the benefits derived from only three hours of sustained activity a week, you'd certainly think that lots of us would choose to be active. It hasn't happened. In fact, as we related in chapter 12, about 67% of adults are sedentary or seldom active. Half of teens and young adults are inactive and our children become less and less active with each new generation. Our overall level of activity and fitness continues to decline. Although you may not fully realize it, we've already answered why this is occurring. It's neither laziness nor lack of will-power. The cause is the complex interaction of our basic survival genetics with our technological environment of increased food abundance and increased leisure time. Somewhere, buried in our genetics, is the biological and psychological tendency to conserve energy whenever we can. Both our body and mind are programmed to take advantage of periods of abundance and leisure. This genetic programming can be overcome, paradoxically, through use of will-power and making healthy choices.

In terms of employing exercise as an obesity treatment, two equally true yet seemingly contradictory statements could be made. These two statements are the quotes at the beginning of this chapter:

> ## Overall, exercise is of marginal benefit in the treatment of obesity.[1]
>
> and
>
> ## Exercise during and after dieting is one of the few predictors of successful long-term weight loss.[2]

In the obesity chapter of the 1998 medical text, *Williams Textbook of Endocrinology*,[1] it is acknowledged that exercise is quite appropriate and necessary as an obesity treatment component. Yet, the reality of obesity treatment outcome reveals that very few obese people actually succeed in establishing and maintaining regular exercise routines. Thus, based on the failure of obese people to actually do it, it is validly concluded that exercise is "of marginal benefit in the treatment of obesity."

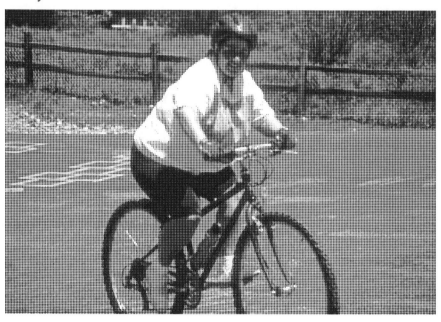

Myers' 1992 *Psychology* text,[2] reviews the behaviors associated with successful long-term weight loss in obese and overweight people. As we have related earlier, about 95% of people who diet and exercise to lose weight will regain the weight within 5 years. Myers' focus was on the 5% who maintained their weight loss. Research shows that these people established a regular but modest exercise program and they stayed on it indefinitely.

Williams Textbook of Endocrinology[1] renders a harsh analysis of why obese people fail to exercise. There are high dropout rates in all obesity treatment programs. But dropout from exercise is especially high. Drastically changing an inactive life-style to one that includes regular and sustained exercise requires "tremendous dedication." This much dedication to change is simply absent.[1]

How Well Does Exercise Work For Weight Loss?

The 1998 federal obesity standards panel[5] (discussed in earlier chapters) reviewed 23 rigorous studies published in the scientific literature that evaluated the effects of exercise on body fat reduction. They found that exercise, in and of itself, results in very modest fat loss. However, the panel reviewed another 23 rigorous studies that evaluated adding exercise to reduced-calorie diets. The combined results of these studies showed a higher, but still rather modest weight and fat loss. An additional 36 scientific studies were reviewed wherein exercise, restricted-calorie diets, and behavioral and life-style change approaches were all incorporated into the treatment program. This more comprehensive approach produced significantly more fat and weight loss and sustained that weight loss over a much longer period of time. The key factor in maintaining the weight loss was remaining in a long-term behavioral support program that provided accountability and motivation. Under this ongoing support condition, many people are able to sustain the "tremendous dedication" required to continue participating in an exercise program.

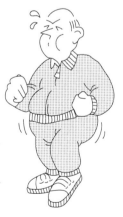

Why Exercise Is Necessary For Maintaining Fat Loss

Many obese patients are willing to go on calorie-restricted diets and take medication. However, a great deal of resistance is encountered when exercise is recommended. It is true that a substantial amount of weight can be lost without exercise. But a large proportion of the "lost weight" is muscle tissue, water, and can even include some bone density. Perhaps even worse is the fact that substantial weight loss without exercise could actually raise body fat percentage if muscle is lost faster than fat. This may contribute to an increase in some health risks. The most health benefits are seen when fat loss comes from a consistent effort over time that includes both calorie reduction and exercise. The following sections show the processes involved in both healthy and unhealthy weight loss.

Calorie Basics

The basics of weight loss and weight gain are simple. Your body consumes energy constantly — primarily consuming the simple sugar, glucose, and, occasionally, free fatty acids. As it consumes the glucose, the body's cells produce heat. The process of energy consumption in cells

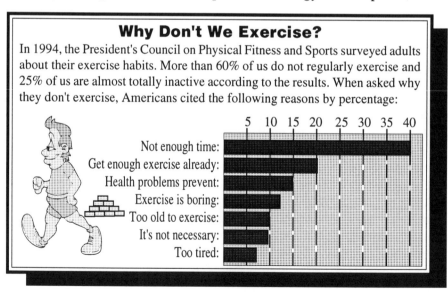

Why Don't We Exercise?

In 1994, the President's Council on Physical Fitness and Sports surveyed adults about their exercise habits. More than 60% of us do not regularly exercise and 25% of us are almost totally inactive according to the results. When asked why they don't exercise, Americans cited the following reasons by percentage:

	5	10	15	20	25	30	35	40
Not enough time:								
Get enough exercise already:								
Health problems prevent:								
Exercise is boring:								
Too old to exercise:								
It's not necessary:								
Too tired:								

is complicated, but the simplest way to understand it is that we "burn" the energy. As you are aware, oxygen is required to burn anything, so we have to breathe in order to supply every cell in the body with the required oxygen. When you exercise, you get hot. This heat is generated by the cells burning more energy. You breathe faster and harder during exercise because you have to take in extra oxygen to keep the "fires" going. You sweat during exercise to lower your body temperature to normal levels.

The energy (glucose) burned by cells comes from the food you eat. The specific amount of energy that various foods can produce is measured in units called *calories*. In the United States, what we commonly call **a food calorie** (actually a kilocalorie in science) is the amount of heat required to raise the temperature of 2.2 pounds of water by 1.8 degrees Fahrenheit.

How the number of calories in different foods is determined is remarkably simple. Calorimetric scientists place carefully measured amounts of a specific food into a special, insulated container that also contains a specific amount of water. The oxygen level in the container is enriched and the food is burned. The heat from the fire is absorbed by the water. Then the water temperature is measured and compared to the starting temperature. The increase in water temperature determines the number of calories in the food.

Calories And Body Fat

If a person takes in more food calories than are needed for fuel, the excess calories are converted to fat. Fat is an efficient form of stored energy. If you regularly use more calories than you consume in food, the body converts some of your stored fat into usable energy and burns it. Under this condition, you'll lose fat. Each pound of body fat stores about 3,500 calories.

The Problem With Dieting Alone
To Reduce Body Fat

As discussed in chapter 8, the regulation of glucose transport into the body's cells, the storage of energy as fat, and the conversion of body fat into energy are regulated by several pancreatic hormones. Insulin and glucagon are the two major hormones involved in maintaining this energy balance.

When blood sugar levels fall because of a diet or fast, glucagon is released. The glucagon immediately signals the liver to produce glucose from its own energy stores and from amino acids it obtains from muscle tissues. Glucagon also activates enzymes in fat cells that begin releasing free fatty acids into the bloodstream for use as energy. Some weight loss on diets comes from a loss of muscle mass — not just burned fat. Proteins in muscle fibers are broken down and converted into glucose. High protein diets attempt to counteract the muscle loss, but some muscle tissue is still burned as energy. (One of the major problems associated with very-low-calorie diets is significant muscle loss.)

Muscle and lean-body mass burn more calories to simply maintain basic survival while body fat is relatively inert. This essential rate of mandatory, baseline energy consumption is called *Basal Metabolic Rate*. As muscle tissue decreases, the body's basal metabolic rate lowers. Thus, after the dieter loses weight by only severely restricting calorie intake, she is forced to stay on a restricted calorie diet to maintain the loss. The body's setpoint mechanism, regulated by various neurochemicals and hormones, was discussed in chapters 7 and 8. Setpoint processes will activate a cascade of events to increase hunger and put into motion various physiological processes that facilitate the regain of weight as fat.

It is known that long periods of severely restricted diets or fasting can reduce the basal metabolic rate by as much as 45%. A great deal of this lowered energy usage comes from a declining body mass and a rapid reduction in physical activity that occurs because of fatigue and various physiological processes that conserve energy. However, 15% of the lowered basal metabolic rate reduction comes from a decrease in the rate at which the body's cells consume energy.[6,7]

Weight Cycling

A great deal of attention has been focused on "weight cycling" because of the observed reduction in basal metabolic rates during diets and after diets. Weight cycling is the repeated loss of and regain of body weight through dieting. It is also known as "yo-yo" dieting.

Research on the effects of weight cycling is inconclusive. Some people do increase body fat percentage with repeated dieting attempts while others don't. There is inconclusive evidence that yo-yo dieters have higher mortality rates, but most research results don't indicate that each attempt at weight loss becomes more difficult due to weight cycling. It is known that metabolic rate declines steadily with age. This could be a contributing factor to a lowered metabolic rate with each dieting cycle.[8]

Exercise Is The Only Sure Way To Maintain Muscle Mass And Increase Both Basal Metabolic Rate & Energy Expenditure

As related earlier in this chapter, muscle and lean tissue require more calorie usage, pound for pound, than does fat tissue for its basic survival. The only way to maintain muscle mass during fat reduction dieting is to exercise and also eat sufficient proteins to supply the amino acids necessary to rebuild muscles. Past chapters have stressed the necessity for increased physical activity, in part, because the old saying, "use it or lose it," is absolutely true with muscle tissue. Any physical activity is helpful, but it should be obvious to you that some forms of exercise are more helpful than others. Duration of exercise is also important. During the first 20 minutes of moderate exercise, the body relies on stored energy in muscles and the liver. After 20 minutes of exercise, the fat cells begin releasing free fatty acids for energy consumption.

Some non-intense forms of exercise (such as walking or simple movements) retain muscle mass and also utilize energy. During a diet when the basal metabolic rate typically declines, regular but short

Two Types Of Exercise

The two types of exercise recommended as part of a comprehensive health fitness program — not just for people trying to manage weight, but everyone — are called aerobic and anaerobic exercise.

Aerobic exercise is a continuous form of exercise that allows your body to consistently replenish oxygen to your working muscles. It is performed at a low to moderate intensity and is endurance-oriented by nature. Aerobic exercise includes walking, jogging, cycling, swimming, running, and dancing. Aerobic training can improve cardiorespiratory endurance and burns fat.

Anaerobic exercise utilizes oxygen at a faster rate than your body can replenish it in the exercising of muscles. By nature, this type of exercise is usually intense and short in duration. Moving weights through repetitive motions is anaerobic. It burns fat and builds muscle mass.

periods of walking or other activity can ensure a higher energy expenditure. Even after exercise ends, the basal metabolic rate will be elevated. A single period of vigorous exercise can increase the basal metabolic rate for up to 24 hours.[6]

Increasing Muscle Mass Leads To Increased Energy Expenditure

The basal metabolic rate (BMR), as described earlier in this chapter, is the amount of energy consumed to maintain life during sleep

Both Types Of Exercise Are Critical Components To Permanent Weight Loss And Health

Approximately 70% of our daily energy expenditure (the burning of calories) comes from basal metabolic rate. Thermogenesis (the production of body heat due to food intake, cold, stress, and food) uses approximately 15% of our daily energy expenditure. The remaining 15% of energy use comes from physical activity. Exercise increases the burning of calories by raising both basal metabolic rate and increasing energy expenditure caused by muscle movement. Resistance training to increase muscle mass boosts energy expenditure by raising basal metabolic rate (due to muscle tissues higher energy needs) and by using energy during the exercise period itself. Both types of exercise lead to reduced body fat percentage as well as maintenance of weight loss when they are used as part of a comprehensive fat reduction plan.

Source of Daily Energy Expenditure
(How Calories Are Typically Used)

PHYSICAL ACTIVITY (Utilizes 15% of energy)	Physical activity and exercise: energy expenditure can be increased by exercise and increased activity or decreased by inactivity.
THERMOGENESIS (Utilizes 15% of energy)	Facultative Obligatory (These are the two primary types of body heat generation.)
BASAL METABOLIC RATE (Utilizes 70% of energy)	Maintenance of basic life-sustaining processes.

Adapted from Bray, G.A., & Bray, D.S. (1988)
Obesity: Part I - pathogenesis. *Western Journal of Medicine*, 149, 429-441.

and wake cycles. Increasing muscle mass will raise the BMR, because muscle is more metabolically active and requires more energy for essential life functions. Therefore, increasing muscle mass results in the expenditure of more energy even when you sit.[7] Thus, increasing muscle mass should be included as a weight loss and fitness goal. Since muscle tissue is enlarged by "resistance" and "strength building" exercise, muscles must be worked by moving weight. Some resistance to movement is required to force the muscle into growing. A person does not have to do serious weight lifting to increase muscle mass. The use of low weights with many repetitions is all that is required.

Coping With Exercise — The Fourth Piece Of The Obesity Puzzle

Regardless of whether you intend to lose weight or not, exercise can lead to substantial health benefits. In addition, exercise impacts all of the other areas of the complex obesity puzzle including biological, psychological, life-style, and diet making it progressively easier to maintain weight loss. The establishment of regular exercise is often the most difficult behavioral change for obese patients. Yet without some form of regular physical activity increases (exercise) the vast majority of dieters and people taking medication for obesity will be doomed to failure.

Exercise Effects All The Puzzle Pieces: A Brief Summary
Exercise triggers the release of a type of brain transmitters called endorphins. Endorphins (meaning *endogenous morphine* because they are

---

Basal Metabolic Rate Declines With Age — But It Doesn't Have To

From adulthood on, basal metabolic rate declines about 2% each decade. In other words, the 65-year old will tend to burn about 8% less calories than he or she did at age 25. Unless this person steadily decreases food intake or increases activity level, a creeping weight gain will occur. This, in fact, is observed in almost everyone as they age. The reason for this decline in basal metabolic rate has long been debated. It is now known that a gradual loss of muscle mass accounts for the decline. In short, as people age, they use their muscles less and less. With the declining work load placed on muscles, they lose mass. Research shows that even minimal resistance training to maintain muscle mass will keep basal metabolic rate from declining.[3]

naturally occurring in the brain and work in a manner similar to narcotic painkillers) can produce a calming, almost euphoric effect. Some research[9] implicates the release of endorphins as the source of what is often described as "runner's high." It is a sense of exhilaration that can occur in people after prolonged, difficult exercise. It is not known whether endorphins actually produce the effect, but it is known that endorphins are released in most people after sustained exercise.[10, 11] Endorphins are linked to the body's own ability to reduce physical pain. For example, you may have experienced minor pain or irritation after cutting a finger. After a period of time, you seem to better tolerate the irritation and will even forget that it is there. If you squeeze the cut or focus your attention on it, you quickly realize that it still hurts a little. But the pain can quickly subside and slip out of your mind. This pain reduction effect may be due to endorphins.[12] A host of research studies have shown that exercise produces beneficial effects on mood. Anxiety, tension, anger, depression, and confusion are all lessened by exercise.[13, 14]

It has been questioned whether exercise itself produces improved mood or whether people with particular mood states are drawn toward activity or inactivity. For example, it is well known that depressed people tend to be inactive. Substantial psychological research has directly addressed this issue. This research confirms that it is the exercise itself that produces beneficial effects on mood.[15] Research has shown that a simple 10-minute walk produces improved energy levels and less anxiety for up to two hours after the walk.[16] As prior chapters have stressed, the psychological and biological aspects of obesity are intimately connected. *We know of no behavioral method more effective than exercise in positively effecting overall mood and reducing obesity.*

Establishing regular exercise habits impacts all other areas of lifestyle. People tend to become health conscious and more active in all areas of living when they exercise. Smoking, dietary habits, and overall motivation are more often considered and addressed by people who exercise.[4]

As related at the beginning of this chapter, there are numerous physical health benefits to exercise. Exercise also reduces insulin resistance and lowers insulin levels while facilitating glucagon release. These factors result in loss of body fat.[3] Exercise is one of the most important treatment components in patients with type 2 diabetes as well as with obese patients and people with cardiovascular heart disease. Most chronic health problems can be improved through exercise.[3, 4, 17, 18]

Coping With The Obesity Puzzle: You Must Increase Muscle Mass And Increase Metabolic Rate Through Exercise

Exercise is a critical component of the obesity puzzle. You must establish an exercise routine lasting at least 30 minutes for 5 or 6 day a week. This component:

Boosts Basal Metabolism
Increases Fat Loss
Prevents Muscle Loss
Builds Muscle Mass
Increases Self-Esteem
Increases Feelings of Control

Any increase in physical activity is helpful to weight loss. However, regular periods of sustained activity combined with resistance training to build muscle mass will result in obvious benefits.

BIOLOGICAL FACTORS

DIET FACTORS

EXERCISE FACTORS

ENVIRON-MENTAL FACTORS

PSYCHO-LOGICAL & SOCIAL FACTORS

Getting Started

Begin by understanding that **any physical activity is better than none.**[19] If you have been inactive, you should start slowly and gradually build activity levels. Check with your physician before starting to discuss health conditions that could restrict the level of activity you can perform. You may not realize this, but you will expend just as many calories by casually walking a mile than by running it. So don't be concerned if you initially move slowly and have to periodically rest.

Develop an initial plan. The plan should be suited to your current physical condition, interests, environment, resources, and social support. Even the weather has to be considered. Your plan should be written down. It does not have to be extensive, but writing down daily progress and activities clearly facilitates your compliance with your chosen exercise goals.[20] We recommend that a continuous health journal be kept (discussed in the prior chapter). A pedometer is highly recommended for obese patients and others trying to lose body fat. This enables both exercise time and distance to be monitored accurately to assess progress.

It May Not Be Fun — At First

The primary reason that many people stop exercising or fail to even initiate it is simple. When a sedentary person begins exercise, it can be experienced as unpleasant. For some people, any form of activity — even a 10 minute stroll — can be aversive. The answer to this is just as simple. **You have to do it regardless of how you might feel.** You have the choice to take charge of your health by becoming more active or to keep things as they are and accept the consequences. If you fail to exercise because you don't like it, you are choosing to remain in your present condition. With time and continued exercise, it will become less aversive.

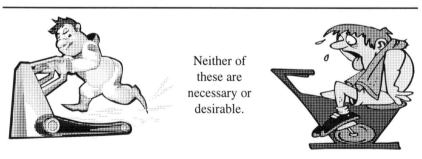

Neither of
these are
necessary or
desirable.

The majority of people who establish regular exercise periods come to enjoy them and even look forward to them. But the only way this is discovered is by actually exercising in spite of a mental urge to stop. By starting slowly and gradually building up longer exercise periods, you can increase the odds that you will continue to exercise.

Make It As Pleasant As Possible

You can do many things to make exercise more enjoyable. With today's small radios, tapes and CD players, you can listen to anything you desire during walks. One good suggestion would be to listen to some weight-loss motivation tapes as you walk. We have developed some of these and many others are available at good bookstores, health stores, and elsewhere.

Find a comfortable place such as a mall where you can pleasantly and safely walk in any weather. Many walkers can be found in almost every mall in the United States at any time of day or night. Many malls open their doors early specifically for people who want to walk in them.

Take walks in parks, around lakes, or other areas in nature. You will find that there are many people who would likely accompany you. Having some social support is one of the prime factors associated with continued exercise. A "buddy" system of exercise, in which you routinely walk or exercise with others, makes exercise more enjoyable, safer, and practical.

What To Ask Before Starting Exercise

Answer the following questions before you begin exercising.

1. Has a doctor ever said you have heart problems?
2. Do you frequently suffer from chest pains?
3. Do you often feel faint or have dizzy spells?
4. Has a doctor ever said you have high blood pressure?
5. Has a doctor ever told you that you have a bone or joint problem, such as arthritis, that has been or could be aggravated by exercise?
6. Are you over the age of 65 and not accustomed to exercise?
7. Are you taking prescription medications, such as those for high blood pressure?
8. Is there a good medical reason, not mentioned here, why you should not exercise?

If you answered "yes" to any of these questions, you should see your doctor before you begin an exercise program.

Source: National Institute of Diabetes, Digestive, and Kidney Diseases (1999)

A treadmill is a very useful piece of equipment for walking. Most treadmills have timers and heart rate monitors and will measure the distance you walk. In addition, treadmills are adjustable and you can easily change the incline to increase or decrease the level of difficulty. In this way you can easily raise your heart rate. In addition, treadmills are used indoors in any weather. You can make it a habit to watch a specific television program while walking on a treadmill or listening to music.

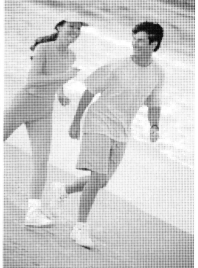

Forming A Successful Physical Activity Program

Adapted from: National Institute of Diabetes, Digestive, and Kidney Diseases (1999)

The "buddy" system of exercise helps keep you on track. When you don't feel like exercise, your buddy will "shame" you into performing, and vice-versa. Your buddy will keep you honest.

• Follow a gradual approach to exercise to get the most benefits with the fewest risks. If you have not been exercising, start at a slow pace and as you become more fit, gradually increase the amount of time and the pace of your activity.

• Choose activities that you enjoy and that fit your personality. For example, if you like team sports or group activities, choose things

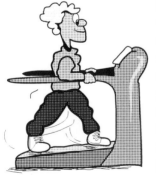

such as soccer or aerobics. If you prefer individual activities, choose things such as swimming or walking. Also, plan your activities for a time of day that suits your personality. If you are a morning person, exercise before you begin the rest of your day's activities. If you have more energy in the evening, plan activities that can be done at the end of the day. You will be more likely to stick to a physical activity program if it is convenient and enjoyable.

• Exercise regularly. To gain the most health benefits it is important to exercise as regularly as possible. Make sure you choose activities that will fit into your schedule.

• Exercise at a comfortable pace. For example, while jogging or walking briskly you should be able to hold a conversation. If you do not feel normal again within 10 minutes following exercise, you are exercising too hard. Also, if you have difficulty breathing or feel faint or weak during or after exercise, you are exercising too hard.

• Maximize your safety and comfort. Wear shoes that fit and clothes that move with you, and always exercise in a safe location. Many people walk in indoor shopping malls for exercise. Malls are climate controlled and offer protection from bad weather.

• Vary your activities. Choose a variety of activities so you don't get bored with any one thing.

• Encourage your family or friends to support you and join you in your activity. If you have children, it is best to build healthy habits when they are young. When parents are active, children are more likely to be active and stay active for the rest of their lives.

• Challenge yourself. Set short-term as well as long-term goals and celebrate every success, no matter how small.

• Pace yourself and don't get injured!

Setting Goals For Regular Exercise

Physical activity does not need to be strenuous to promote weight loss or produce health benefits. However, there is a growing consensus among researchers and clinicians indicating the minimal level of activity you should eventually try to attain. The majority of health benefits are achieved when you engage in 30 minutes of moderate-intensity exercise 5 to 6 days each week.[20] One way to assess "moderate intensity" walking is the "conversation test." If you are breathing so hard that conversation is difficult, you are probably exercising at levels above the moderate level. This procedure for gauging walking speed is very practical — especially in the beginning phase of establishing a regular walking routine. You will find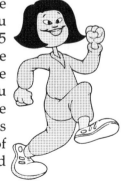

that as time goes by, and you have walked regularly for a few weeks, conversation will be easier. This means you should increase your walking speed.

Warm-Up

Prior to any exercise you should warm-up. The best way to warm-up is to do the planned exercise lightly (i.e., walk slowly for a few minutes). Warm-ups are recommended to last 5 to 15 minutes depending on what you are planning on doing. Warm-ups increase blood flow and reduce strain on the heart.

Warm-Downs

Warm-downs are also called cool-downs. This is a 5 to 15 minute time period following an exercise routine when you can gradually lower the physical intensity. For example, if you take a 30 minute walk, you can walk the last 5 minutes slower to allow your heart rate to gradually decline. Walking, stretching, and minor movements can be utilized as cool-down activities.

Target Heart Range

Maintaining *target heart rate* is recommended as the most accurate way of assessing whether you are exercising in the "moderate-intensity" range. As you exercise, your heart rate and breathing rate increase. The general rule is that you want to eventually exercise at about 60%-70% of your maximal heart rate,[3] but, initially, keeping it above 50% is adequate.[4] This range (50% to 70%) of heart rate is easy to calculate and is based on your age.

Figure Your Target Heart Rate

To calculate your target heart range, you begin by estimating your maximum heart rate. This is done by subtracting your age from 220.

220 - _____ = _____
Place your age here.

Multiply the above number by .5 = _____
Multiply the above number by .7 = _____

Your target 50% to 70% heart range is between the two numbers you just calculated.

To calculate target heart range, you begin by estimating your maximum heart rate. This is done by subtracting your age from 220. If, for example, you are 45 years old, your maximum heart rate is 175 (220 - 45 = 175). The 50% to 70% target heart range is then estimated by multiplying the maximum by first 50% and then by 70%. Thus, the target heart range for our 45-year-old example is about 87 to 122 (.5 x 175 = 87.5; .7 x 175 = 122.5). This means that the person should engage in physical activity that keeps his or her heart rate between 87 and 122.

With the improvements that come from regular exercise, people employing the target heart range method will find that they will have to walk faster and for a longer time to reach target range. As fitness continues to improve, exercise should be increased in intensity to keep the heart rate elevated, and, the goal should be closer to the 70% level.

There are several methods to determine heart rate during exercise. With practice, you should be able to take your pulse on the side of your neck or at your wrist. You will have to stop exercising a few moments to do this. Several small commercial devices are available that have both a stopwatch and a pulse counter. This device conveniently hangs around your neck, and can show accurate pulse rate and elapsed time.

Calories Consumed During Exercise

It's true that exercise burns calories. However, the effect of moderate exercise on producing fat loss is not dramatic. Exercise is best viewed as an essential component of a comprehensive fat loss plan that has overall improvements in health and fitness as a goal. Moderate, sustained exercise in and of itself is estimated to produce weight loss in the range of 4 to 7 pounds after a few months in obese people who consistently engage in it.[20] However, with improvements in insulin resistance, decreased appetite, and overall activity increases resulting from improved mood, regular exercise will result in greater fat loss.

The number of calories expended by exercise depends on the type of exercise itself, its intensity, how long it is performed, and the weight of the individual. The exact number of calories a given exercise uses can be precisely measured, but what is required to make these calculations is complicated. The Calorie Control Council (www.caloriecontrol.org) gives the following calorie usage estimates of various activities.

Activity	150 Pound Person Calories Used In 30 Minutes	300 Pound Person Calories Used In 30 Minutes
Ballroom Dancing	62-155	125-310
Canoeing (slowly)	90-100	180-200
Cooking	92-100	185-200
Walking Slowly (2.5 mph)	105-115	210-230
Cleaning	117-177	235-355
Brisk Walking (4 mph)	125-172	250-345
Golf	150-175	300-350
Jogging (6 mph)	157-240	315-480
Cycling (9 mph)	157-240	315-480
Tennis	157-240	315-480
Skating	160-200	320-400
Gardening (heavy)	225-262	450-525
Basketball	240-312	480-625
Aerobic Dancing	240-312	480-625
Swimming	240-312	480-625
Cross Country Skiing	240-312	480-625

Exercise Videotapes & Television Fitness Programs

With cable television now reaching almost every American home, chances are quite good that you have seen several aerobic and fitness programs as you surf the channels. These tend to be shown at the same time every day, so if you find one that suits your level of fitness, available time, and musical tastes use that 30 minutes as your exercise period. You can participate in your living room or anywhere else you can set up a television. Move a chair out of the way. Get a large rubber backed mat and exercise on it. Step aerobics can be especially beneficial. You are already paying for cable, so why not take advantage of it?

Exercise videotapes are a huge market. There are so many exercise videos available that a review of them is impractical. When you purchase one, what you get is what you are stuck with. Rather than buying a tape, we suggest renting it at a video store first and trying it out. Many libraries also have them for rent. One consistent observation made with people who use exercise videotapes is that they buy a lot of them. This occurs because listening and exercising to the exact same routine over and over gets boring. Try to get a tape that is consistent with your philosophy and goals. For example, Richard Simmons' tapes tend to appeal to people who have been severely obese for the majority of their lives. We recommend them especially for people just starting to increase physical activity. You certainly won't feel as if you are the only "large" person trying to exercise when you watch them. It is probably better if you like the person who is leading the exercise and it seems that Simmons produces an immediate "love him or hate him" reaction. Whatever you might think about him, our observations (we don't know him) from his books, tapes, appearances, and shows is that he is quite genuine. His tapes also stress simple dancing and body movements especially to songs from the '60s, '70s, and '80s. He has an excellent motivational style and he has been obese himself. Richard Simmons maintains a large web site with a "club," social support chat rooms, and products. The web address is www.richardsimmons.com

A lot of the celebrity tapes are technically good, but you have to realize that not all of these gorgeous people have had weight problems. As we related in the beginning of this book, actresses get paid huge sums

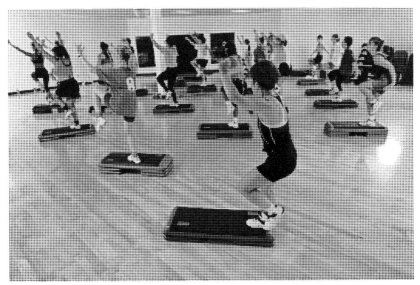

of money to stay slim. So, their knowledge of the struggles obese people continuously face is probably limited. However, if you feel drawn to one of these tapes because the individual appeals to you, try it out. The object here is to establish regular exercise.

The final format of exercise tapes is put out by fitness experts. These tend to be technically correct and can be very useful. You may find a beginner's level video useful especially when you start a strength building routine.

Establishing A Strength Building Program

Muscle mass burns energy simply by being there — even when you are resting. (Remember that all body tissue uses energy to sustain life.) Since muscle has the highest BMR, the more muscle mass you have, the more energy (calories) your body will consume to maintain it. Muscle burns more calories pound for pound than does fat, so the object of building muscle is to increase metabolism, burn fat, and enhance fitness. Muscles are built by resistance training. The repetitive movement of weights is the best way to build muscles.

Weight lifting to build muscle mass does not have to be exhausting nor unpleasant, nor does it have to be of long duration. You can obtain all of the equipment you need inexpensively at a local department store. The major problem with using your own weights as opposed to going to a gym or health club is that the equipment you have at home may well be unused. Eventually you may put it away in a hidden, out-of-the-way closet. (Out of sight, out of mind.) In addition, the types of movements you can perform are limited by the "free" weights typically used in homes. (Free weights are unattached to a machine.) Modern resistance machines allow the full range of movements and allow you to exercise all muscle groups and decrease the chances of injury.

The choice as to whether you will join a club is left up to you, but being in a club can increase motivation and provide you with professional as-

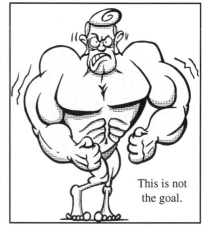

This is not
the goal.

sistance. Spend some time at a club to get a feel for it before you join. It's a good idea to have someone you know at the club to provide support. If you are there often enough, you will develop friends with similar goals and body size. Club members more easily establish a particular time when they will exercise than do people who aren't in clubs. The establishment of a regular exercise time can increase the probability of continuing the exercise routine.

For the vast majority of obese people, obtaining a few "dumbbells" of varying weights (and following the manual of exercises coming with them) can be a sufficient beginning. You have to find your own "beginning level" to determine what you need. You might start by buying three sets of dumbbells. One set could be 10 pounds, another 15, and the third 20 or 25 pounds. You must determine the appropriate weights for you, so a good idea is to go into the store and test them. Frequently, an informational brochure accompanying the weights can give a lot of information on their use.

Goals When Starting Resistance Training

Beginners are in a starter phase that lasts 3 weeks or so. The goals are to build your strength gradually without developing too much muscle soreness or injury.[4] You should only use light weights during this phase. Do each specific muscle exercise 10 to 15 times. Each full movement is called a *repetition*. The number of repetitions done per cycle is called a *set*. For example, you might begin with 10 repetitive arm curls with the right arm. (That is a completed set.) Then move to the left arm. When you have completed exercising all of the muscle groups (a full set with each) you have completed a full circuit. You should then repeat the circuit. You should do this form of weight lifting approximately 2 times a week in the beginning. Always allow a

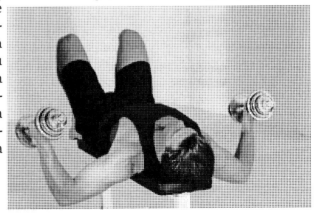

An example of chest and shoulder exercise with dumb-bells.

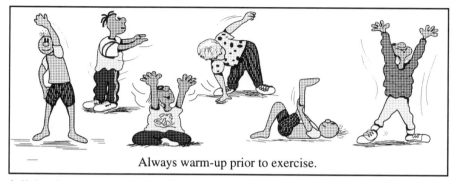

Always warm-up prior to exercise.

full day between working the same muscle groups. You should however, perform your regular exercise (such as walking for 30 minutes) every day. You will notice strength improvements quickly. You might also find that your weight doesn't fall as rapidly or it may even slightly increase. This is due to the addition of muscle. Do not be disappointed. You are likely to note that clothing fits better. Remember that fat is fluffy and occupies more space than does muscle.

Strength Building Phase

After you have completed the 3 week starter phase, you can slowly increase the intensity of the weight lifting. This strength building phase lasts 4 to 20 weeks. You can carefully increase the amount of weight lifted, the number of repetitions, and the number of sets. Do your weight lifting 3 times a week ensuring that you leave a day of rest between each. (But still do your regular aerobic exercise 5 or 6 days a week.) The goal of this phase is to increase your strength, endurance, and muscle mass to a desirable level. You will find that in only 5 or 6 weeks you will develop a noticeable increase in muscle size and strength in a more compact body. Set your goals carefully and remember what your initial motivations were. We aren't trying to turn anyone into a Charles Atlas. But some increase in muscle mass is necessary for continuing a healthy battle against body fat.

Maintenance Phase

Maintaining muscle mass and strength is a life-long process. This means that weight lifting (resistance training) has to become a permanent part of your life. **However, you do not have to work as hard to maintain**

muscles as it takes to develop them.
Working out two times a week without
increasing the weight or repetitions is
all that is required. Once you reach the
level of strength and muscle size you
feel comfortable with, continue the same
routine twice a week, altering the type of
exercise every three months.

Minimal Weight Lifting

This is unwise.
Never combine
weights with
aerobics because
it increases the
work load of the
heart too much.

If you use a gym or fitness club, establish a resistance training
routine based upon their recommendations. Equipment will be available
that can work every muscle group. Be cautious about doing too much too
fast and expect some muscle soreness. You will be working some muscle
areas that have long been unused.

For those who want to develop a minimal resistance training
program at home, we offer a few suggestions. First, you must warm-up
for 5 minutes or so by stretching, bending, and walking. You could
perform your weight lifting after taking a 30 minute walk, but you still
have to stretch some. When you don't have equipment that allows a full-
range of exercises, a few low-grade calisthenics should be used to work
some muscle groups.

Bent knee crunches will work your abdominal muscles. These are
done by lying flat on your back with your knees raised and the bottom
of your feet on the floor. Start with 10 crunches or so and try to eventually
raise the number of repetitions to 25 or more. Place your hands across

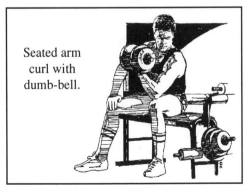

Seated arm
curl with
dumb-bell.

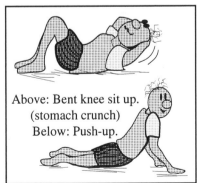

Above: Bent knee sit up.
(stomach crunch)
Below: Push-up.

your chest with your left hand on your right shoulder and right hand on left shoulder. Your wrists will be touching your neck. Without pulling your head forward, use your lower abdominal muscles to lift your upper back a few inches off the floor. Hold your stomach in while you do this and breathe out when you lift each time.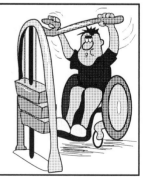

If you don't have a weight bench, push-ups will work chest and shoulder muscles. These are done by lying on your stomach and knees. Don't try doing push-ups on your toes, but simply try to push your chest off the floor. *Always breath out when you push.* You may find these muscles to be very weak so be careful about muscle strain.

In reality, your weight training plan has to be formed based on your current level of fitness. If all you have are a few dumbbells or a barbell with weights, your ability to build muscle strength will usually be limited to your arms and upper body. You should start with 10 repetitions of an exercise for each muscle group (one set), and go through your circuit again. **(Remember to breathe out as you make the movement.)** Then increase the weight and do the entire circuit again. When you buy your weights try to obtain a manual that shows the possible exercises. You local library will also have many books that demonstrate weightlifting routines. You need to exercise your upper arms, shoulders, back muscles, chest, buttocks, and legs. You will find that if you carefully choose an exercise circuit of about 10 exercises, you can work all of these body areas. Each circuit will probably last 10 minutes or so meaning you

Yoga

Yoga is great relaxation, but it isn't exercise.

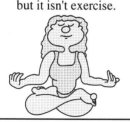

Handicapped Exercise

Most fitness clubs have established resistance training routines for handicapped people. Various machines can easily be adapted to just about any physical challenge.

could complete the entire routine in 20 minutes. Just remember to avoid injury — don't try to much.

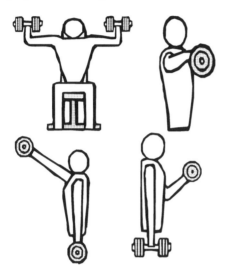

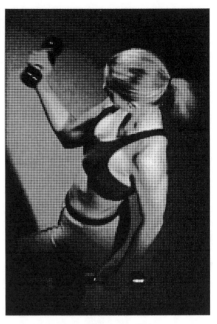

Common Exercises With Dumbbells
Working the biceps, shoulders, triceps, chest, back, and legs.

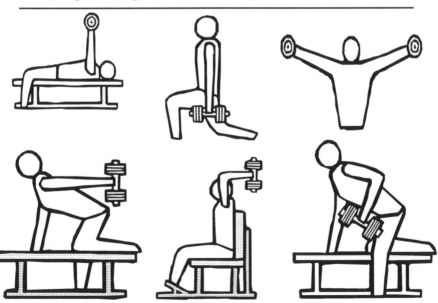

Chapter References & Notes

[1] Flier, J. S., & Foster, D. W. (1998) Eating disorders: obesity, anorexia nervosa, and bulimia nervosa. In: J. Wilson, D. Foster, H. Kronenberg, & P. Larsen (Eds.) *Williams Textbook of Endocrinology: 9th Edition*. Philadelphia: Saunders.

[2] Myers, D. G. (1992) Psychology. New York: Worth Publishers.

[3] McArdle, W. D., Katch, F. I., & Katch, V. L. (1991) *Exercise Physiology: Energy, nutrition, and human performance*. Malvern, PA: Lea & Febiger.

[4] Powers, S. K., & Dodd, S. L. (1996) *Total Fitness*. Needham Heights, MA: Allyn & Bacon.

[5] National Institutes of Health (1998) *Clinical Guidelines on the Identification, Evaluation, and Treatment of Overweight and Obesity in Adults*. Washington, D.C.

[6] Flatt, J. P. (1992) The biochemistry of energy expenditure. In: P. Bjorntorp, & B. N. Brodoff (Eds.) *Obesity*. Philadelphia: Lippincott.

[7] McArdle, W. D., Katch, F. I., & Katch, V. L. (1991) *Exercise Physiology: Energy, nutrition, and human performance*. Philadelphia: Lea & Febiger.

[8] Weight Control Information Network. (1999) *Weight Cycling*. Washington, D. C.: National Institute of Diabetes and Digestive and Kidney Diseases.

[9] Rahkila, et. al. (1987) Response of plasma endorphins to running exercises in male and female endurance athletes. *Medicine & Science In Sports & Exercise*, 19, 451.

[10] Aforzo, et. al. (1986) In vivo opioid receptor occupation in the rat brain following exercise. *Medicine & Science In Sports & Exercise*, 18, 380.

[11] Carr, D. B., et. al. (1981) Physical conditioning facilitates exercise induced secretion of beta-endorphins and beta-lipotrophin in women. *New England Journal of Medicine*, 305, 560.

[12] Little, G. L. (1997) *Psychopharmacology*. Memphis: Advanced Training Associates.

[13] Morgan, W. P. (1985) Affective beneficence of vigorous physical activity. *Medicine & Science In Sports & Exercise*, 17, 94.

[14] Yates, A., et. al. (1983) Running — an analogue of anorexia. *New England Journal of Medicine*, 308, 251.

[15] Myers, D. G. (1992) *Psychology*. New York: Worth Publishers.

[16] Thayer, R. E. (1987) Energy, tiredness, and tension effects of a sugar snack versus moderate exercise. *Journal of Personality and Social Psychology*, 52, 119-125.

[17] O'Keefe, J. H., et. al. (1999) Improving the adverse cardiovascular prognosis of type 2 diabetes. *Mayo Clinic Proceedings*, 74, 171-180.

[18] American Diabetes Association (1997) Consensus development conference on insulin resistance. *Diabetes Care*, 21 (2), 310.

[19] Anderson, D. A., & Wadden, T. A. (1999) Treating the obese patient. *Archives of Family Medicine*, 8, 156-167.

[20] American Association of Clinical Endocrinologists and The American College of Endocrinology (1998) *AACE/ACE Position statement on the prevention, diagnosis and Treatment of Obesity*. AACE/ACE.

Chapter 15
THE FINAL PIECE OF THE OBESITY PUZZLE: FORMING A LIFE-LONG FOOD PLAN

Let thy food be thy medicine, and thy medicine be thy food.
— **Hippocrates**

Summary—Diet advice can be confusing and contradictory. Dieters will try almost any new approach in a desperate attempt to find the magical blend of foods that will make fat disappear from their bodies. But it's a battle that is inevitably lost as the dieter slips and relapses. Diets don't work for permanent body fat loss, yet much of the diet industry continues to tell us that their "novel" approach is the only way.

Dieters often feel engaged in a struggle of wills against their own bodies. It *is* an internal war because our genetic predispositions are dictating body weights to ensure survival. The only **smart choice** is to work with our nature by establishing a life-long food plan as part of an overall health plan including appropriate medication, life-style changes, stress reduction, and exercise.

The diet industry has offered lots of approaches to dieting ranging from the truly dangerous to workable plans. Fasting, protein diets, liquid diets, single food diets, low and zero carbohydrate diets, no-fat and ultra-low-fat diets are all drastic approaches. They are, at best, temporary approaches. The most workable food plans stress maintaining a balance among food groups and adjusting the consumption of specific foods to correct for insulin resistance. These food plans also stress making a permanent commitment to healthy eating.

A life-long food plan must be healthy, the foods in it must be appealing and satisfying, and it must be something you can and will live with the rest of your life. In forming a food plan, calories should be counted. The simple scientific truth is that calories determine whether you gain, lose, or maintain weight.

Our food plan recommendations are anchored by a set of conclusions based upon the biological and genetic research on obesity and insulin resistance. Overweight and obese people should: avoid simple carbohydrates (sugars); limit intake of starch (e.g., potatoes, corn); increase intake of fiber-based carbohydrates (e.g., fruits, many vegetables, beans); control intake of fat and reduce saturated fat (substituting olive or canola oil); increase fish intake; increase intake of protein. We recommend (especially for those with insulin resistance) forming a food plan in which 40% of calories come from protein, 30% from fat, and 30% from carbohydrates.

To depict this 40% protein, 30% fat, 30% carbohydrate approach, we utilize a **Food Diamond.** Foods are judged by their effect on insulin secretion after they are ingested. Foods that produce lower insulin responses should be chosen. Some foods, such as bananas, potatoes, bread, carrots, crackers, pretzels, and most cereals should be avoided. There are excellent substitutes for all of these foods and, with careful and selective shopping, even palatable (high fiber) bread can be found.

To form a long-term food plan, you must become a smart consumer. Learn to read and understand the nutrition labels on food packages. Many "healthy" frozen food meals can be utilized to make your plan easier and more enjoyable. The majority of the work in developing eating plans is at the beginning. Write down planned meals and calculate calories, fat, protein, and carbohydrate totals. As you form a workable food plan and become accustomed to the serving sizes and calorie totals, the work load will drop considerably.

• • •

Diets can be confusing, contradictory, enticing, and downright dangerous. The unrelenting pursuit of thinness, driven by unreasonable social and psychological pressures, will cause people to try almost anything to become more physically appealing. Few dieters are motivated by the desire to improve physical health. The struggle to be thin usually stems from rejection — real or imagined — by others or self.

Dieting is sometimes viewed as a struggle with oneself. It is a battle of wills where neither side wins. A dieter often feels that his body seems to have a will of its own. This struggle causes hunger, cravings, and food obsessions and eventually precipitates a relapse back to prior eating habits. A dieter is led to believe that the body has to be resisted through sheer force of conscious will-power, self-deprivation, and a host of tricks that might occasionally overcome nearly unbearable urges to eat. In the inevitable moments of letdown, it all crashes. Soon, the dieter is back to the beginning once again. *Diets don't work, and it's time all of us, including those of us in the medical profession, admit it.*

Your Body Has A Will Of Its Own

Your body does have a will of its own. If you think about it for a moment, you'll realize that your body has to automatically perform a lot of functions — without your conscious involvement. If you had to consciously control everything happening in your body, you'd be dead. Your heart beats, you breathe, digest food and have an incredible number of essential, life-sustaining activities going on in every nook and cranny of your body without you ever thinking about them. If you had to consciously make your heart beat every second and consciously force yourself to breathe, as soon as your attention got diverted, you'd drop over. You'd never be able to sleep. Nature was wiser than we realize in removing physiological functioning from our conscious control. If we had the ability to control how much fat would be stored on our bodies, how many of us today would select a "healthy range" of 15% to 26%? Only a few. We live in a society which praises ultra-thin, body-fat free people.

The "will" of the body is programmed into you through the basic genetics that produced the incredible structures of the brain and human body. Nature has programmed us for survival. We may be fatter than ever before in human history, but it isn't nature which has gone haywire. In industrialized societies, we have altered our natural environment. We can now store food, so famines are no more — and we keep developing labor saving devices so that we no longer have to physically exert ourselves. When you diet, you are fighting nature.

Nature loses few battles — if any. If you are in a quest to defeat your nature, you probably won't win. We earlier stated that you probably will never reach the level of thinness you desire. We say this because we have found that, in our modern world, few of our patients are able to reach or maintain a "perceived" ideal weight. Nature has established a setpoint for your weight, and, the lower your weight goes, the greater the resistance.

The Smart Choice
Is To Work With Nature

There are smart choices you can make — not to battle nature, but to work with it — in the quest for fat loss and health. We have already discussed the use of medications to alter some of nature's biological dictates, addressed stress and personal issues that effect eating and mood, looked at adjustments you can make in how you live in your environment, and shown the importance of increasing physical activity (through exercise) to accomplish health goals. The final piece of the complex puzzle of obesity is responsible eating. *You have to establish a life-long food plan* (not to be confused with a "diet") that works with your biological predispositions while satisfying your urges and tastes. It is easier than it appears, but it takes some work and planning.

Our Food Can Be Poison

One of the first things you must do in forming your food plan is accept that some foods are simply not appropriate. Diabetics come to understand this quickly. Poisonous substances are toxic — they endanger health. Food can be toxic. Too much fat is toxic. Our genetic programming isn't well adapted to a lot of the foods in our modern world. Refined, bleached flour, cremes, sugar, nitrite laden sugar cured meats, and cheeseburgers (dripping in fat and mayonnaise) dominate our lifestyle. Our physiological responses to the continued ingestion of these once rare treats is easy to see: increased obesity, diabetes, cancer, heart disease, and even some mental disorders.

It has long been recognized that what we eat is a major component in obesity and that certain foods are unhealthy. However, the diet industry has long given impractical and unhealthy advice to people with misguided goals. In many ways the diet industry takes advantage of the desperation of the obese. The focus has been on "rapid weight loss to look better" — not to become healthier through gradual loss of body fat and increased fitness. So many "natural" diet aids are available today making impossible claims and promises. Chapter 17 reviews some of these; but, you have got to realize that these promises are empty and set you up for failure.

Things Are Changing Bit By Bit

The history of diets for "weight loss" shows how fanatical and even gullible a portion of society is. Fad diets come and go and come back again. We live in world expecting a "quick fix" for problems. So when a diet or supplement touts that you'll lose 10 pounds in only 5 days, a lot of us will try it.

In recent years, the government, medical associations, various fitness experts, and nutritionists have attempted to give us reliable information on appropriate eating. *The Food Guide Pyramid* is the result of this effort. The food choices in it are a vast improvement over past recommendations and it certainly is better than fad diet plans. However, for the increasing numbers of overweight and obese people we believe the pyramid's recommendations are inadequate and impractical. We believe that some people, especially the obese with insulin resistance and type 2 diabetics, have an underlying biological nature that requires modifications to the pyramid's food plan.

Hype & Real Help In The Diet Industry

A few of the most popular diets for weight loss are discussed below. These range from the truly dangerous to programs that are of real help. Many are contradictory. *Appendix B* provides a brief summary and analysis of commercial programs. *Appendix C* lists university based programs and treatment centers for children and adults as a resource for those who have more serious problems.

Fasting

Over the years, various diet fads have emerged. Fasting to lose weight became a fad in the 1920s and 1930s. In the 1950s a series of studies were conducted on hospitalized obese patients to appraise how well fasting worked as a method for weight loss. Everyone knew that eating nothing (essentially drinking only water) would result in weight loss, but the physiologic repercussions to the person fasting were unknown.

Fasting patients reported feelings of well-being and euphoria and stated they weren't hungry except for the first day. The analysis of physiological dysfunction was, however, alarming. Results showed large fluid losses, acidosis, muscle breakdown, vitamin and mineral deficiencies, and elevations of uric acid in the blood. Effects on the heart indicated rhythm disturbances and loss of heart muscle. More recent research shows that fasts are ineffective over the long term.[1] "When you hear someone recommend a diet solely on the basis of how it makes you feel — remember this lesson."[2]

High Protein Diets - Liquid Protein Diets

Medical researchers tried modifications to fasts noting that the major problems occurred from muscle loss. Researchers began by giving injections of glucose—but it didn't work to reduce the muscle loss. Next, low-calorie protein supplements were added. The muscle loss stopped, but high levels of ketones were found in the blood. Adding glucose to the protein supplement reduced the ketones. The level of protein was gradually increased to stop muscle loss.

Throughout the 1970s various research groups began utilizing protein-glucose mixtures with obese patients on an out-patient basis. Liquid protein diets quickly followed. The 1976 book, *The Last Chance Diet*, lived up to its title for some people who tried it. The book advocated the use of specific protein supplements during fasts, but the lack of glucose produced ketosis. Many people subsequently developed heart arrhythmias and nearly 60 people died.[1]

Protein-Sparing Modified Fasts (PSMF) are still around. They tend to be high protein, low carbohydrate plans encouraging a liquid "protein shake" or supplement with at least one regular meal daily. Medical supervision is required for these diets. Problems occur with increased ketone levels and potassium depletion.[1]

Single Food Diets

Diets that focus on a single food have long circulated among people wanting to lose weight fast. They are nutritionally unbalanced, but easy to do. They do tend to produce weight loss early in the diet (much of which is water), but typically result in rapid weight regain. There are many variations. The so-called grapefruit diet began in the 1930s as *The Hollywood Diet*. It combined a few vegetables with grapefruit. The cabbage soup diet has many variations including the addition of a few vegetables and meats as time passes. Similar diets are based on rice, beans, apples, and other low-calorie foods.

Low Carbohydrate Diets

The diet industry constantly bombards us with "new and revolutionary" miracle approaches to weight loss. Book jackets tell us that everything they know about dieting is wrong and to use the new approach discovered after decades of research or analysis by "so and so."

Eat all you want and forget about calories is often touted as a revolutionary concept.

In 1961, physician Herman Taller published *Calories Don't Count* in which he described obesity as a metabolic disorder. There were three ways the metabolic disorder manifested: 1. The body produced fat at a higher than normal rate; 2. The body stores fat at a higher than normal rate; and, 3. The body releases fat for metabolism at a slower than normal rate. (This was a remarkable insight for his time, although, some of his assumptions were incorrect.) Taller proposed that a by-product of carbohydrates, pyruvic acid, serves as an inhibitor of the body's ability to burn stored fat. In addition, pyruvic acid is itself converted into fat. He recommended maintaining a fat-equilibrium by limiting carbohydrate and saturated fat intake while increasing unsaturated fat intake. Taller's low carbohydrate, high-fat and high-protein diet became very popular and has been recycled in various forms.

Irwin Stillman's 1967 book, *The Doctor's Quick Weight Loss Diet*, also proposed a low carbohydrate diet. Stillman believed that protein was difficult for the body to digest and that by consuming lots of protein (with the fat usually accompanying it) and restricting carbohydrates, lots of body fat would be lost. Cardiologist Robert Atkins' series of books, including his 1992 book *Dr. Atkin's New Diet Revolution*, recommend low (or zero) carbohydrate intake meaning that fat and protein are the primary (or only) foods consumed.

The low carbohydrate diets are appealing to a lot of people because meat, cheese, cream, eggs, and other high-fat foods are both satisfying and tasty. The diet results in a rapid loss of weight — water. It tends to lack nutrients, produces high ketone levels, and is not healthy for diabetics or people with heart conditions.[1] People on zero carbohydrate diets often discover that the most difficult part is the total elimination of bread (no sandwiches), cereals and grains, and pasta.

Another low carbohydrate diet is based on the possibility of *carbohydrate addiction*. The concept of carbohydrate addiction comes from observations of binge eaters and others having cravings for foods rich in carbohydrates. The term was coined by Kemp in 1963. The symptoms are said to include obsessive thinking about food, the feeling of hunger or dissatisfaction even after eating, fatigue after eating, feelings of anger or anxiety that seem to come from nowhere, and an overall heightening of emotionality. Carbohydrate addiction is believed to be caused by an overrelease of insulin after the consumption of carbohydrates. The Hellers' 1991 book, *The Carbohydrate Addict's Diet*, outlines this idea. The concept, we now know, is linked to insulin and insulin resistance.

Low Fat, No-Fat Diets With High Carbohydrates

In 1955 at the age of 40, Nathan Pritikin took his first stress test. He had serious heart disease, cholesterol levels of 280, and was told to avoid exertion. Pritikin had come to believe that the American diet was too high in fat and too low in fruits, vegetables, and grains. Pritikin also believed that the usual advice doctors gave heart patients about avoiding exertion was unhealthy. So he began jogging. His cholesterol levels went down to just over 100. In 1966, Pritikin took another stress test with the same doctor who had told him 11 years earlier to avoid exertion. The test showed no signs of heart abnormality.

In 1975, Pritikin began offering classes to various patients including those with heart disease, diabetes, and high blood pressure. In 1979, the *Pritikin Program for Diet and Exercise*, outlined his low-fat/exercise approach. One of the cardiologists that took an interest in Pritikin was a young Dr. Dean Ornish. In 1985, Pritikin committed suicide after being hospitalized in the final stages of terminal leukemia. The autopsy showed virtually no artery clogging or heart disease.

In the November 1995 issue of *American Health*, free-lance writer Peter Hellman told about his experience attending the 13-day program at Pritikin's Longevity Center in Santa Monica, CA. Hellman states that over 60,000 people have attended either a 7, 13, or 26-day Pritikin program since 1975. Hellman paid $6,409 for 13 days. Returnees get a 20% discount.

The day begins with an (optional) 6 a.m. stretching class followed by a 6:30 exercise class lasting 75 minutes. A 45-minute treadmill work-out is followed by 15 minutes of circuit training in a weight room. A tag is worn showing target pulse rate range. The afternoon activities include various exercise options.

Hellman states that the key concept is that you cannot keep weight off if you have hunger pangs. Three large meals are served along with two snack times. In addition, apples, oranges, and air-popped popcorn are almost always available. Each day, various 50-minute lectures are held designed to educate and convince attendees to follow the regimen after they return to home. The program also provides many other activities including taking participants into the community and on shopping trips as well as viewing nightly movies.

Ornish's 1993 book, *Eat More, Weigh Less*, recommends that fat calories should be 10% or less of daily consumption. His early research showed how heart disease could be reversed by diet, exercise, and stress reduction, and he now recommends that *everyone* use the approach. A strict diet of low fat, low-cholesterol, and high-fiber is included with meditation, exercise, and stress reduction techniques. It is a sound approach for some people, especially those with heart disease. Restrictive eating is a major drawback and water retention remains a problem, especially in the start of the diet.[1]

Susan Powter, who touts a low-fat diet, represents a new breed of fitness guru for women touting low-fat diets. Her enthusiastic, in-your-face style is aggressive and leads to one of two probable reactions: you either love her, or hate her. She probably wouldn't have it any other way. Her 1993 book *Stop the Insanity* begins with the words, "I'm not angry, damn it. I'm passionate."

Her message to women is simple and effective. She believes that women should stop dieting for men. They should lose weight and get into shape to empower themselves. The yo-yo dieting patterns seen in so many women and the starvation diets promoted by the diet industry are "insane." Powter promotes a low-fat diet (despite saying she's anti-diet) combined with exercise. Her 1995 book *Food* details her recommended diets, advice on eating out, preparing food, and trying to deal with guilt and fear.

Less Drastic Approaches

If you carefully observe him, it's difficult to dislike Richard Simmons. He's for real and he truly cares about obese people. Like most of the diet gurus, Simmons has been there. In his 1980 book, *Never Say Diet*, Simmons relates his transformation from fat to thin. He was born in New Orleans in 1948 and quickly became the "fat kid" who was the brunt of everyone's jokes. At age 8 he tried his first weight-loss gimmick — sheets of plastic wrap held around the waist and arms with rubber bands. At age 11, a sixth grade girl turned down his dance date request telling him he was "obese." He had to get a dictionary to look the word up.

Immediately after graduating high school he went to Italy on a scholarship (his weight was 214). He relates that while in a restaurant he was approached by an agent who subsequently had him star in television commercials: for husky clothes, candy bars, meatballs — anything related to fat. Simmons became extremely well-known throughout Italy — and he became increasingly fat. In 1968 he made a personal appearance at a supermarket. When he went back to his car he found a note on the windshield. The unsigned note stated: "Fat People Die Young; Please Don't Die."

The note produced instant shock and paranoia in Simmons. He checked into a hospital where he was told that he was a "walking time bomb." Simmons immediately began a series of failed diets and fads. Then he just quit eating and joined a gym to exercise. In less than three months he lost 112 pounds, but he became weak and sick and returned to the hospital. The 1993 book, *Richard Simmons' Never Give Up*, goes into some additional details about his diet enlightenment. He began to read countless books on diet, exercise, and nutrition, but one public school textbook provided the key for Simmons' diet formula: "the balance of correct portions of all the food groups is the secret to health" — **balance and portions** was the secret. Simmons pieced together a three-pronged approach to weight loss: a balance of diet, exercise, and the right mental attitude. He moved to California, and, after a brief period as the maitre d' at a restaurant where he observed the way Americans eat, Simmons opened a restaurant with an adjacent exercise studio. His restaurant *"Ruffage"* focused on an enormous salad bar (and no fat entrees) and his outrageous style of interacting with guests became a hit. Soon, a host of celebrities and others were coming to his restaurant and studio. During this time, Simmons collected 72,368 eating habits/weight/exercise questionnaires from people.

Simmons' *Deal-A-Meal* and *Food Mover* methods stem from his earlier understanding of the important of balance and right portions. They are simple approaches appropriate for obese people who need help keeping up with daily eating and exercise. He focuses on a life-long battle with fat and feeling better about self. Thus, the approach also incorporates social support and self-esteem issues. Simmons believes that all fat people are unhappy and can't really start living until they lose weight. He has an extremely high-energy, fun, personable approach that is obvious in his *Sweating to the Oldies* video work-out tapes. Simmons appears to be a source of inspiration, hope, encouragement, and unconditional love for the overweight. He has a gentle yet prodding humorous style that is adored by many. His diet tends to follow the guidelines in the Food Guide Pyramid.

A "New" Zone

In 1995 a new set of books proposing high protein diets emerged. These included the Eades's *Protein Power*, Puhn's *5 Day Miracle Diet*, and Barry Sears' *The Zone. Sugar Busters!* followed not long afterward. All recommend that carbohydrate intake should be reduced and that some carbohydrates are better than others. Insulin resistance, aggravated by the ingestion of certain carbohydrates, is cited as the primary causal factor in the growing rate of obesity.

The Zone proposes controlling food intake at every meal to produce a specific level of insulin that promotes maximum calorie utilization and fat burn. The basics are given in the numbers 40-30-30. Each meal (and snack) must consist of 40% carbohydrate, 30% protein, and 30% fat. The amount of lean body mass determines the amount of protein you should eat every day.

The Zone and *Sugar Busters!* distinguish between good and bad carbohydrates based on the insulin response they produce. This is called the glycemic index. Some fruits (such as bananas) and vegetables (carrots) are not permitted due to their stimulation of insulin (these have a high glycemic index).

There is no doubt that insulin resistance is related to obesity and that many foods stimulate high insulin release. The "glycemic" index of carbohydrates is also useful. However, maintaining the 40-30-30 distribution with each meal and snack is complicated and difficult.

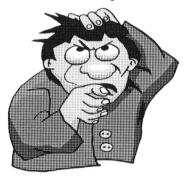

Forming A Life-Long Food Plan

The scientific meaning of **diet** is different from the definition commonly used. Most people use the word diet to describe a *temporary, self-imposed restriction of eating* to lose weight. *Scientifically, a diet is the food and drink a person regularly consumes.* The word diet has a Greek origin and means the manner in which one leads life. Rather than *going on diets* for weight loss, you must restructure the way you think about the word diet. Your diet is what you eat — not something you do temporarily. Temporary changes in diet seldom produce the desired effect. What you must do is form a permanent, life-long food plan that produces a healthy, beneficial effect. There are three major considerations that are necessary in forming a successful food plan:

It must be healthy from a nutritional perspective.
The foods included in it should be satisfying and, as much as possible, appeal to you
It must be a plan you can live with the rest of your life.

Forming A Healthy Food Plan

The typical "healthy" diet (like that proposed in the *Food Guide Pyramid*) recommends that food intake should be composed of 58% carbohydrates, 30% fat, and 12% protein.[3] Carbohydrates supply the majority of the energy utilized by the body. Fats are utilized for essential cell functions, the transport of some essential vitamins, and contribute to feelings of satiation.[1] (Body fat also serves to protect vital organs and provided insulation as well as storing needed energy reserves.) Proteins serves as the "building blocks" for muscle and other tissues as well as being utilized in cell functions. Protein can also be utilized as fuel when necessary. The number of calories contained in a gram of carbohydrates, fat, and protein are different. In addition, the calories contained in protein and carbohydrate are not *exactly* 4 as is commonly reported (they are actually about 5% higher). The approximate calorie yields are:

> **1 gram of carbohydrate = 4 calories**
> **1 gram of fat = 9 calories**
> **1 gram of protein = 4 calories**

Why Calories?

Despite some claims that counting fat grams, or carbohydrate grams, or servings is all that's required to lose weight, the scientific facts remain unchanged. Calories determine whether you gain, lose, or maintain body fat (visit the Calorie Control Council's web site for information: www.caloriecontrol.org).

Your body burns energy scientifically measured in standard units (calories). Decreasing your daily caloric intake below the level of calories consumed results in fat loss. Whenever you ingest more calories than your body uses, the result is fat gain. From a purely scientific perspective, it doesn't matter to the body's energy system what supplies the calories. You could lose weight by eating nothing but 1000 calories a day of pure fat. (This would be stupid.) It does matter from a scientific *health* viewpoint where your calories come from. Using the caloric value of foods is the only reliable way to develop a workable food plan. After you become accustomed to eating on your food plan, you can become less calorie conscious as long as you maintain the basics of your plan.

Restrictive "diets" based on the counting of grams of carbohydrates or fat ultimately are effective or ineffective based on one factor: calories consumed.

Carbohydrates

There are two major types of carbohydrates. **Simple carbohydrates** are made up of one or two simple sugars. Table sugar (called sucrose), made up of glucose and fructose, is a simple carbohydrate. Fructose (found primarily in fruits), maltose (malt sugar), lactose (milk sugar), and galactose (found in breast milk) are other examples of simple carbohydrates. Simple sugars are rapidly absorbed into the bloodstream and precipitate a high insulin release. *Overweight and obese people should avoid simple carbohydrates.*

Complex carbohydrates not only contain sugars (glucose) but also have micronutrients (vitamins and minerals) in them. There are two types of complex carbohydrates: starches and fiber. **Starches** are composed of long chains of sugar. Foods that supply starches include corn, grain, beans and peas, and potatoes.

Starches are rapidly absorbed in the first 18 inches of intestine. The rapid rise in blood sugar causes a demand for insulin, thus, the pancreas secretes a heavy load of insulin. These peak levels of insulin, in turn, can cause increased fat storage and a drop in blood sugar, stimulating more hunger. (This is the model proposed for hypoglycemia.) We believe that lowering the intake of starch and sugar products decreases this reaction and reduces insulin resistance.

Fiber is indigestible carbohydrate. Some starchy foods, such as potatoes, can be eaten raw without producing the insulin response. However, when potatoes are cooked, the heating breaks down the fiber bonding allowing the digestion of the starch. For people with insulin resistance, this is like taking a sugar pill. Whole grains, most vegetables, and many fruits provide a lot of fiber. When starch is consumed with fiber, the absorption seems to be slowed and peak insulin levels are thusly lower. As a result, less fat is stored and more fat is burned. The "bulk" of fiber can produce a sensation of fullness, and high levels of ingested fiber are associated with reduced risk of developing colon cancer, breast cancer, and heart disease. *Overweight, obese, and type 2 diabetics should limit starch and increase the intake of fiber.*

Fat

The total elimination of dietary fat is not desirable. **Essential fatty acids** are needed for healthy skin and normal cell growth. Some dietary supplements for essential fatty acids are available, but the regulation and guarantee of what is actually in these supplements is up to the manufacturer.

Triglycerides are the primary fat source consumed in diet. Triglycerides are made from fatty acids. Two types of fatty acids exist: **saturated fat** and **unsaturated fat. Saturated fats** come from meat and animal products as well as coconut oil. (The tastiest "movie popcorn" is popped in coconut oil.) Saturated fats are associated with high cholesterol levels and heart disease. Obese and overweight people should avoid saturated fats.

Unsaturated fats are commonly called "cooking oils" and are derived from plants. The least harmful (and sometimes even beneficial) unsaturated fats are called monounsaturated fat. **Olive oil** and **canola oil** are the best of these.

Also important are **omega-3 fatty acids**. These beneficial fats are found primarily in fish (but not canned fish). They result in lower blood levels of cholesterol and triglycerides. One or two weekly servings of fish are strongly recommended to decrease the risk of heart disease.[4]

Overweight and obese people should control the intake of fat and reduce dietary saturated fat. Olive oil or canola oil should be used as a substitute for other oils. Fish intake should be increased.

Proteins

Proteins are critical for numerous bodily functions. Meats, fish, dairy products, nuts, and beans have protein. The problem with many protein sources is that they come with **compound fats**. Compound fats are combinations of protein, triglycerides, and cholesterol. Selecting protein products low in fat (such as lean meat and nonfat milk) is very important. **Proteins** are constructed from chains of amino acids. The recommended daily allowance (RDA) of protein is easy to estimate. Take your body weight in pounds and divide it by 2.2 (this converts your weight in pounds to kilograms). Adult males then multiply the number of kilograms of body weight by .9 and females multiply it by .8. For example a 220 pound man weighs 100 kilograms (220 ÷ 2.2 = 100). The 100 is then multiplied by .9 yielding 90. The 90 represents the number of grams of protein recommended per day. *Overfat and obese people should increase protein intake. Protein should be the primary source of calories. Proteins should come from lean meats, skim milk, nuts, and beans, however, compound fats should be monitored. The use of the drug orlistat can help decrease compound fat absorption.*

How Many Calories Should You Eat Each Day?

There are many methods used to estimate the number of calories an overweight or obese person should eat each day. The ultimate decision is up to you. Chapters 12 and 13 gave some hints and we offer a few specific guidelines below.

Keep in mind that we are trying to teach you how to form a life-long food plan — not a "diet." Thus, you should choose to consume enough calories to fulfill all of your nutritional needs, keep you feeling satisfied, yet still produce a healthy level of fat loss. A daily multi-vitamin can be helpful to ensure you receive all of the necessary require-ments. Remember, also, that exercise is an essential component in a comprehensive health plan.

A simple formula for determining a daily target level for calories can be used. This formula is designed for overweight and obese people who are engaging in some form of exercise. The formula begins with a realistic, desirable body weight. Chapter 4 can help you determine a body weight that is reasonable (see BMI chart, page 46). Remember that you may have an unrealistic expectation about how thin you want to be, so set the initial weight goal higher than your "fantasy" goal.

The next step is easy, but you have to make a decision about how much exercise you are actually getting. Multiply your desired weight by one of three numbers:

10 if you are doing low amounts of exercise (walking 3 hours a week).

11 if you are engaging in moderate exercise (walking 4-5 hours a week).

12 if you are engaging in both aerobic exercise (4 + hrs/week) and resistance training.

The number you calculate by multiplying your desired body weight by 10, 11, or 12 is your daily calorie target. For example, a woman

---

Calculating Your Target Goal For Daily Calories

Begin by listing your *reasonable desired* weight below:

_____

Multiply the above number by:

    x 10 if you exercise 3 hours a week
    x 11 if you exercise 4-5 hours a week
    x 12 if you exercise 4+ hours and do resistance training

   = _____

The product above is your daily calorie goal.
(You can adjust this number small amounts.)

If You Are A Couch Potato

How do you set a daily calorie goal if you are inactive? First, we've already stressed that some exercise is necessary. Only 5% of people who "diet" will be successful. Plus, without exercise, you're likely to lose some of the muscle you have remaining. If you insist on using this *un*smart method of trying to lose weight, multiply your desired body weight by 7, 8, or 9 to get your daily calorie target.

sets an initial weight goal of 140 pounds. She is moderately exercising and walks 6 days a week for 45 minutes each day. Multiplying her desired weight (140) by the number 11 yields 1,540. Thus, she should form a food plan based on a daily intake of 1,540 calories. A woman who desires to weigh 160 pounds (who is heavily exercising) would set a daily calorie plan based on 1,920 calories (160 x 12 = 1,920). A man who was engaged in light exercise who wants to weigh 200 pounds would form a plan based on 2,000 calories (200 x 10 = 2,000).

Determining What To Eat

Since insulin resistance plays a crucial role in the development and maintenance of obesity (as well as diabetes and metabolic syndrome), foods that produce a large insulin response should be avoided. We recommend that 40% of daily calories come from protein, 30% from fat, and 30% from complex carbohydrates. If you take orlistat you may more easily decrease fat ingestion. If you take prescription sugar or starch blockers, it may help with the insulin peak that comes from eating sugar.

> **40% of calories should come from protein**
> **30% from fat**
> **30% from complex carbohydrates**

Why 40-30-30?

The dietary recommendation of 40% protein, 30% carbohydrate, and 30% fat for people who are obese and type 2 diabetics is based on the underlying genetics of thrifty genes in the modern world. Our ancestors began life as hunters. Gradually, they learned to gather some grain, fruits, and vegetables from the bounty of the land. Sugars, refined flour, and processed and preserved foods — virtually all of the foods we take for granted — were simply not available to them. Diabetes and obesity (except in a select few) were rare. In short, their genetic predispositions were designed for survival in a harsh, unpredictable world in which the "thrifty" conservation of energy was an advantage.

From a long-term historical perspective, the emergence of our current industrialized society is of very recent origin. The ability to produce and process ample food, store it indefinitely, and easily and rapidly transport it has been present in our society less than 100 years. The wide-spread use of modern, labor-saving conveniences (automobiles, planes, household & work conveniences) is also less than 100 years old. From an evolutionary viewpoint, *modern diet and habits of inactivity are a sudden and dramatic change.*

Some people obviously have a genetic constitution that has allowed them to easily adapt to these sudden changes in diet (they remain thin and eat anything they want). But over half of us retain the thrifty genes to some degree or other (as evidenced by 55% of us being classified as overweight). Obese people, who make up almost half of those who are overweight, probably are at least moderately influenced by thrifty genes. Type 2 diabetics and people with insulin resistance appear strongly influenced by genetics. Severely obese people and culturally identifiable groups, like the Pima Indians, appear to have the strongest genetic influence.

It is likely that the Pimas would return to their prior physical condition of health and fitness if they returned to the harsh life-style of their hunter-gatherer-farmer ancestors. (**Appendix F** shows a sample "ancient Native American" diet.) The same is probably true for most obese people. Of course, none of us are going to do that nor do we want to do that. *What we can do is to live our lives in the modern world in ways that are in harmony with our basic nature.* Increasing physical activity and attending to stress are a start. Making changes in our daily diet is the final step toward working within our underlying nature.

The 40% protein diet more closely resembles the diet of our naturally thin ancestors. It is hard to maintain high levels of body fat when utilizing this diet. It isn't difficult to make food plans based on the 40-30-30 recommendation, and a wide variety of food choices is available with it. However, in the very beginning stage of formulating a food plan, some work is necessary.

Formulating A Food Plan

We do not think it is essential that each meal and snack be precisely 40-30-30. The percentages should be viewed as overall target ranges. Try to keep each day's food consumption close to these ranges. Diabetics and people with insulin resistance should make a concerted effort to avoid eating simple carbohydrates. Starchy carbohydrates, especially, should be avoided.

The Food Diamond

The Food Guide Pyramid is at variance with the 40-30-30 target listed in this chapter. We agree, in principle, with others (e.g. *The Zone*) who recommend decreased intake of some carbohydrates (starchy and simple), increased intake of protein, and carefully chosen fats. We have made a visual representation of this recommendation which we term *The Food Diamond*. For most people, it will be impractical to consistently match the 40-30-30 range. American foods are heavily carbohydrate based or have too much fat. But the type of carbohydrate is important, as we have already stated. If you can get close to the range (for example, 35-35-30), it will be adequate for most people. It's worth noting that some of the labels on foods are inaccurate, misleading, and sometimes difficult to decipher. Different brands of the exact same product can have vastly different "numbers." Portions are also different. Thus, forming a food plan does take some work.

In making your food plan, calculate the caloric values of various foods you choose. Total up the calories (each day) from carbohydrate, fat, and protein to ensure that you approximate the 40-30-30 range. Most of your foods should be fresh, not cooked in oil. Always measure portions. The foods we recommend in the **Food Diamond** are based, in part, on their effect on insulin resistance. Some foods, like bananas, potatoes, most bread products, crackers, chips, and cereals (starchy carbohydrates and sugar) are best avoided. You may use some carefully chosen "healthy" frozen food meals. During your trip to the grocery store, spend some time in the frozen food section studying labels. Identify those frozen meals that fit into the 40-30-30 plan. Weight Watchers®, Healthy Choice®, and some other brands produce many acceptable products, but read the label. Don't judge these meals by calories alone. Calories say nothing about fat and sugar content. A properly chosen frozen meal can be a God-send for people with time management problems. You must formulate your own food plan, but the foods recommended by the **Food Diamond** are wide ranging and satisfying. The next page shows the **Food Diamond** with recommended food choices.

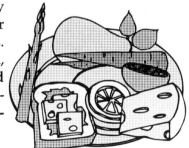

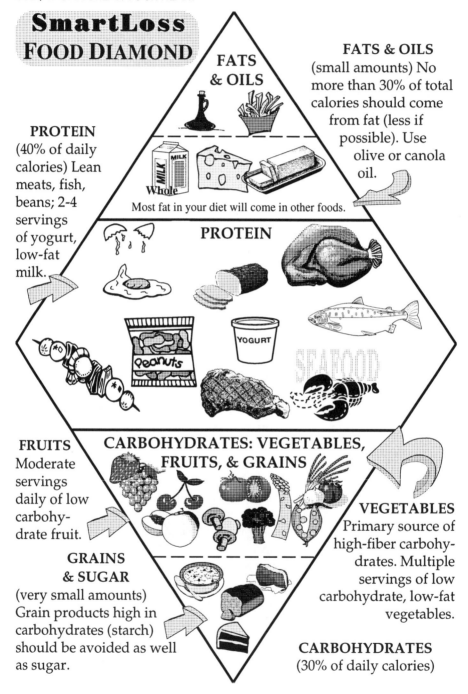

SmartLoss FOOD DIAMOND

FATS & OILS

FATS & OILS (small amounts) No more than 30% of total calories should come from fat (less if possible). Use olive or canola oil.

Most fat in your diet will come in other foods.

PROTEIN (40% of daily calories) Lean meats, fish, beans; 2-4 servings of yogurt, low-fat milk.

PROTEIN

YOGURT

Peanuts

FRUITS Moderate servings daily of low carbohydrate fruit.

CARBOHYDRATES: VEGETABLES, FRUITS, & GRAINS

VEGETABLES Primary source of high-fiber carbohydrates. Multiple servings of low carbohydrate, low-fat vegetables.

GRAINS & SUGAR (very small amounts) Grain products high in carbohydrates (starch) should be avoided as well as sugar.

CARBOHYDRATES (30% of daily calories)

Proteins — Protein should constitute about 40% of your daily calorie intake. Consumption of some high protein foods as snack foods (such as sliced turkey) relieve hunger well, but read labels. Many protein containing foods also have high fat content. Carefully check food labels and serving sizes to ensure that you can calculate your actual portion size. Remember that most products include protein, fat, and carbohydrate. Some products (such cheese and eggs) should be eaten in small quantities. The most acceptable protein foods include:

Dairy:	*Nuts:*	*Beans:*	*Meats & Fish:*
Fat Free Milk		Soy Beans	Fresh Fish
Yogurt,	Peanuts	Black beans	(broiled, baked, grilled)
Low Fat, No Sugar Added	Peanut Butter	Black Eyed Peas	All Meats
Ice Cream, Fat Free, No	(Natural, No Sugar)	Lentils	(lean, fat trimmed, baked,
Sugar Added	(Use nuts sparingly,	Kidney Beans	broiled, grilled)
Eggs (Including Fat Free	They all have high fat.)	Lima Beans	
Frozen)			

Carbohydrates—Complex carbohydrates, especially those high in fiber, should form the basis of 30% of your total caloric intake. Whole grains, vegetables, and some whole fruits provide variation and bulk to your diet. A smart idea is to use artificial sweeteners in place of sugar for all cooking and baking. **Appendix A** contains a section on artificial sweeteners. Check the product label for added sugar content. Avoid products with added sugar. The most acceptable carbohydrate foods include:

Vegetables:	*Fruits:*	*Grains:*	*Cereals:*
Tomatoes	Cherries	Soy Bread (Bürgen)	
Cauliflower	Grapefruit	Oat Bran Bread	Fiber One
Onions	Pears	(Bürgen)	All Bran
Peppers	Strawberries	Pumpernickel Bread	Bran Chex
Cabbage	Plums	Barley, pearled	Oat Bran
Sweet Potatoes	Apples	Bulgar	Oatmeal
Yellow Squash	Apricots (dried)	Rice, Brown	Special K
All Green Vegetables	Grapes	Whole Grain Pasta	
	Oranges	Vermicelli	
	Peaches		

Fat — You should keep dietary fat to 30% or less of your daily calories. Many foods typically contain fat. For example, most meats supply protein but also contain a lot of fat (well-marbled beef, labelled *Prime*). Much of your fat will come from protein and carbohydrate sources. Use all oil sparingly. Olive oil should be used for baking and cooking. Olive oil and vinegar is the recommended salad dressing. If you monitor your calories, the occasional, sparing use of dressings (such as bleu cheese) can be acceptable.

The First Week

The smart way to approach making a food plan is to develop a complete one week plan. Incorporate the food plan into your **health journal**. Write down what you eat every day and total the calories. You should become a knowledgeable consumer. Read and understand nutrition labels. Measure servings and portions carefully. Avoid impulse buying. Eat before you go grocery shopping. As you move into the first week, evaluate how well you are doing with the foods you selected, including how satisfied you feel. Then, plan for the second week. Within the first month of creating a food plan, you will find certain foods you truly like and foods you clearly should avoid. Some foods that have "binge potential" for you should not be present, or even easily available to you (like in a closet or behind the onions in the fridge).

Appendix F presents an example of food plan meals and various calorie-controlled recipes. Increase or decrease the calories according to your specific daily calorie goal. **Appendix D** presents the approximate calorie, fat, carbohydrate, and protein values of many common foods. You should calculate carefully according to weights, size, or serving indicated. **Appendix E** shows the calories, fat, carbohydrate, and protein in many common fast food items. There are a few fast food restaurants where the only healthy item available is a diet drink. If you must eat fast food, at least choose the healthiest alternatives you can.

The U.S. government maintains a massive data base of nearly 6,000 foods showing composition and nutritional values. The web address is: www.nal.usda.gov/fnic/foodcomp

Reading The Labels

All of the foods you purchase at grocery stores must have a standardized label. We have reproduced a U.S. FDA label for reference. The top lines give you the all-important **Serving Size** and the total number of **Servings Per Container** or package. The label shown indicates that the package has four servings each one-half of a cup.

The **Amount Per Serving** shows, first, how many total **Calories** are in each half-cup serving and how many of these calories come from **Fat**. Each serving of this food has 90 calories with 30 (33%) of these calories coming from fat (90 total calories ÷ 30 = 33%). Using our 30% calories from dietary fat recommendation, this food is in the desired range. If you ate the entire package, you'd consume 360 calories (4 x 90 = 360). The fat percentage would remain at 33%.

The left side of the label indicates **Total Fat** grams and **Saturated Fat**. Remember that saturated fat is associated with high cholesterol and heart disease so you want to look for foods that are low in saturated fat totals. One thing you should notice is that each serving of this product has 3 grams of fat. If you multiply the 3 fat grams by the 9 calories contained in each fat gram, you'll come up with 27 calories. But the product label indicates that 30 calories come from fat. Why? The answer is because the food values are averages and rounded off.

Cholesterol and **Sodium** content should be taken into account. Try to avoid high cholesterol and high sodium products.

The **Total Carbohydrate** grams for each serving of this product is 13. If we multiply the 13 grams by 4 calories, carbohydrate provides a total of 52 calories per serving. Thus, carbohydrate calories comprise 58% of all the calories in this product. This is more than the 30% we recommend, but in a meal, a balance could be made by also including a high protein, low-fat meat. **Dietary Fiber** grams are also shown. The RDA of dietary fiber is 25-30 grams per day, but we recommend a higher level. **Sugars** indicates how many grams of the total carbohydrates come from sugar products and is useful information for diabetics and obese people trying to reduce insulin resistance.

The **Protein** grams per serving in this product are 3. Since each protein gram has 4 calories, 12 calories (13%) of the calories in this product come from protein.

If we total the calories from the three sources (fat, carbohydrate, and protein) it comes to 82 calories (30 + 52 + 12 = 94). This is fairly close to the product's stated 90 calories. In going over hundreds of labels, we

NUTRITION FACTS

Serving Size 1/2 cup (114g)
Serving Per Container 4

Amount Per Serving

Calories 90 — Calories from Fat 30

	% Daily Value*
Total Fat 3g	5%
Saturated Fat 0g	0%
Cholesterol 0mg	0%
Sodium 300mg	0%
Total Carbohydrate 13g	13%
Dietary Fiber 3g	4%
Sugars 3g	12%
Protein 3g	

Vitamin A	80%	•	Vitamin C	60%
Calcium	4%	•	Iron	4%

* Percent Daily Values are based on a 2,000 calorie diet. Your daily values may be higher or lower depending on your calorie needs.

		Calories	2000	2500
Total Fat	Less than		65g	80g
Sat Fat	Less than		20g	25g
Cholesterol	Less than		300mg	300mg
Sodium	Less than		2400mg	2400mg
Total Carbohydrate			300g	375g
Fiber			25g	30g

Calories per gram:
Fat 9 • Carbohydrates 4 • Protein 4

discovered that some products *include* the indigestible fiber in total carbohydrates — while other's don't. Unless you have a lot of time, a calculator, and a good understanding of fiber, the best approach is to simply go with the label's stated grams.

The bottom of the label is confusing to most people and can be ignored if you stay within your calorie limits and the 40-30-30 range. The percentages on the right hand side of the label are also confusing. They are based on the *Food Guide Pyramid's* recommendations and can be ignored if you adhere to your food plan. You should try to ensure that you consume sufficient vitamins while restricting sodium and cholesterol.

WHAT COUNTS AS A SERVING?		
Food Groups		
Bread, Cereal, Rice, and Pasta		
1 slice of bread	1 ounce of ready-to-eat cereal	1/2 cup of cooked cereal, rice, or pasta
Vegetable		
1 cup of raw leafy vegetables	1/2 cup of other vegetables, cooked or chopped raw	3/4 cup of vegetable juice
Fruit		
1 medium apple, banana, orange	1/2 cup of chopped, cooked, or canned fruit	3/4 cup of fruit juice
Milk, Yogurt, and Cheese		
1 cup of milk or yogurt	1-1/2 ounces of natural cheese	2 ounces of process cheese
Meat, Poultry, Fish, Dry Beans, Eggs, and Nuts		
2-3 ounces of cooked lean meat, poultry, or fish	1/2 cup of cooked dry beans or 1 egg counts as 1 ounce of lean meat. 2 tablespoons of peanut butter or 1/3 cup of nuts count as 1 ounce of meat.	

Serving Sizes

Food labels indicate serving sizes for the vast majority of products. With some foods, however, such as fruits, vegetables, or meats it can be difficult to know a serving size. The Food Guide Pyramid gives an excellent synopsis of serving sizes. We have reprinted their chart.

Chapter References & Notes

[1] McArdle, W. D., Katch, F. I., & Katch, V. L. (1991) *Exercise physiology: Energy, nutrition and human performance.* Malvern, PA: Lea & Febiger. This massive medical text gives excellent reviews of research on numerous diets.

[2] Eades, M. R. (1989) *Thin So Fast.* New York: Warner Books.

[3] Powers, S. K., & Dodd, S. L. (1996) *Total Fitness: exercise, nutrition, and wellness.* Needham Heights, MA: Allyn & Bacon.

[4] Kromhout, D., Bosschiefer, E. B., & Lezenne-Coulander, C. (1985) The inverse relation between fish consumption and 20-year mortality from coronary heart disease. *New England Journal of Medicine, 312,* 1205-1209.

Chapter 16
SOLVING THE OBESITY PUZZLE WITH SMARTLOSS

Never does nature say one thing and wisdom another.
— **Juvenal**

Summary — The Developmental Model of Obesity gradually outlined in this book demonstrates the complexity of this disease. The subtle interconnections among the components of obesity require that a sincere and simultaneous effort be made with each piece of the obesity puzzle. We call this approach *SmartLoss*.

Individuals struggling with obesity should begin by analyzing past life-style, behaviors, beliefs, and attitudes about obesity. Most people will fit into one of four possible positions: 1. *Yo-Yo Dieting* wherein the individual is actively fighting out-of-control issues while only erratically responding to things under his control; 2. *Unresponsive Worrying* wherein the individual worries about obesity and makes half-hearted efforts while blaming others for failures; 3. *Fat Acceptance* characterized by acceptance of obesity and the conscious choice to embrace living; and, 4. *SmartLoss* wherein the individual makes a simultaneous and systematic effort to address all of the components of obesity. We see only two rational choices that can lead to a genuine sense of serenity — Fat Acceptance or SmartLoss.

The SmartLoss approach begins with a complete health evaluation and appropriate medications based on individual need. In session one, a plan for managing all components of the obesity puzzle is devised and initiated. Individuals with serious personal issues contributing to obesity are referred for individual psychological counseling. All clients should participate in weekly, structured groups (preferably cognitive-behavioral) where personal issues, life-style, environmental responses, exercise, and nutrition are addressed. The group is designed to provide emotional and social support as well as introduce specific information and tools effective in fat reduction. Stress and relaxation coping skills are taught and demonstrated, small life-style adjustments made, and exercise planned. A health journal and structured workbook is utilized.

Clients develop an ongoing program of exercise with a minimal achievement goal of 6 days of 30-minute exercise periods. In addition, three days of moderate, light weight resistance training is required. Exercise is entered into the health journal.

Food Plans are formed immediately based on the client's tastes and caloric needs. Clients are encouraged to write down everything they eat and calculate the total daily calories within their health journal. An immediate shopping trip to a grocery store — spending time reading food labels — is highly recommended. After one and two months on the initial food plan, adjustments are made and the client should be prepared to maintain the eating plan.

Finally, SmartLoss stresses that coping with obesity is a never-ending task. This task can never be made pain-free, but for the sake of health, it must be done!

• • •

Most of us who have struggled with obesity have gone in circles our entire lives. We've lost lots of weight and been momentarily pleased by our reflections in the mirror. The compliments from others are briefly appreciated. But then something inexplicable goes wrong. Our resolve seems to break and weight returns. We usually try to regain control of the situation, but soon everything collapses. Others are often silenced by our relapse and soon the return to our prior condition is complete until something motivates us to try again.

In this book we've tried to explain why this repetitive cycle happens. We believe the analogy of being trapped in the river is an excellent representation of the complex processes involved in obesity. We won't summarize it again, but it's worth repeating that obesity is a multifactorial disease. The chart showing the "Developmental Model of Obesity" depicts the complicated, often self-reinforcing processes in-volved. The implications of this are rather deep. All of the important factors of the disease have to be simultaneously ad-dressed or a permanent change is unlikely. Furthermore, we have to develop the wis-dom to identify the factors we can control as well as those we can't. SmartLoss is learning from our failures, emphasizing what works, and dealing with our inner selves so we don't quit.

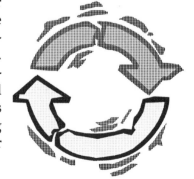

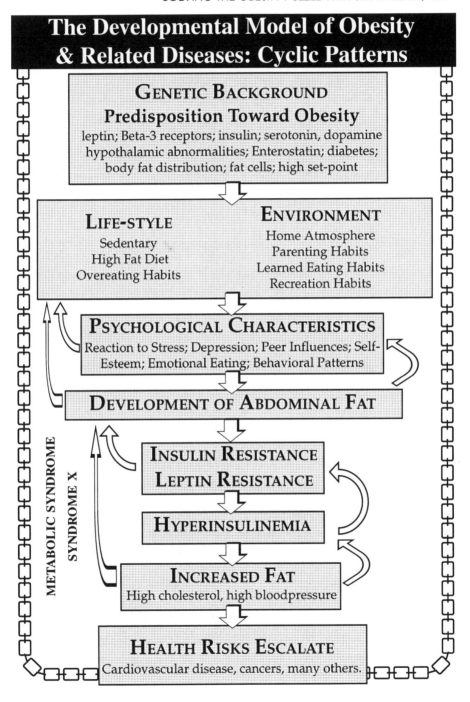

The Developmental Model of Obesity & Related Diseases: Cyclic Patterns

GENETIC BACKGROUND
Predisposition Toward Obesity
leptin; Beta-3 receptors; insulin; serotonin, dopamine
hypothalamic abnormalities; Enterostatin; diabetes;
body fat distribution; fat cells; high set-point

LIFE-STYLE
Sedentary
High Fat Diet
Overeating Habits

ENVIRONMENT
Home Atmosphere
Parenting Habits
Learned Eating Habits
Recreation Habits

PSYCHOLOGICAL CHARACTERISTICS
Reaction to Stress; Depression; Peer Influences; Self-
Esteem; Emotional Eating; Behavioral Patterns

DEVELOPMENT OF ABDOMINAL FAT

INSULIN RESISTANCE
LEPTIN RESISTANCE

HYPERINSULINEMIA

INCREASED FAT
High cholesterol, high bloodpressure

HEALTH RISKS ESCALATE
Cardiovascular disease, cancers, many others.

METABOLIC SYNDROME
SYNDROME X

Making Choices About Worry

We expect that you have already made choices about your health and fitness, but we want to clarify one choice you should consciously make. Most obese people worry about their condition. Their behavior is erratic, inconsistent, contradictory, and moves from one extreme to another. We offer two simple explanations for these responses. First, those who worry and take drastic actions lack fundamental acceptance of their nature and the fact that some things are beyond personal control. Secondly, they fail to exert control over all of the things that they can change in their lives (as well as trying to change some things that are not controllable). Thus, the moods most often seen in these people are anxiety and stress.

There are two rational, alternative positions that can lead to a sense of serenity. You can come to accept obesity (or fatness, if you prefer) and move on with your life. You can be more active, cope with stress issues, develop a social support system, and cope with health issues if and when they arise. People who consciously choose this course of action essentially quit waging a war on fat and just accept it as a fact of nature.

The other rational position is *SmartLoss*. This position also leads to serenity by accepting things that are beyond control. However, it also actively exerts control over all of the things that can be changed. This book has covered the five primary pieces of the obesity puzzle and tried to demonstrate how each can be managed. In this chapter, we'll present a unified, but brief, approach to implementing *SmartLoss*.

The positions regarding worry are outlined on pages 312-313 entitled, "The Four Primary Life-Style & Attitude Positions." You may find it useful to examine the characteristics shown in each position and identify those most common in your past efforts at weight loss. You may uncover some important explanations regarding your past failures and successes. A brief summary of each position is presented.

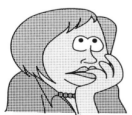
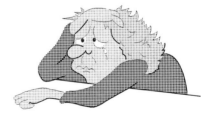

PUTTING TOGETHER THE OBESITY PUZZLE: THE FIVE COMPONENTS OF

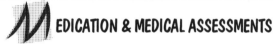

SmartLoss™

MEDICATION & MEDICAL ASSESSMENTS

EXERCISE

FOOD PLAN

Medication designed to address your health risks and needs.

Exercise tailored to your life-style, condition, and motivation.

Food Plan tailored to your individual life-style and tastes.

Psychological issues explored and social support provided through counseling and support groups.

Environmental and Life-Style issues impacting stress levels and obesity identified and modified.

PSYCHOLOGICAL & SOCIAL SUPPORT

ENVIRONMENT & LIFE-STYLE

The Four Primary Life-Style & Attitude Positions Commonly Encountered In Obese People

There are four primary life-style/attitude positions obese people commonly take. One position results in long-term fat loss and increased health: **SmartLoss**. Those who come to understand and accept what *is* and *is not* under personal control can develop serenity. The **SmartLoss** position manages controllable issues and accepts those that can't be changed. The **Fat Acceptance** position is the only other rational choice that can lead to serenity. This position accepts things that can't be changed and makes conscious choices to control some things that are under control. The other two positions are the most common. They are irrational, lead to erratic, inconsistent behavior, and produce chronic worry and stress. There are some variations and combinations possible between positions.

SmartLoss
Accepts things out-of-control.
Changes things under control.
Serenity

ACCEPTANCE
USES NEEDED MEDICATION
CHOOSES EATING PLAN
REGULAR EXERCISE
ACTIVE LIFE-STYLE
EFFECTIVE STRESS COPING
STEADY FAT REDUCTION

Fat Acceptance
Accepts things out-of-control.
Changes *some* things under control
by conscious choice.
Serenity

ACCEPTANCE
MINIMAL MEDICATIONS
LOVES & ACCEPTS FOOD
NO REGULAR EXERCISE
ACTIVE LIFE-STYLE
EFFECTIVE STRESS COPING
FAT ACCEPTANCE

WORRIES
NO MEDICATION
DRASTIC DIETS
ERRATIC EXERCISE
HIGH STRESS LIFE-STYLE
POOR STRESS COPING
WEIGHT CYCLING

WORRIES
USES MEDICATION
ERRATICALLY DIETS
NO EXERCISE
HIGH STRESS LIFE-STYLE
POOR STRESS COPING
STEADY WEIGHT GAIN

Yo-Yo Dieter
Battles out-of-control issues.
Erratically responds to
things under control.
Anxiety & Stress

Unresponsive Worrier
Worries about out-of-control issues.
Worries about things under control.
Erratic behavior — blames others.
Anxiety & Stress

The Yo-Yo Dieter

The yo-yo dieter is motivated to lose weight for others. Being in love, wanting to be attractive, seeking acceptance, or trying to please a spouse are a few reasons for losing weight. The individual mistakenly believes that weight loss will solve all her other problems. The weight cycler is rewarded for losing weight by the comments and compliments received from others. But the compliments are short-lived. Eventually the person finds that being thinner fails to resolve personal problems and the rewards for being thin seem few. Motivation wanes and weight returns. The food is rewarding and provides a comforting solace, but eventually some critical event occurs and she becomes motivated to lose weight again. Yo-yo dieters tend to be miserable when they are fat and miserable when they are thin. A "spoof" title of a country song, "I'm so miserable when you're gone, it's like you're still here," applies to a lot of people who stay in this life-style/attitude position.

Unresponsive Worrier

The Unresponsive Worrier will say, "I'm trying to lose weight, but it's not working." Medication will be accepted and used, but this person won't make any other changes. The person will "try" to diet and exercise, but he will have countless excuses for failing to do them. The coping strategy typically employed is to blame others, circumstances, or stress. Rather than cope with stress, people in this life-style & attitude position use stress as an excuse for inaction. Avoidance of reality is an underlying issue, and, chronic worry results.

Fat Acceptance

Accepting obesity as a natural circumstance of one's nature is a rational life-style & attitude position that leads to a form of serenity. The most rational behaviors in this position are to become physically active by seeking social involvement, effectively deal with stress and personal issues, and remain aware of health risks and problems. As health problems arise, they are addressed medically. People who accept the fat acceptance position simply cease trying to lose fat. While some obesity treatment specialists and fitness gurus may be repelled by this position, those who are truly in the fat acceptance position embrace life and try to enjoy it to the fullest despite limitations.

SmartLoss

People who take the SmartLoss position gather information about all of the wide-ranging factors that contribute to obesity. They organize a reasonable but comprehensive life-long plan of action with the goal of actively changing all of the issues and problems that can be changed. They also accept certain issues and problems as a reality of nature. They cease worrying and develop serenity because they are essentially doing everything they can reasonably do. A strong sense of personal identity forms from these efforts.

SmartLoss: Summary Of Actions

As reviewed in this book, a comprehensive approach to obesity requires several simultaneous actions aimed at impacting all of the obesity puzzle's components. These components are medication, psychological & social issues, life-style habits, exercise, and food planning. The first step in beginning SmartLoss is to have a thorough medical examination by a competent physician practicing obesity medicine. **Appendix A** provides an overview of how to choose a health care provider for obesity, questions to ask, and how to spot ineffective (even fraudulent) providers.

If you have an initial plan of action, and choose the correct program provider, you can immediately put into motion actions that impact all of the obesity components. All of these actions demand a long-term, sustained effort. But all of them should be put into place immediately.

Medications & Medical Assistance

Your medical doctor needs a thorough understanding of your health condition and background to determine which medications are best for you. The choice to accept these medications is up to you, but by being an informed consumer, you can make intelligent decisions. Weigh the risks and benefits of any medications recommended. If you are obese, have insulin resistance, a high risk of developing diabetes, or other obesity-related health risks you should seriously consider medication. The fat blocker orlistat, for example, appears to be so free of serious side effects that it may eventually become an over-the-counter drug.

Take medications as directed. Remember that medications help to reduce the pain of reducing and are only a single, but significant, component to treating obesity. Report side-effects and problems to your physician promptly.

Research shows us that people undergoing treatment for obesity should be seen frequently. Less knowledgeable physicians may schedule your next visit several months away. In truth, you need to be seen at least once monthly — probably even more. (This may last indefinitely.) The SmartLoss approach strongly urges patients to be seen by staff every week during the first three months. Physicians are typically too busy to see patients as often and for as long as they would like, however, appropriate obesity treatment programs will provide frequent health screenings (including your weight, blood pressure check, body fat percentage, and a brief series of questions regarding exercise, diet, stress, and medication) between your visits with the physician. This should be coordinated with a comprehensive program of other services explained to you at your initial visit. You should be asked to participate in several ongoing activities. These include nutrition classes, support groups, stress management, evaluation of environment and life-style confrontation, and forming exercise and eating plans. An ideal way to address all of these components is in a structured, cognitive-behavioral workbook used in weekly groups. (Cognitive-behavioral approaches focus on changing behavior and thinking; the **Glossary [Appendix G]** contains more information.) We have developed a 12-week *SmartLoss Group Workbook* to accomplish this task, but there are other programs that can accomplish the same goal. For reasonable success, you must participate in all program components.

Psychological & Social Support

Chapter 11 reviewed various ways of addressing individual psychological and social support needs. In your initial session, you will be asked several personal questions and will probably complete a wide-ranging questionnaire. Based on your responses, the treatment provider may decide to ask you to participate in some form of psychological counseling. Childhood abuse, emotional problems, personal stress issues, and serious conflicts should initially be handled individually. You may also be prescribed an antidepressant for stress, anxiety, depression, or obsessive-compulsive behavior.

You should be provided with a health journal (or a "diet and feelings diary" at a minimum) and given some instruction on its use. It is used to record eating, exercise, feelings, and other significant events. The journal should be used to chart your progress and should be utilized by all of the program's staff at different times. You should also receive some additional materials (such as a group workbook, tapes, information brochures, etc.).

SmartLoss recommends that all obesity patients enter an ongoing counseling program that sequentially addresses all of the components of the obesity puzzle. You will be offered a place in a weekly counseling/education group. This ongoing weekly group program is typically completed in 12 weeks. Several different groups, each meeting at different times, allow patients the latitude to attend a meeting most convenient to them. The groups are typically facilitated by staff trained in the method that is employed. The facilitators should be able to handle basic counseling needs and have sufficient knowledge in exercise, nutrition, stress management, and obesity medications. Our program format is organized into a 12-session cognitive-behavioral workbook. There are other behavioral and cognitive-behavioral programs on the market that are adequate and effective.

The group should provide basic counseling, lead to some insights, and provide social support. You may be encouraged to attend other support meetings. Stress-reduction and basic relaxation techniques should be demonstrated and taught. You may be asked to listen to tapes that relate to relaxation, stress, coping with binges, exercise, or other issues.

Environmental & Life-Style Component

The ongoing group program should enable you to objectively evaluate your environment and how it impacts your life-style. What do you really do with your time? When can you free yourself for a 10 or 15 minute walk. How can you reduce fast food consumption, and how can you choose the right foods at restaurants? What do you do during your leisure time? What small changes can you make in your day-to-day life that could lead to large changes over time? How do you handle the stress from your overall environment?

You should begin examining your environment and life-style within 2 weeks of entering a program. You should identify behavioral areas that can and should be modified and make specific plans to change them. The group should be used as a gauge to identify progress and reformulate plans as necessary. The program relies on encouragement and reward, not shame and guilt!

The degree of stress in your environment and how it impacts you should be a consideration. You should be taught to employ effective stress management techniques. The program should offer you the tools and support needed to overcome these obstacles. The essential goal of the environmental and life-style program component is to increase overall physical activity and reduce stress through exercise and appropriate behavioral responses. We recommend the use of a pedometer to monitor physical activity with the results recorded in the health journal.

Exercise

SmartLoss demands regular periods of sustained exercise. A minimum of 3 hours per week of some type of exercise is the eventual goal. Ideally, the 3 hours would be spent over 6 days for 30 minutes each day. Walking is sufficient for this exercise component, but finding another enjoyable form of individual exercise (e.g., using a dance videotape) is acceptable. In the beginning, you should gradually build up to the 30 minute period by taking several 5 or 10 minute walks during the day. Increasing regular exercise above the 30 minute daily minimum is very beneficial to both fat reduction and health. All exercise should be documented in your health journal. Avoid injury!

SmartLoss strongly encourages some muscle-building resistance training. The eventual goal is to perform low weight, high repetition resistance training 2-3 days each week. You should follow the recommendations given in the exercise chapter. With the careful choice of a series of appropriate weight exercises, you could fulfill this 3-time-a-week requirement in 20-40 minutes per session. Feelings, observations about increased strength, and specific weight lifting exercise should be recorded in the health journal. Don't get injured.

Forming A Healthy Food Plan

Forming a healthy food plan begins with calculating your daily calorie goal. (In your initial meeting with the program, a calorie total may be recommended to you.) Next, you should choose a starter menu (for about one week) that allows you to stay within the daily caloric limits. Rid your home of all inappropriate food items (unless children's needs dictate otherwise). Take a shopping trip to a large grocery store (after eating) and plan on spending some time looking at food labels. While we recommend that obese and overweight people should try to get 40% of their calories from protein, it isn't always necessary to do so if you can stay within the calorie goal. Your tastes and medical conditions can greatly impact what you can and should eat. The primary goal is to reduce your total calorie intake to a healthy level in a way that appeals to you so that you don't feel deprived. This will increase the chances that you can successfully follow your plan.

During the first one to two months, record everything you eat in your health journal and total the calories, fat, protein, and carbohydrates. As you become accustomed to staying within the calorie limits, you will more easily form an ongoing food plan. Remember that you are forming a life-long eating plan. Your real goal is to develop new eating behaviors that are permanent.

It's A Life-Long Issue

Obesity is a life-long issue that can't be avoided. Every day you gaze into a mirror and are confronted with a choice. Each day you stand at a choice point on your path through life. This shouldn't be seen as a misfortune; after all, health is a life-long issue for everyone. With diligence and effort, you can learn to balance the components of your obesity problem. Most of the work is on the front end of this effort. Which fork in the road you decide to take will impact your health. Should you choose to traverse the road to health, you will learn powerful new behaviors. You will also discover that you are able to enjoy many activities that you previously avoided. You can teach yourself good habits. You can learn to enjoy a lot of things you have been avoiding. But you have to choose and choose wisely.

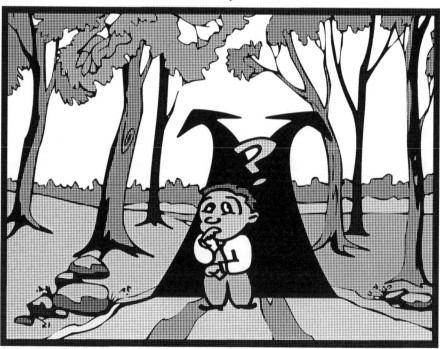

Special Issues: Children, Weight Surgery, Medication Complications, Smoking, Choosing A Commercial Program, Very Low Calorie Diets, Dietary Supplements, Artificial Sweeteners, & Fat Replacers

Portions of this appendix have been adapted from various government sources.

Children's Issues

In the United States at least one child in five is overweight and the number of overweight children continues to grow. Over the last 2 decades, this number has increased by more than 50 percent, and the number of "extremely" overweight children has nearly doubled (*Archives of Pediatric & Adolescent Medicine* [1995] 149, 1085-91). Although children have fewer weight-related health problems than adults, overweight children are at high risk of becoming overweight adolescents and adults.

What Causes Children to Become Overweight?

Children become overweight for a variety of reasons. The most common causes are genetic factors, lack of physical activity, unhealthy eating patterns, or a combination of these factors. In rare cases, a medical problem, such as an endocrine disorder, may cause a child to become overweight. Your physician can perform a careful physical exam and some blood tests, if necessary, to rule out this type of problem. Another cause relates to social influence, especially from parents.

Life-style

A child's total diet and his or her activity level both play an important role in determining a child's weight. The increasing popularity of television and computer and video games contributes to children's inactive life-styles. The average American child spends approximately 24 hours each week watching television — time that could be spent in some sort of physical activity. A 1998 study evaluated the television viewing time of 4,063 children aged 8-16 years. Boys and girls who watched television for 4 hours or more a day were the most likely to be overweight. (Anderson, R. E., et. al. [1998] *Journal of the American Medical Association*, 279, 938-942).

Ways To Help An Overweight Child

Be Supportive

One of the most important things you can do to help overweight children is to let them know that they are okay whatever their weight. Children's feelings about themselves often are based on their parents' feelings about them. If you accept your children at any weight, they will be more likely to accept and feel good about themselves. It is also important to talk to your children about weight, allowing them to share their concerns with you. Your child probably knows better than anyone else that he or she has a weight problem. For this reason, overweight children need support, acceptance, and encouragement from their parents.

Focus On The Family

Parents should try not to set children apart because of their weight, but focus on gradually changing their family's physical activity and eating habits. Family involvement helps to teach everyone healthful habits and does not single out the overweight child.

Increase Your Family's Physical Activity

Regular physical activity, combined with healthy eating habits, is the most efficient and healthful way to control your weight. It is also an important part of a healthy life-style. Some simple ways to increase your family's physical activity include the following:

• Be a role model for your children. If your children see that you are physically active and have fun, they are more likely to be active and stay active for the rest of their lives.

• Plan family activities that provide everyone with exercise and enjoyment, like walking, dancing, biking, or swimming. For example, schedule a walk with your family after dinner instead of watching TV. Make sure that you plan activities that can be done in a safe environment.

• Be sensitive to your child's needs. Overweight children may feel uncomfortable about participating in certain activities. It is important to help your child find physical activities that they enjoy and that aren't embarrassing or too difficult.

• Reduce the amount of time you and your family spend in sedentary activities, such as watching TV or playing video games.

• Become more active throughout your day and encourage your family to do so as well. For example, walk up the stairs instead of taking the elevator, or do some activity during a work or school break-get up and stretch or walk around. The point is not to make physical activity an unwelcome chore, but to make the most of the opportunities you and your family have to be active.

Teach Your Family Healthy Eating Habits

Teaching healthy eating practices early will help children approach eating with the right attitude — that food should be enjoyed and is necessary for growth, development, and for energy to keep the body running. The best way to begin is to learn more about children's nutritional needs by reading or talking with a health professional and then to offer them some healthy options, allowing your children to choose what and how much they eat.

Helping Children Develop Good Attitudes About Eating

Don't place your child on a restrictive diet. Children should never be placed on a restrictive diet to lose weight, unless a doctor supervises one for medical reasons. Limiting what children eat may be harmful to their health and interfere with their growth and development.

To promote proper growth and development and prevent overweight, parents should offer the whole family a wide variety of foods from each of the food groups. If you are unsure about how to select and prepare a variety of foods for your family, consult a physician or registered dietitian for nutrition counseling.

Reduce Fat

Reducing fat is a good way to cut calories without depriving your child of nutrients. Simple ways to cut the fat in your family's diet include eating lowfat or nonfat dairy products, poultry without skin and lean meats, and lowfat or fat-free breads and cereals. Making small changes to the amount of fat in your family's diet is a good way to prevent excess weight gain in children: however, major efforts to change your child's diet should be supervised by a health professional. In addition, fat should not be restricted in the diets of children younger than 2 years of age. After that age, children should gradually adopt a diet that contains no more than 30 percent of calories from fat by the time the child is about 5 years old. Don't overly restrict sweets or treats. While it is important to be aware of the fat, salt, and sugar content of the foods you serve, all foods-even those that are high in fat or sugar-have a place in the diet, in moderation.

Other Hints

Guide your family's choices rather than dictate foods. Make a wide variety of healthful foods available in the house. This practice will help your children learn how to make healthy food choices. Encourage your child to eat slowly. A child can detect hunger and fullness better when eating slowly. Eat meals together as a family as often as possible. Try to make mealtimes pleasant with conversation and sharing, not a time for scolding or arguing. If mealtimes are unpleasant, children may try to eat faster to leave the table as soon as possible. They then may learn to associate eating with stress. Involve children in food shopping and preparing meals. These activities offer parents hints about children's food preferences, teach children about nutrition, and provide children with a feeling of accomplishment. In addition, children may be more willing to eat or try foods that they help prepare.

Plan for snacks. Continuous snacking may lead to overeating, but snacks that are planned at specific times during the day can be part of a nutritious diet, without spoiling a child's appetite at mealtimes. You should make snacks as nutritious as possible, without depriving your child of occasional chips or cookies, especially at parties or other social events. Below are some ideas for healthy snacks.

Healthy Snacks

Fresh, frozen, or canned vegetables and fruit served either plain or with lowfat or fat-free cheese or yogurt. Dried fruit, served with nuts or sunflower or pumpkin seeds. Breads and crackers made with enriched flour and whole grains, served with fruit spread or fat-free cheese. Frozen desserts, such as nonfat or lowfat ice cream, frozen yogurt, fruit sorbet, popsicles, water ice, and fruit juice bars. Children of preschool age can easily choke on foods that are hard to chew, small and round, or sticky, such as hard vegetables, whole grapes, hard chunks of cheese, raisins, nuts, and seeds, and popcorn. Its important to carefully select snacks for children in this age group.

Discourage Eating Meals Or Snacks While Watching TV

Try to eat only in designated areas of your home, such as the dining room or kitchen. Eating in front of the TV may make it difficult to pay attention to feelings of fullness, and may lead to overeating.

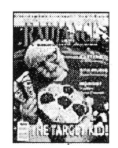

Don't Use Food To Punish Or Reward Your Child

Withholding food as a punishment may lead chil-dren to worry that they will not get enough food. For example, sending children to bed without any dinner may cause them to worry that they will go hungry. As a result, children may try to eat whenever they get a chance. Similarly, when foods, such as sweets, are used as a reward, children may assume that these foods are better or more valuable than other foods. For example, telling children that they will get dessert if they eat all of their vegetables sends the wrong message about vegetables.

Set A Good Example

Children are good learners, and they learn best by example. Setting a good example for your kids by eating a variety of foods and being physically active will teach your children healthy life-style habits that they can follow for the rest of their lives.

Multigenerational Issues

In Exodus 20:1-5, Moses was given the first three commandments. "Thou shalt have no other gods before me. Thou shalt not make unto thee any graven image... Thy shalt not bow down thyself to them, nor serve then: for I the Lord thy God am a jealous God, visiting the iniquity of the fathers unto the children unto the third and fourth generation..."

Obesity runs in families. Children learn eating habits from parents, including what foods are eaten, where and when eating takes place, and how much is eaten. Parents with poor eating habits tend to pass them on to their children, who, in turn, pass them on.

Radiance Magazine Kids Project!

Radiance Magazine has developed an ongoing project to "help children of all ages feel seen, loved, and valued for who they are, whatever their size or shape." Parents' teenagers, and professionals who work with children should take a look at their project: www.radiancemagazine.com

Surgery For Weight Loss

Severe obesity is a chronic condition that is very difficult to treat. Surgery to promote weight loss by restricting food intake or interrupting digestive processes is an option for severely obese people. A body mass index (BMI) above 40 — which means about 100 pounds of overweight for men and about 80 pounds for women — indicates that a person is severely obese and therefore a candidate for surgery.

Surgery also may be an option for people with a BMI between 35 and 40 who suffer from life-threatening cardiopulmonary problems (for example, severe sleep apnea or obesity-related heart disease) or diabetes. However, as in other treatments for obesity, successful results depend mainly on motivation and behavior.

The Normal Digestive Process

Normally, as food moves along the digestive tract, appropriate digestive juices and enzymes arrive at the right place at the right time to digest and absorb calories and nutrients. After we chew and swallow our food, it moves down the esophagus to the stomach, where a strong acid continues the digestive process. The stomach can hold about 3 pints of food at one time. When the stomach contents move to the duodenum, the first segment of the small intestine, bile and pancreatic juice speed up digestion. Most of the iron and calcium in the foods we eat is absorbed in the duodenum. The jejunum and ileum, the remaining two segments of the nearly 20 feet of small intestine, complete the absorption of almost all calories and nutrients. The food particles that cannot be digested in the small intestine are stored in the large intestine until eliminated.

How Does Surgery Promote Weight Loss?

The concept of gastric surgery to control obesity grew out of results of operations for cancer or severe ulcers that removed large portions of the stomach or small intestine. Because patients undergoing these procedures

tended to lose weight after surgery, some physicians began to use such operations to treat severe obesity. The first operation that was widely used for severe obesity was the intestinal bypass. This operation, first used 40 years ago, produces weight loss by causing malabsorption. The idea was that patients could eat large amounts of food, which would be poorly digested or passed along too fast for the body to absorb many calories.

The problem with this surgery was that it caused a loss of essential nutrients and its side effects were unpredictable and sometimes fatal. The original form of the intestinal bypass operation is no longer used.

Surgeons now use techniques that produce weight loss primarily by limiting how much the stomach can hold. These restrictive procedures are often combined with modified gastric bypass procedures that somewhat limit calorie and nutrient absorption and may lead to altered food choices.

Two ways that surgical procedures promote weight loss are:

1. By decreasing food intake (restriction). Gastric banding, gastric bypass, and vertical-banded gastroplasty are surgeries that limit the amount of food the stomach can hold by closing off or removing parts of the stomach. These operations also delay emptying of the stomach (gastric pouch).

2. By causing food to be poorly digested and absorbed (malabsorption). In the gastric bypass procedures, a surgeon makes a direct connection from the stomach to a lower segment of the small intestine, bypassing the duodenum, and some of the jejunum.

Although results of operations using these procedures are more predictable and manageable, side effects persist for some patients.

What Are the Surgical Options?

Restriction Operations

Restriction operations are the surgeries most often used for producing weight loss. Food intake is restricted by creating a small pouch at the top of the stomach where the food enters from the esophagus. The pouch initially holds about 1 ounce of food and expands to 2-3 ounces with time. The pouch's lower outlet usually has a diameter of about 1/4 inch. The small outlet delays the emptying of food from the pouch and causes a feeling of fullness.

After an operation, the person usually can eat only a half to a whole cup of food without discomfort or nausea. Also, food has to be well chewed. For most people, the ability to eat a large amount of food at one time is lost, but some patients do return to eating modest amounts of food without feeling hungry.

Restriction operations for obesity include gastric banding and vertical banded gastroplasty. Both operations serve only to restrict food intake. They do not interfere with the normal digestive process.

• Gastric banding. In this procedure, a band made of special material is placed around the stomach near its upper end, creating a small pouch and a narrow passage into the larger remainder of the stomach. In the future, it may be possible to perform gastric banding with smaller incisions through a laparoscope, a flexible fiberoptic tube and light source through which some surgical instruments may be passed. Laparoscopic gastric banding has not yet been approved by the Food and Drug Administration.

• Vertical banded gastroplasty (VBG). This procedure is the most frequently used restrictive operation for weight control. Both a band and staples are used to create a small stomach pouch.

Restrictive operations lead to weight loss in almost all patients. However, weight regain does occur in some patients. About 30 percent of persons undergoing vertical banded gastroplasty achieve normal weight, and about 80 percent achieve some degree of weight loss. However, some patients are unable to adjust their eating habits and fail to lose the desired weight. In all weight-loss operations, successful results depend on your motivation and behaviors.

A common risk of restrictive operations is vomiting caused by the small stomach being overly stretched by food particles that have not been chewed well. Other risks of VBG include erosion of the band, breakdown of the staple line, and, in a small number of cases, leakage of stomach juices into the abdomen. The latter requires an emergency operation. In a very small number of cases (less than 1 percent) infection or death from complications can occur.

Gastric Bypass Operations

Gastric bypass operations combine creation of small stomach pouches to restrict food intake and construction of bypasses of the duodenum and other segments of the small intestine to cause malabsorption.

• Roux-en-Y gastric bypass (RGB). This operation is the most common gastric by-

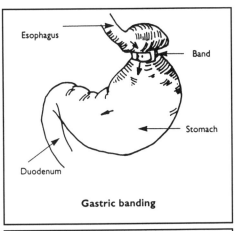

Gastric banding

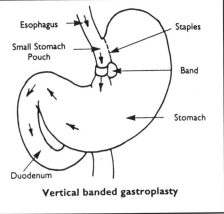

Vertical banded gastroplasty

pass procedure. First, a small stomach pouch is created by stapling or by vertical banding. This causes restriction in food intake. Next, a Y-shaped section of the small intestine is attached to the pouch to allow food to bypass the duodenum (the first segment of the small intestine) as well as the first portion of the jejunum (the second segment of the small intestine). This causes reduced calorie and nutrient absorption.

• Extensive gastric bypass (biliopancreatic diversion). In this more complicated gastric bypass operation (figure 5), portions of the stomach are removed. The small pouch that remains is connected directly to the final segment of the small intestine, thus completely bypassing both the duodenum and jejunum. Although this procedure successfully promotes weight loss, it is not widely used because of the high risk for nutritional deficiencies.

Gastric bypass operations that cause malabsorption and restrict food intake produce more weight loss than restriction operations that only decrease food intake. Patients who have bypass operations generally lose two-thirds of their excess weight within 2 years.

The risks for pouch stretching, band erosion, breakdown of staple lines, and leakage of stomach contents into the abdomen are about the same for gastric bypass as for vertical banded gastroplasty. However, because gastric bypass operations cause food to skip the duodenum, where most iron and calcium are absorbed, risks for nutritional deficiencies are higher in these procedures. Anemia may result from malabsorption of vitamin B12 and iron in menstruating women, and decreased absorption of calcium may bring on osteoporosis and metabolic bone disease. Patients are required to take nutritional supplements that usually prevent these deficiencies.

Gastric bypass operations also may cause "dumping syndrome," whereby stomach contents move too rapidly through the small intestine. Symptoms include nausea, weakness, sweating, faintness, and, occasionally, diarrhea after eating, as well as the inability to eat sweets without becoming so

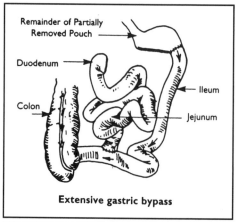

Extensive gastric bypass

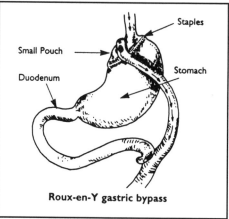

Roux-en-Y gastric bypass

weak and sweaty that the patient must lie down until the symptoms pass.

The more extensive the bypass operation, the greater is the risk for complications and nutritional deficiencies. Patients with extensive bypasses of the normal digestive process require not only close monitoring, but also life-long use of special foods and medications.

Explore Benefits and Risks

Surgery to produce weight loss is a serious undertaking. Each individual should clearly understand what the proposed operation involves. Patients and physicians should carefully consider the following benefits and risks:
Benefits

• Immediately following surgery, most patients lose weight rapidly and continue to do so until 18 to 24 months after the procedure. Although most patients then start to regain some of their lost weight, few regain it all.

• Surgery improves most obesity-related conditions. For example, in one study blood sugar levels of most obese patients with diabetes returned to normal after surgery. Nearly all patients whose blood sugar levels did not return to normal were older or had diabetes for a long time.

Risks

• Ten to 20 percent of patients who have weight-loss operations require follow-up operations to correct complications. Abdominal hernias are the most common complications requiring follow-up surgery. Less common complications include breakdown of the staple line and stretched stomach outlets.

• More than one-third of obese patients who have gastric surgery develop gallstones. Gallstones are clumps of cholesterol and other matter that form in the gallbladder. During rapid or substantial weight loss a person's risk of developing gallstones is increased. Gallstones can be prevented with supplemental bile salts taken for the first 6 months after surgery.

• Nearly 30 percent of patients who have weight-loss surgery develop nutritional deficiencies such as anemia, osteoporosis, and metabolic bone disease. These deficiencies can be avoided if vitamin and mineral intakes are maintained.

• Women of childbearing age should avoid pregnancy until their weight becomes stable because rapid weight loss and nutritional deficiencies can harm a developing fetus.

Is the Surgery for You?

For patients who remain severely obese after nonsurgical approaches to weight loss have failed, or for patients who have an obesity-related disease, surgery may be the best next step. But for other patients, greater efforts toward weight control, such as changes in eating habits, behavior modification, and increasing physical activity, may be more appropriate. Answers to the following questions may help in your decision to undergo surgery for weight loss. Are you:

• unlikely to lose weight successfully with (further) nonsurgical measures?

• well informed about the surgical procedure and the effects of treatment?

• determined to lose weight and improve your health?

• aware of how your life may change after the operation (adjustment to the side effects of the surgery, including need to chew well and inability to eat large meals)?

• aware of the potential for serious complications, the associated dietary restrictions, and the occasional failures?

• committed to lifelong medical follow-up?

Do you:

• have a BMI of 40 or more?

• have an obesity-related physical problem (such as body size that interferes with employment, walking, or family function)?

• have high-risk obesity-related health problems (such as severe sleep apnea or obesity-related heart disease)?

Remember: There are no guarantees for any method, including surgery, to produce and maintain weight loss. Success is possible only with your fullest cooperation and commitment to behavioral change and medical follow-up — and this cooperation and commitment should be carried out for the rest of your life.

Liposuction

Liposuction essentially removes fat cells beneath the skin. It is considered to be cosmetic surgery rather than a weight loss technique. Liposuction typically removes 5 or 6 pounds of fat per surgery. Modern liposuction is accomplished by making a series of small (less than an inch long) incisions through the skin. It can take 6 months or so for the results of the surgery to be seen because swelling occurs. The procedure causes a fair amount of tissue trauma.

People who have liposuction can regain all of the fat removed by the surgery — but not in the fat cells removed through the liposuction. The weight is gained elsewhere.

About half of all fat storage is internal, thus, those who gain weight after liposuction will regain some of it internally.

Liposuction can be a fairly safe procedure, however, you should carefully check out the clinic and doctor doing the procedure. The relevant point (in accordance with this book's topic) is that liposuction is not a weight loss surgery.

Obesity Treatment & Other Medications

Obese patients are sometimes taking a host of medications. These can include blood pressure medicines, antidepressants, thyroid medicines, and over-the-counter preparations. When obesity medications are also being considered, it is very important to inform your doctors of all medications you take. Some medicines may interact with obesity medications or be counterproductive to reducing fat. Only your doctor (or a pharmacist) can help you make informed decisions.

Drugs To Avoid — Or May Be Counterproductive

An exhaustive review of all drugs is impractical. In order for you to understand the necessity of informing your health care providers about your medications, a brief overview is provided.

Diuretic drugs and beta-blockers (blood pressure medicines) should be avoided if at all possible. Calcium channel blockers, ACE inhibitors, and angiotensin II receptor blockers (Diovan) should be substituted for other blood pressure medications. Some antidepressants (especially the MAO-I and tricyclics) should be avoided. Some Tricyclics can cause weight gain: (e.g., imipramine [Tofranil & Janimine], desipramine [Norpramin & Pertofrane], amitriptyline [Elavil & Endep], nortriptyline [Pamelor], doxepin [Sinequan & Adapin], trimipramine [Surmontil], and maprotiline [Ludiomil]. MAO-I antidepressants (monoamine oxidase inhibitors) are contraindicated for most obesity drugs. Lithium (used for cyclical manic-depression - bipolar affective disorder) leads to weight gain. If lithium has stabilized your mood, however, you should probably remain on it. In general, thyroid medicines do not cause any problems when taken in conjunction with obesity medications.

Phenylpropanolamine (PPA) is an over-the-counter weight loss drug. PPA can result in modest short-term weight loss, but typically the user rapidly develops tolerance to the drug's effect. PPA can cause increased blood pressure and heart palpitations. Many decongestants contain PPA. PPA should be avoided when using other obesity medications.

Smoking & Weight

If you want to stop smoking but are worried about gaining weight, this section may help. Many ex-smokers do gain a few pounds, but only a few gain a lot of weight. You can substantially improve your health if you quit smoking. Smoking is very harmful to your health. Making some simple changes, like developing healthier eating and physical activity habits, should help you control your weight gain when you quit smoking.

Will I Gain Weight if I Stop Smoking?

Not everyone gains weight when they stop smoking. On average, people who quit smoking gain only about 10 pounds. You are more likely to gain weight when you stop smoking if you have smoked for 10 to 20 years or smoked one or more packs of cigarettes a day. You can control your weight while you quit smoking by making healthy eating and physical activity a part of your life. Although you might gain a few pounds, remember you have stopped smoking and taken a big step toward a healthier life.

What causes weight gain after quitting?

Nicotine is a powerful stimulant found in tobacco. Nicotine is highly addictive. When you quit smoking you may experience:

• Short-term weight gain. The nicotine kept your body weight low, and when you quit smoking, your body returns to the weight it would have been had you never smoked. You can, however, control this by watching what you eat, exercising, and by seeking medical assistance. Several medications are available that greatly assist with the transition from smoking.

• You might gain 3 to 5 pounds due to water retention during the first week after quitting.

• A need for fewer calories. After you stop smoking, you may use fewer calories than when you were smoking.

Will This Weight Gain Hurt My Health?

Smoking causes more than 400,000 deaths each year in the United States. You would have to gain about 100 to 150 pounds after quitting to make your health risks as high as when you smoked. The health risks of smoking and the benefits of quitting are listed below.

The Health Risks of Smoking

When you smoke...

• Your heart rate increases.

• You expose yourself to some 4,000 chemicals in cigarette smoke and 40 of these chemicals cause cancer.

• You are much more likely to get lung cancer than a nonsmoker. Men are 22 times more likely to develop lung cancer, while women who smoke are 12 times more likely.

• You are twice as likely to have a heart attack as a nonsmoker.

• You increase your risk for heart disease, stroke, some types of cancer, emphysema, chronic bronchitis, and other lung diseases.

• You are hurting not only your own health, but the health of anyone who breathes the smoke, including nonsmokers.

The Benefits of Quitting

When you quit smoking...

• Your body begins to heal from the effects of the nicotine within 12 hours after your last cigarette.

• Your heart and lungs start repairing the damage caused by cigarette smoke.

• You breathe easier and your smoker's cough starts to go away.

• You lower your risk for illness and death from heart disease, stroke, chronic bronchitis, emphysema, lung cancer, and other types of cancer.

• You contribute to cleaner air, especially for children who are at risk for illnesses because they breathe others' cigarette smoke.

What Can You Do to Avoid Gaining Weight When You Quit Smoking?

To avoid gaining weight when you quit smoking, you need to become more physically active and improve your eating habits before you stop. Physical activity helps to control your weight by increasing the number of calories your body uses. Making healthy changes to your eating habits will prevent weight gain by controlling the amount of calories you eat. Try to gradually improve your eating habits. Changing your eating habits too quickly can add to the stress you may feel as you try to quit smoking. Eating a variety of foods is a good way to improve your health. To make sure you get all of the nutrients needed for good health, choose a variety of foods from each group. The Nutrition Facts Label that is found on most processed food products can also help you select foods that meet your daily nutritional needs.

When You Are Ready to Quit Smoking

Pick a day to quit smoking during a non-stressful period. For example, try not to quit smoking during holiday seasons when you might be tempted to eat more. Quitting during a stressful time at work or at home might cause extra snacking or a smoking relapse. Try to focus on quitting smoking and healing your body. Your first goal should be to quit smoking and let your body heal from the effects of nicotine. After you feel better and are not smoking, work harder on improving your eating and physical activity habits to help you lose any weight that you might have gained.

After You Quit

Learn how to reduce cravings for both cigarettes and food. Once you stop smoking, it is important to learn how to handle cravings for cigarettes and food. Remember, a craving only lasts about 5 minutes. Consider these actions to help deal with your cravings.

• Replace smoking with other activities. Snack on fruit or sugarless gum to satisfy any sweet cravings. Keep your hands busy. Replace the action of holding cigarettes with activities like doodling, working puzzles, knitting, twirling a straw, or holding a pen or pencil.

• Drink less caffeine. Try to avoid drinking beverages that contain caffeine, such as sodas. Nicotine withdrawal will make you feel jittery and nervous, and the caffeine may only make nicotine withdrawal worse.

• Get enough sleep. When you feel tired, you are more likely to crave cigarettes and food.

• Reduce tension. To help relieve tension, relax by meditating, taking a walk, soaking in the tub, or taking deep breaths. Find something that will help you relax and replace the urge to smoke.

• Get support and encouragement. You need a lot of support when you quit smoking. Talk to a friend when you get the urge to smoke or join a support group such as Nicotine Anonymous. You can also participate in workshops offered by health care providers that will help you quit smoking. If you can, find a friend to quit with you for mutual support.

• Talk to your doctor about nicotine replacement. If you have significant withdrawal symptoms or are concerned about weight gain, talk to your doctor. Some nicotine replacement products, formerly available by prescription only, are now available over the counter. Using nicotine gum or a nicotine patch, along with improved eating habits and physical activity, will help you reduce your risk of a smoking relapse. Nicotine gum has been shown to delay weight gain after quitting. You may also want to talk to your doctor about prescription medications that are available to help you quit smoking.

• Try not to do things that tempt you to smoke or eat when you are not hungry. Keep a journal of where and when you feel most tempted to smoke and avoid these situations. Substitute healthy activities for smoking to help you avoid the urge to smoke or eat when you are not hungry.

• Try not to panic about modest weight gain. Accept some weight gain as a normal result of the nicotine leaving your body. Know that quitting smoking is the best thing that you can do for you and those around you. Improving your life-style as you stop smoking can help you prevent a large weight gain and become a healthy nonsmoker.

Choosing A Commercial Program

Almost any of the commercial weight-loss programs can work, but only if they motivate you sufficiently to decrease the amount of calories you eat or increase the amount of calories you burn each day (or both). What elements of a weight-loss program should an intelligent consumer look for in judging its potential for safe and successful weight loss?

Do diet programs work?

Approximately 8 million Americans a year enroll in some kind of structured weight-loss program involving liquid diets, special diet regimens, or medical or other supervision. In 1991, about 8,500 commercial diet centers were in operation across the country, many of them owned by a half-dozen or so well-known national companies.

Before you join such a program, you should know that according to published studies relatively few participants succeed in keeping off weight long-term. Recently, the FTC brought action against several companies challenging weight-loss and weight-maintenance claims. Unfortunately, some other companies continue to make overblown claims.

The FTC stopped one company from claiming its diet program caused rapid weight loss through the use of tablets that would "burn fat" and a protein drink mix that would adjust metabolism. The FTC also took action against three major programs using doctor supervised, very low-calorie liquid diets, and they agreed to stop making claims unless they could back them up with hard data.

Before you sign up with a diet program, you might ask these questions:

• What are the health risks?

• What data can you show me that proves your program actually works?

• Do customers keep off the weight after they leave the diet program?

• What are the costs for membership, weekly fees, food, supplements, maintenance, and counseling? What's the payment schedule? Are any costs covered under health insurance? Do you give refunds if I drop out?

• Do you have a maintenance program? Is it part of the package or does it cost extra?

• What kind of professional supervision is provided? What are the credentials of these professionals?

• What are the program's requirements? Are there special menus or foods, counseling visits, or exercise plans?

What are some clues to weight loss fraud?

It is important for consumers to be wary of claims that sound too good to be true. When it comes to weight-loss schemes, consumers should be particularly skeptical of claims containing words and phrases like:

easy
effortless
guaranteed
miraculous
magical
breakthrough
new discovery
mysterious
exotic
secret
exclusive
ancient

A Responsible and Safe Weight-Loss Program

A responsible and safe weight-loss program should be able to document for you the five following features:

1. The diet should be safe. It should include all of the Recommended Daily Allowances (RDAs) for vitamins, minerals, and protein. The weight-loss diet should be low in calories (energy) only, not in essential foodstuffs.

2. The weight-loss program should be directed towards a slow, steady weight loss unless your doctor feels your health condition would benefit from more rapid weight loss. Expect to lose only about a pound a week after the first week or two. With many calorie-restricted diets there is an initial rapid weight loss during the first I to 2 weeks, but this loss is largely fluid. The initial rapid loss of fluid also is regained rapidly when you return to a normal-calorie diet. Thus, a reasonable goal of weight loss must be expected.

3. If you plan to lose more than 15 to 20 pounds, have any health problems, or take medication on a regular basis, you should be evaluated by your doctor before beginning your weight-loss program. A doctor can assess your general health and medical conditions that might be affected by dieting and weight loss. Also, a physician should be able to advise you on the need for weight loss, the appropriateness of the weight-loss program, and a sensible goal of weight loss for you. If you plan to use a very-low-calorie diet (a special liquid formula diet that replaces all food intake for I to 4 months), you definitely should be examined and monitored by a doctor.

4. Your program should include plans for weight maintenance after the weight loss phase is over. It is of little benefit to lose a large amount of weight only to regain it. Weight maintenance is the most difficult part of controlling weight and is not consistently implemented in weight-loss programs. The program you select should include help in permanently changing your dietary habits and level of physical activity, to alter a life-style that may have contributed to weight gain in the past. Your program should provide behavior modification help, including education in healthy eating habits and long-term plans to deal with weight problems. One of the most important factors in maintaining weight loss appears to be increasing daily physical activity, often by sensible increases in daily activity, as well as incorporating an individually tailored exercise program.

5. A commercial weight-loss program should provide a detailed statement of fees and costs of additional items such as dietary supplements.

What is a Very Low-Calorie Diet (VLCD)?

VLCDs are commercially prepared formulas of 800 calories or less that replace all usual food intake. VLCDs are not the same as over-the-counter meal replacements, which are meant to be substituted for one or two meals a day. VLCDs, when used under proper medical supervision, effectively produce significant short-term weight loss in moderately to severely obese patients.

Who Should Use a VLCD?

VLCDs are generally safe when used under proper medical supervision in patients with a body mass index (BMI) greater than 30. BMI is a mathematical formula that takes into account both a person's height and weight. To calculate BMI, a person's weight in kilograms is divided by height in meters squared. Use of VLCDs in patients with a BMI of 27 to 30 should be reserved for those who have medical complications resulting from their obesity. VLCDs are not recommended for pregnant women or breast-feeding women. VLCDs are not appropriate for children or adolescents, except in specialized treatment programs. Very little information exists regarding the usage of VLCDs in older individuals. Because individuals over 50 already experience normal depletion of lean body mass, use of a VLCD may not be warranted. Additionally, persons over 50 may not tolerate the side effects associated with VLCDs because of preexisting medical conditions or need for other medications. Therefore, a physician, on a case by case basis, must evaluate increased risks and potential benefits of drastic weight loss in older individuals. Additionally, people with significant medical problems or who are on medications may be able to use a VLCD, but this too must be determined on an individual basis by a physician.

Health Benefits Associated With a VLCD

A VLCD may allow a severely to moderately obese patient to lose about 3 to 5 pounds per week, for an average total weight loss of 44 pounds over 12 weeks. Such a weight loss can improve obesity-related medical conditions, including diabetes, high blood pressure, and high cholesterol. Combining a VLCD with behavioral therapy and exercise may also increase weight loss and may slow weight regain. However, VLCDs are no more effective than more modest dietary restrictions in the long-term maintenance of reduced weight.

Adverse Effects Associated With a VLCD

Many patients on a VLCD for 4 to 16 weeks report minor side effects such as fatigue, constipation, nausea, and diarrhea, but these conditions usually improve within a few weeks and rarely prevent patients from completing the program. The most common serious side effect seen with VLCDs is gallstone formation. Gallstones, which often develop in obese people, anyway, (especially women), are even more common during rapid weight loss. Some research indicates that rapid weight loss appears to decrease the gallbladder's ability to contract bile. But, it is unclear whether VLCDs directly cause gallstones or whether the amount of weight loss is responsible for the formation of gallstones.

Overview of Dietary Supplements

What is a dietary supplement?

A dietary supplement is any product taken by mouth that contains a so-called "dietary ingredient" and its label clearly states that it is a dietary supplement. The "dietary ingredients" in dietary supplements may include vitamins, minerals, herbs, and amino acids as well as substances such as enzymes, organ tissues, metabolites, extracts or concentrates. Dietary supplements can be found in many forms such as pills, tablets, capsules, liquids or powders. They must be identified on the label as a dietary supplement.

How are dietary supplements regulated?

The label of a dietary supplement must contain enough information about the composition of the product so that consumers can make informed choices. The manufacturer must make sure the label information is truthful and not misleading. The manufacturer is also responsible for making sure that all the dietary ingredients in the supplements are safe. Manufacturers and distributors do not need to register with FDA or get FDA approval before producing or selling dietary supplements.

How do I report a problem or illness caused by a dietary supplement?

FDA can be contacted to report general complaints or concerns about food products, including dietary supplements. You may telephone or write to FDA. If you think you have suffered a serious harmful effect or illness from a dietary supplement, your health care provider can report this by calling FDA's MedWatch hotline at 1-800-FDA-1088.

Are advertisements for dietary supplements regulated by FDA?

No. The Federal Trade Commission (FTC) handles advertising for dietary supplements and most other products sold to consumers. FDA works closely with FTC in this area, but their work is directed by different laws.

Does FDA routinely analyze the content of Dietary Supplements?

FDA has limited resources to analyze the composition of food products, including dietary supplements. So, FDA focuses first on public health emergencies and products that may have caused injury or illness. Then products thought to be fraudulent or in violation of the law are analyzed. FDA uses the remaining funds for routine monitoring of products pulled from store shelves. FDA does not analyze supplement products before they are sold to consumers. The manufacturer is responsible for ensuring that the ingredient list is accurate and that the ingredients are safe. They are also required to make sure that the content matches the amount declared on the label. There are no rules that limit a serving size or the amount of nutrients in any form of dietary supplements. This decision is made by the manufacturer and does not require FDA review or approval. For one dietary ingredient, ephedrine alkaloids, FDA has proposed to permit serving sizes of 8 mg or less.

What kinds of claims can be made on the labels of Dietary Supplements?

As with other food products, the manufacturer can put certain claims on the product label. These claims tell consumers about the nutritional value of the product. Claims defined by FDA to describe the nutrient content of a product, like "good source" or "high", can appear on the label if one serving meets the definition. There are specific rules as to which substances can be listed using these nutrient content claims. Manufacturers can also put FDA-approved "health claims" on a product label. Health claims describe the connection between a nutrient or food substance and a disease or health-related condition. Claims about these diet/disease relationships can appear on the label if the content of the product meets the FDA requirements and if the claim is one of the approved health claims.

Why do some supplements have wording that says: "This statement has not been evaluated by the FDA. This product is not intended to diagnose, treat, cure, or prevent any disease"?

Certain statements may be included on the label that give the manufacturer's description of the role of the dietary supplement. These statements are not authorized by FDA. The manufacturer is responsible for ensuring that these statements are accurate and truthful. For this reason, the law says that if a dietary supplement label includes this information, it must also state that FDA has not evaluated the statement.

What are some of the questionable weight loss products?

Some dieters peg their hopes on pills and capsules that promise to "burn," "block," "flush," or otherwise eliminate fat from the system. But science has yet to come up with a low-risk "magic bullet" for weight loss. Some pills may help control the appetite, but they can have serious side effects. Other pills are utterly worthless.

The Federal Trade Commission (FTC) and a number of state Attorney General have successfully brought cases against marketers of pills claiming to absorb or burn fat.

The Food and Drug Administration (FDA) has banned 111 ingredients once found in over-the-counter diet products. None of these substances, which include alcohol, caffeine, dextrose, and guar gum, have proved effective in weight-loss or appetite suppression. Beware of the following products that are touted as weight-loss wonders:

• Diet patches, which are worn on the skin, have not been proven to be safe or effective. The FDA has seized millions of these products from manufacturers and promoters.

• "Fat blockers" purport to physically absorb fat and mechanically interfere with the fat a person eats.

• "Starch blockers" promise to block or impede starch digestion. Not only is the claim unproven, but users have complained of nausea, vomiting, diarrhea, and stomach pains.

• "Magnet" diet pills allegedly "flush fat out of the body." The FTC has brought legal action against several marketers of these pills.

• Glucomannan is advertised as the "Weight Loss Secret That's Been in the Orient for Over 500 Years." There is little evidence supporting this plant root's effectiveness as a weight-loss product.

• Some bulk producers or fillers, such as fiber-based products, may absorb liquid and swell in the stomach, thereby reducing hunger. Some fillers, such as guar gum, can even prove harmful, causing obstructions in the intestines, stomach, or esophagus. The FDA has taken legal action against several promoters containing guar gum.

• Spirulina, a species of blue-green algae, has not been proven effective for losing weight.

Phony weight-loss devices range from those that are simply ineffective to those that are truly dangerous to your health. At minimum, they are a waste of your hard-earned money. Some of the fraudulent gadgets that have been marketed to hopeful dieters over the years include:

• Electrical muscle stimulators have legitimate use in physical therapy treatment. But the FDA has taken a number of them off the market because they were promoted for weight loss and body toning. When used incorrectly, muscle stimulators can be dangerous, causing electrical shocks and burns.

• "Appetite suppressing eyeglasses" are common eyeglasses with colored lenses that claim to project an image to the retina which dampens the desire to eat. There is no evidence these work.

• "Magic weight-loss earrings" and devices custom-fitted to the purchaser's ear that purport to stimulate acupuncture points controlling hunger have not been proven effective.

Brief Review Of Weight-Loss Supplements

For some odd reason, the terms "natural" and "all natural" have become synonymous with "healthy." Nature is full of poisons. Nicotine is "all natural." Cyanide is found in nature. Dirt is natural, too. A substance that is advertised as "all natural" is not necessarily safe. In fact, many of the "all natural" products sold for weight loss are not only dangerous, they are useless, and cost even more than effective prescription medications. Little is known about many of them. We recommend that obese people refrain from using these supplements.

Ephedra

Many "weight loss" products sold in health food stores as fat burners contain *ma huang*, an ancient Chinese herbal remedy for asthma. In the 1920s, a pharmacologist isolated ephedrine from ma huang. Amphetamines were subsequently synthesized in an attempt to create more effective asthma drugs.

Ephedra is linked to hundreds of adverse reactions including sudden increases in blood pressure, headaches, irritability, heart irregularities, and even heart attacks and death. Liver problems have also occurred in users.

The exact amount and quality of ephedra in ma huang supplements may be unknown. The FDA has recommended that people take no more than 8 milligrams a day for one week maximum. However, most users far exceed the dosage and time limits.

St. John's Wort

Herbal fen-phen usually contains ma huang and St. John's Wort. St. John's Wort is a low grade inhibitor of serotonin reuptake. Mild depression is sometimes relieved by St. John's Wort and the combination with ma haung is an attempt to duplicate phentermine and Prozac. St. John's Wort is not increased in effectiveness with increased doses and the quality and quantity of the products are difficult to know.

Senna

Senna is a frequent ingredient in "weight loss teas." It produces weight loss (water) because it is a laxative.

Guarana & Kola

Lots of weight loss supplements contain guarana and kola. Both essentially contain caffeine.

How do you recognize quackery?

• Be wary if immediate, effortless or guaranteed results are promised.

• Look for telltale words and phrases such as "breakthrough," "miracle," "secret remedy," "exclusive," and "clinical studies prove that..."

• Beware of promotions for a single product claimed to be effective for a wide variety of ailments.

• Don't forget that, unlike scientists and health professionals, quacks do not subject their products to the scrutiny of scientific research. The quack simply thrusts a product onto the market in order to get your money.

• Be cautious of money-back guarantees, for a guarantee is only as good as the company that backs it.

• If it sounds too good to be true — it probably is.

Using Low-Calorie Sweeteners: Benefits of Use

Adapted from Calorie Control Council © 1999 by permission: www.caloriecontrol.org

SWEET CHOICES:

Why do people crave sweetness?

Research shows that people have an inborn desire for sweet taste, one of the four fundamental taste sensations. Newborn infants have been observed to react positively to sweetness. Also, studies with adults, as well as infants, have demonstrated that the pleasant response to sweet solutions is a reflex, innate reaction, rather than a learned response. Historical evidence, such as a 20,000-year-old cave painting of a neolithic man robbing a wild bees' nest, indicates that humans may always have had a preference for sweets. It also is likely that sweetness was used in early times as an indicator of safety in selecting foods. This phenomenon may have led to the search for sources of additional sweetness (sweeteners) to make foods more palatable.

How is the desire for sweetness satisfied?

Honey and fruits have long been sought out for their sweet taste; however, since it was first refined some 600 years ago, table sugar (sucrose) has been the standard for sweetness. Until recent decades, sucrose was virtually the only sweetener in general use. Currently, in the U.S., low-calorie sweeteners such as aspartame, saccharin, acesulfame potassium and sucralose provide alternatives to sucrose.

These sweeteners contribute few or no calories to the diet and are the primary sweetening agents for low-calorie and sugar-free foods and beverages. In addition, polyols, or "sugar alcohols," are appropriate for use in reduced-calorie products since they have caloric values which are lower than sucrose. Various caloric alternatives to sucrose also are being used in dietary foods and beverages, such as crystalline fructose and high fructose corn syrups. These sweeteners, however, contribute calories and may not always be suitable for various dietary and health needs.

What is the ideal sweetener?

The ideal sweetener is as sweet or sweeter than sucrose and has a pleasant taste with no aftertaste. Consumer acceptance of a sweetener is closely linked to how similar its taste is to sugar. The ideal sweetener also is colorless, odorless, readily soluble, stable, functional, economically feasible and does not promote dental cavities. It is nontoxic and is either metabolized normally or excreted from the body unchanged without contributing to any metabolic abnormalities, such as diabetes. Currently, the availability of a variety of low-calorie sweeteners allows the use of sweeteners either alone or in combination to achieve the requirements of the ideal sweetener.

What is a "low-calorie" sweetener?

A low-calorie sweetener provides consumers with a sweet taste without the calories or carbohydrates that come with sugar and other caloric sweeteners. Some low-calorie sweeteners, such as aspartame, are "nutritive," but are low in calories because of their intense sweetness. For example, because aspartame is 180 times sweeter than sucrose, the amounts needed to achieve the desired sweetness are so small that aspartame is considered virtually non-caloric. Many non-nutritive sweeteners, such as saccharin, are non-caloric because they are not metabolized and pass through the body unchanged. Currently, acesulfame potassium, aspartame, saccharin and sucralose are the only available low-calorie sweeteners in the United States.

Is there a need for low-calorie sweeteners?

Without low-calorie sweeteners, many of the reduced-calorie and light products that are in such great demand today would not be possible. A recent national consumer survey shows that more than 144 million Americans age 18 and over consume low-calorie/sugar-free foods and beverages — nearly double the number a decade ago. This wave of calorie consciousness has resulted in an exploding demand for low-calorie foods and beverages — what has been referred to as the "light revolution." Manufacturers currently are providing consumers with an increasing variety of low-calorie food and beverage choices.

What are the benefits and limitations of aspartame?

In addition to being low in calories, aspartame tastes very similar to sugar. It is 180 times sweeter than sugar and is appropriate for many food applications. Aspartame also enhances some flavors, and when combined with other sweeteners, it has a synergistic sweetening effect (the combination of the sweeteners is sweeter than the sum of the individual sweeteners). Aspartame loses sweetness with prolonged exposure to high temperatures of oven or range heat and over an extended period of time in liquids. However, it can be added successfully to recipes and an encapsulated form is now available for commercial baking.

Is aspartame safe?

Aspartame has been extensively studied in animals and humans for more than two decades in more than 100 studies. When FDA approved aspartame, it noted: "Few compounds have withstood such detailed testing and repeated, close scrutiny, and the process through which aspartame has gone should provide the public with additional confidence of its safety." Persons born with a rare genetic disease called phenylketonuria (PKU), numbering about 15,000 in the total U.S. population, know to restrict their intake of phenylalanine from all dietary sources. Because aspartame-containing products are a source of phenylalanine in the diet, they carry the labeling, "Phenylketonurics: Contains Phenylalanine." It should be noted, however, that phenylalanine is found in much greater quantities in meats, milk and other protein foods. In addition to the FDA, the Joint Expert Committee on Food Additives of the World Health organization, the Scientific Committee for Food of the European Union, and regulatory agencies in more than 100 countries have reviewed aspartame and found it safe for use. Additionally, a number of health groups, including the American Medical Association, the American Diabetes Association and the American Academy of Pediatrics Committee on Nutrition, have issued statements in support of aspartame.

What are the benefits and limitations of saccharin?

Saccharin, the oldest of the approved low-calorie sweeteners, continues to be important for a wide range of food and beverage applications. It is a very stable sweetener allowing for good product shelf life and, like aspartame, has a synergistic sweetening effect when combined with other sweeteners. Also, saccharin is 300 times sweeter than sucrose and is relatively inexpensive to manufacture. A slight aftertaste is perceived by some people. However, combining saccharin with another low-calorie sweetener helps eliminate any aftertaste.

Is saccharin safe?

Nearly a century of use in the food supply has allowed studies to determine if saccharin poses a risk to humans. More than 30 human studies have been completed and overwhelmingly support saccharin's safety. One study, of 9,000 individuals conducted by the National Cancer Institute, concluded that there was "no evidence of increased risk with the long-term use of artificial sweeteners (saccharin and cyclamate) in any form or with use that began decades ago." Saccharin is approved in more than 100 countries and has been determined safe by the Joint Expert Committee on Food Additives (JECFA) of the World Health Organization and the Scientific Committee for Food of the European Union. JECFA noted that the animal data which earlier raised questions about saccharin are not relevant to humans. Additionally, the extensive research on saccharin has been reviewed by many in the scientific community and by national health groups. These reviews have led to significant statements in support of saccharin. the case against saccharin still rests primarily on controversial high-dose rat studies in which a sensitive strain was fed the human equivalent of the sodium saccharin in hundreds of cans of diet soft drink a day for a lifetime. Even then, the tests produced bladder tumors only in some of the male rats at the highest doses. A panel of international scientists, which met at Duke University to review saccharin research, reported that "saccharin administered to the rat at high doses produces profound biochemical and physiological changes which do not occur in humans under normal patterns of use." The panel concluded that "the appearance of tumors in rats seems to be a species-and organ-specific phenomenon for which there is at present no explanation."

An extensive dose-response rat study, sponsored by the Calorie Control Council and conducted at the International Research and Development Corporation (IRDC), has further elucidated saccharin's safety at human levels of use by placing the rat data and its relevance to human health in proper perspective. The Duke panel noted: "The results of the IRDC study, by defining more sharply the dose-response relationship for bladder tumor risk in the rat, support the view that the present level of exposure of humans to saccharin, through its use as a food additive, presents an insignificant cancer risk."

Recent research further demonstrates saccharin is unlikely to cause cancer in humans. Saccharin's effects on the rat bladder relate to the salt form (sodium saccharin), diet, urine pH and sodium levels, protein concentrations and types of proteins, and the sex, age and strain of the rats fed sodium saccharin.

Other research indicates that the bladder tumors developed by male rats fed high doses of sodium saccharin are related to very high doses of the sodium salt and not saccharin per se. Sodium ascorbate (vitamin C) and sodium citrate, found in many foods and beverages, demonstrate similar effects.

What are the benefits and limitations of acesulfame potassium?

Acesulfame potassium (also known as

acesulfame K) was approved by FDA in 1988. It is a non-caloric sweetener and has a clean sweet taste that is 200 times sweeter than sugar. Acesulfame potassium's high degree of stability when exposed to heat and in liquids makes it a versatile sweetener with potential use in a wide range of foods and beverages.

Acesulfame potassium may be combined with other low-calorie sweeteners resulting in synergistic blends that provide improved taste profiles and overcome the slight aftertaste which may be noted otherwise with high concentrations in some products. Such blends also can provide economic and stability advantages.

Is acesulfame potassium safe?

Acesulfame potassium's safety is supported by more than 90 studies conducted over 15 years. In addition to the U.S., it has been reviewed and determined safe by regulatory authorities in about 90 countries — including Canada, the United Kingdom, France, Switzerland, Italy and Belgium — by the Joint Expert Committee on Food Additives of the World Health Organization, and by the Scientific Committee for Food of the European Union.

What about the newest low-calorie sweetener, sucralose?

Sucralose is the only non-caloric sweetener created from sugar. Its unique combination of sugar-like taste and excellent stability allow sucralose to be used as a sugar replacement in virtually every type of food and beverage. It is 600 times sweeter than sugar, so very little is needed to obtain the same sweetness intensity. On April 1, 1998, the U.S. Food & Drug Administration approved sucralose for use in 15 different food and beverage categories. (More information on sucralose.)

Why is there a need for more than one low-calorie sweetener?

The availability of a variety of sweeteners greatly increases low-calorie product choices. With several low-calorie sweeteners available, each can be used in the applications for which it is best suited. Also, by having a variety of sweeteners from which to choose, manufacturers can overcome sweetener limitations by using them in combination. Using the most appropriate sweetener, or combination of sweeteners, for a given product is known as the "multiple sweetener approach."

How does the "multiple sweetener approach" benefit consumers?

The multiple sweetener approach allows the low-calorie food and beverage industry to meet the growing consumer demand for additional good-tasting, reduced-calorie products. A limited choice of sweeteners results in limited options for the consumer. Research has shown that certain low-calorie sweeteners perform better in certain products than in others. A wide variety of low-calorie sweeteners provides products with improved taste, increased stability, lower manufacturing costs, and ultimately more choices for the consumer.

Is there an advantage to using more than one sweetener in a product?

Low-calorie sweeteners are synergistic, meaning that when one sweetener is combined with another, the resulting sweetness is greater than the sum of the individual sweeteners. In certain products, blending sweeteners can provide improved taste as well as economic and stability advantages. Sweetener blends, which were first introduced in the 1960s in diet soft drinks, are currently used in products such as gelatins, puddings, flavored coffees, gum and frozen desserts. Sweetener blends are widely popular in Europe and Canada.

What quantities of low-calorie sweeteners are consumed each year?

The amounts of low-calorie sweeteners consumed per capita are relatively very small, mainly because of their intense sweetness. Statistics from the U.S. Department of Agriculture show that the average combined consumption of low-calorie sweeteners is less than two ounces per person per year. This compares to nearly 150 pounds per capita consumption of sugar and other caloric sweeteners.

How do low-calorie sweeteners receive regulatory approval?

Before a low-calorie sweetener is approved for commercial use, it must undergo extensive testing (which can cost millions of dollars) and years of regulatory scrutiny. U.S. food safety laws prohibit FDA from approving a low-calorie sweetener (or any food ingredient) that has not been shown to be "safe," which the agency defines as "a reasonable certainty in the minds of competent scientists that the substance is not harmful under the intended conditions of use." The burden of demonstrating safety is on the petitioner requesting approval. The petitioner is required to provide FDA with extensive data, including the name, chemical identity and composition of the sweetener, the physical or other technical effects the sweetener is intended to produce, and comprehensive reports of research concerning safety. In addition to scientific evidence, FDA also considers projected consumption levels, as well as specific use levels requested in the petition.

Do consumers want reduced-calorie foods and beverages?

There has been a steady and significant increase in consumer demand for reduced-calorie products. Interestingly, a national consumer survey revealed that, despite the wide variety of reduced-calorie products available, nearly half the consumers of these products would like to see additional low-calorie foods and beverages in the marketplace. The fitness craze, which has grown into a national phenomenon, has brought with it an increasing number of converts to the light market. Also, an estimated 54 million adult Americans are dieting, primarily to control weight. For most dieters, the use of low-calorie food and beverage options is an important element of weight-control strategy.

Why do people consume low-calorie products?

Low-calorie products provide consumers with many benefits. Whether by choice or necessity, millions of Americans restrict their intake of calories, carbohydrates and fats. According to opinion research, most people consume low-calorie products to stay in better overall health, eat or drink healthier foods and beverages, maintain weight, reduce weight or maintain an attractive physical appearance. Most people use low-calorie products as part of an overall healthy lifestyle. Research also shows that health professionals believe low-calorie sweeteners are especially beneficial to obese individuals and those with diabetes. Low-calorie sweeteners also do not promote dental cavities.

Are low-calorie foods and beverages useful in controlling weight?

As part of an overall sensible weight-control program, low-calorie foods and beverages can help consumers control calories and therefore control weight. Health professionals agree that the key to losing weight is to burn more calories than are consumed, either by increasing physical activity or consuming fewer calories — or, preferably, both. Low-calorie foods and beverages provide consumers an alternative to higher-calorie, sugar-sweetened products. Recent studies support the effectiveness of low-calorie sweeteners in controlling caloric intake. In one recent study, researchers at Harvard Medical School concluded that aspartame "is a valuable adjunct to a comprehensive program of balanced diet, exercise and behavior modifications for losing weight."

Health professionals are increasingly reminding Americans that "calories still count" — foods and beverages containing low-calorie sweeteners can increase the variety of reduced-calorie choices in the diet.

Copyright © 1999 Calorie Control Council

Fat Replacers

Adapted from the Calorie Control Council
by permission
www.caloriecontrol.org

New Fat Replacers on the Horizon

Many consumers are striving to meet dietary recommendations to reduce fat and cholesterol intake. With more than twice the calories/gram of sugar, fats are the greatest hidden source of calories in food. (Fat is 9 calories/gram; sugar is 4.) New fat replacers are providing consumers with an expanding number of products that have excellent taste and texture with less fat, cholesterol and calories.

The fat replacers developed to date generally fall into one of three categories: carbohydrate based; protein based; or fat based. Most of the low-fat products introduced in recent years contain arbohydrate-based fat replacers (e.g., cellulose, maltodextrins, gums, modified starches, polydextrose). Carbohydrates have been used safely for many years as thickeners and stabilizers. These ingredients are also effective fat replacers in many formulated foods. They are not suitable for frying foods.

Protein-based fat replacers have received considerable public attention due to FDA's Generally Recognized As Safe (GRAS) approval of microparticulated protein. Protein-based ingredients have tremendous potential for use in a variety of products, especially frozen and refrigerated products. Although protein-based fat replacers are not suitable for frying foods, they can be used in many heat applications (e.g., cream soups, pasteurized products, baked goods).

Scientists have been able to chemically alter fatty acids to provide fewer or no calories, making fat-based fat replacers possible. Some fat-based fat replacers actually pass through the body virtually unabsorbed. These ingredients have the advantage of heat stability and offer excellent versatility, including use in frying. Currently, the availability of fat-based ingredients used in reduced-fat products is limited.

Pursuing the Mystery of Taste and Texture

While a food ingredient's functionality for a given product application may be one of many questions of interest to food technologists, its acceptability to consumers is based primarily on a single question: How does it taste?

The development of low-calorie and low-fat ingredients has been complicated by the fact that scientists really do not know much about the mechanism of taste. Thus it is difficult, if not impossible, to predict how a given ingredient will taste to all individuals.

A significant advantage of a multiple ingredient approach to calorie control is that manufacturers can look for and utilize the best "recipe," i.e., the low-calorie ingredient (or combination of ingredients) that is most pleasing for a given product. The result is a greater variety of low-calorie/low-fat foods and beverages that have the taste, texture and appeal of their traditional counterparts.

More Healthy Choices

Reduced-calorie and reduced-fat foods and beverages will not replace a person's need for moderation and overall good nutrition. However, they do provide palatable alternatives which can make the difficult task of reducing fat and calories in the diet easier. Thus, when incorporated into a nutritionally balanced diet, these products can contribute positively to a healthy lifestyle.

With increased knowledge about taste and technology, the food and beverage industry is on the verge of developing a wider variety of good-tasting, low-calorie and low-fat products to meet the growing needs and demands of American consumers. A limited choice of low-calorie ingredients results in limited options for consumers. On the other hand, a wide variety of low-calorie ingredients provides products with improved taste and texture, increased stability, lower manufacturing costs, and ultimately, more choices for the consumer. And that's good news for the growing number of calorie- and fat-conscious consumers.

Environmental Nutrition's Critique of Popular Weight Loss Programs

Diet Center

(Akron, OH) (800) 333-2581 www.dietcenterworldwide.com

Program Overall Approach: Personalized diet and exercise program, emphasizing healthy body composition. *Exclusively You* option based on supermarket foods; prepackaged cuisine optional. Minimum daily calorie level; 1,200. Vitamin and fiber supplements provided during reducing phase. *Concept 1000* option provides, 1,000 daily calories from three meal replacements (shakes or bars) and one regular meal. Some locations offer phentermine. Body composition analysis at the start and every 4 to 5 weeks.

Healthful Lifestyle Components: *Exclusively Me* behavior management program used in conjunction with one-to-one counseling sessions.

Staffing: Weekly consults with nonprofessional counselors, typically Diet Center graduates. Staff R.D., M.D. and board of health professionals design programs at corporate level.

Cost/Results: Fees average $30-$50/week, plus additional $17.50 a day for food for *Concept 1000* option. Maintenance averages $100/ year. Expected weight loss: no more than two pounds weekly. Length of reducing phase varies; one-year maintenance program recommended.

Pros: Emphasizes body composition, not pounds, as a measure of health. Choice of two diet plans; only Concept 1000 requires Diet Center foods.

Cons: Expensive. No professional guidance. No group support.

Health Management Resources

(Boston) (617) 357-9876 www.yourbetterhealth.com

Program Overall Approach: Makes use of a very-low-calorie diet (VLCD) consisting of fortified, high protein liquid meal replacements (520-800 calories/day) under medical supervision. *Healthy Solutions* plan (1,000-1,600 calories/day) combines meal replacements with regular foods, including optional prepackaged HMR entrees and five servings of fruits and vegetables daily. Mandatory weekly 90-minute group meetings (60 minutes during maintenance). Dieters assigned personal coaches for weekly meetings or calls. Receive health risk appraisal. VCLD requires written approval from an M.D. for patients with certain medical conditions, such as diabetes. Phentermine available.

Healthful Lifestyle Components: Recommends burning minimum of 2,000 calories/week in physical activity. Addresses lifestyle issues in weekly classes and personal counseling.

Staffing: Program developed by M.D.'s R.D.'s, R.N.'s and psychologists. Each location has at least one M.D. and health educator. Dieters of VLCD see M.D. or R.N. weekly.

Cost/Results: VLCD averages $150/week, but may be covered by insurance. *Healthy Solutions* averages $20/week plus cost of products. Maintenance averages $80/month. Expected weight loss: one to five pounds weekly. Reducing phase typically lasts 12-20 weeks; refeeding phase lasts 8. Maintenance recommended for up to 18 months.

Pros: Few eating decisions. Emphasizes exercise. Supervised by health professionals.

Cons: Expensive if not covered by insurance. Requires prepackaged food and strong commitment to exercise. May be difficult to transition to regular foods. Side effects of VLCD include intolerance to cold, constipation, dizziness, dry skin and headaches.

Jenny Craig

(La Jolla, CA) (619) 812-7000 www.jennycraig.com

Program Overall Approach: *ABC (About Better Choices)* program relies on Jenny Craig's Cuisine plus additional supermarket foods. 1,000 to 2,600 calories daily. Optional, weekly *Options Lifestyle* classes and one-to-one counseling. After losing half of goal weight, clients given option to transition to regular foods.

Healthful Lifestyle Components: Emphasizes increased physical activity, changing ingrained habits and balanced eating.

Staffing: Program developed by R.D.'s and psychologists. M.D.'s, R.D.'s and Ph.D's consult on program design. Non-professional staff counsels clients.

Cost/Results: Costs $99 to $299 to join (latter includes unlimited maintenance). *Jenny Craig's Cuisine* averages additional $70/week. Expected weight loss: up to two pounds weekly. Program length varies, depending on weight goal. Maintenance option of one year or unlimited.

Pros: Little food preparation required. Plans available for vegetarians, people with diabetes, breast-feeding moms and those on kosher diets.

Cons: Must rely on prepackaged foods, making dining out and socializing difficult. Lacks professional guidance at client level. Limited maintenance options.

Nutri/System

(Horsham, PA) (215) 442-5300 www.nutrisystem.com

Program Overall Approach: Diet based mostly on Nutri/System prepackaged foods. Reducing diet averages minimum of 1,200 calories/day for women; 1,500 for men. Maintenance diet based on optional purchase of prepackaged fare. Nutri/System's multivitamin/mineral supplement recommended for all dieters, but not included in price. Mostly one-to-one weekly counseling with weigh-in; some centers offer group classes. *Herbal Phen-Fen* and phentermine offered at some centers.

Healthful Lifestyle Components: Clients determine weekly goals with consultants, often focusing on exercise. Brochures on health topics available with three-month and 12 month programs. Exercise video and audio tapes available at extra cost.

Staffing: R.D.'s and health educator develop program. Ph.D. and M.D. consult on program design. L.P.N., R.N. or diet technician acts as personal consultant, providing guidance once a week for 15-20 minutes.

Cost/Results: One-month costs about $99; three months about $269; 12 months about $500. Food costs an additional $49-$69/week. Vitamin/mineral supplements also extra. Expected weight loss: no more than two pounds weekly. Program length varies according to weight-loss goals.

Pros: Few eating decisions.

Cons: Expensive. *Herbal Phen-Fen* can be dangerous. Weak on lifestyle education component. Little contact with health professionals.

Optifast
(Minneapolis) (800) 662-2540 www.optifast

Program Overall Approach: Medically supervised program of for-tified liquid meal replacements or prepackaged foods, eventually including regular foods. Dieters assigned one of three plans: 800, 900, or 1,200 calories daily. Mandatory weekly sessions promote positive eating behaviors. One-to-one counseling available. Some sites offer phentermine.

Healthful Lifestyle Components: Emphasizes changes in behavior and diet planning for "real" foods in group and counseling sessions.

Exercise physiologist available to help design personal exercise plan.

Staffing: Clients assigned a case manager who coordinates care. Dieters seen regularly by M.D., R.N., R.D. and psychologist; consulting exercise physiologist available. Group meeting leaders are psychologist or R.D.'s.

Cost/Results: Costs $1,500 to $3,000 depending on diet and desired weight loss. Price includes maintenance at some centers. Insurance may cover part of cost. Expected weight loss: no more than 2% of body weight weekly. Reducing phase lasts about 13 weeks; transition phase lasts about six. Maintenance begins at week 20 with no time limit.

Pros: Close contact with health professionals. Beneficial for people with serious health problems, who need low calorie level to promote quick weight loss. Few eating decisions.

Cons: Expensive if not covered by insurance. Must rely on Optifast products during much of the reducing phase. May be difficult to transition from liquid diet to regular food.

Overeaters Anonymous

(Rio Rancho, NM) (505) 891-2664 www.overeatersanonymous.org

Program Overall Approach: Nonprofit support group whose members are admitted compulsive eaters. Patterned after the 12-step Alcoholics Anonymous program. Addresses physical, emotional and spiritual aspects of overeating. Members encouraged to seek separate professional help for diet plan and dealing with emotional problems.

Healthful Lifestyle Components: Makes no recommendations for exercise or behavior change.

Staffing: Non-professional group members lead meetings and conduct activities.

Cost/Results: Makes no weight-loss claims. Unlimited length. Self-supporting with member contributions. Optional monthly journal, *Lifeline*, costs $12.99/year in U.S.

Pros: Inexpensive method of group support. No need to follow a specific diet plan. No weigh-ins.

Cons: Lacks professional guidance. OA stopped giving out diets in 1987, but some members still advocate unhealthy eating practices, including avoiding carbohydrates.

Registered Dietitian Consultation

(Milwaukee) (800) 932-8677 www.eatright.org

Program Overall Approach: Provides a personalized approach to weight control that takes into consideration your individual needs, including medical history, family situation, eating and exercise habits and preferences, travel and dining-out routines and budget.

Healthful Lifestyle Components: Exercise strongly encouraged as part of sensible weight control. R.D.'s help client identify barriers to weight loss and maintenance and provide healthy lifestyle education.

Staffing: R.D.'s have degrees in human nutrition or closely related area, plus practical experience, typically a hospital internship. Often have advanced degrees. Must pass accreditation exam and participate in continuing education.

Cost/Results: Costs $35 to $150 per hour; weight-control groups usually cost substantially less. Insurance may pay for visits. Expected weight loss: usually more than two pounds/week.

Pros: Eating prescription adapted to your lifestyle and medical history. Appropriate for any age group and entire families.

Cons: Expensive if not covered by insurance.

TOPS (Take Off Pounds Sensibly)
(Milwaukee) (800) 932-8677 www.tops.org

Program Overall Approach: Nonprofit organization whose members meet weekly in groups. Requires members to submit weight goals and diets in written form from health professionals. Provides peer support. Holds periodic contests and recognition programs for weight loss.

Healthful Lifestyle Components: Makes no specific lifestyle or exercise recommendations.

Staffing: Led by elected volunteer non-health professional who directs and organizes activities for one year. Health professionals may be invited to speak at weekly meetings.

Cost/Results: First visit free. $20 annual fee, which includes monthly *TOPS News*. Local weekly dues set by each chapter-about $5/month. No claims made for weight loss. Unlimited length.

Pros: Inexpensive form of group support. No purchases required. Has potential for long term participation.

Cons: Focuses on weight loss as chief measure of success. Must weigh in weekly. Groups vary widely in approach. Program lacks professional guidance.

Weight Watchers
(Woodbury, NY) (800) 651-6000 www.weight-watchers.com

Program Overall Approach: Emphasizes calorie-controlled, high-fiber eating and healthful lifestyle habits. *1-2-3 Success* program assigns members daily good point allotment, which averages 1,250-1,500 calories/day for women. Weekly group meetings with mandatory weigh-in. Need to lose at least five pounds to join.

Healthful Lifestyle Components: Emphasizes positive lifestyle changes, such as regular exercise. Encourages daily physical activity. *Tools For Living* helps members deal with personal beliefs about being overweight.

Staffing: M.D. and R.D.'s design and direct program. Group leaders are non-health professional program graduates.

Cost/Results: Costs $17-$20 to join, plus $10-$14 weekly, which entitles members to unlimited meetings for that week. Meetings free if you maintain goal weight within two pounds for six weeks. Expected weight loss: up to two pounds weekly.

Pros: Flexible, easy-to-use program offering group support. Plans available for vegetarians, teens and breast-feeding moms.

Cons: Lacks professional guidance at client level. No personalized counseling. Weekly weigh-ins.

Appendix C
Resources For Obesity & Eating Disorder Treatment & University Based Programs & Centers By State

Reprinted from National Institutes of Health Resources.

National Resources & Organizations

National Cancer Institute
Cancer Information Service
Phone: (800)-4-CANCER
E-mail: cis@icic.nci.nih.gov
Web: www.nci.nih.gov

National Heart, Lung, and Blood
Institute Information Center
P.O. Box 30105
Bethesda, MD 20824-0105
Phone: (301) 251-1222
E-mail: nhlbiic@dgsys.com
Web: www.nhlbi.nih.gov/nhlbi/nhlbi.htm

Office on Smoking and Health Centers
for Disease Control and Prevention
Mail Stop K-50
4770 Buford Highway, NE
Atlanta, GA 30341-3724
Phone: (770) 488-5705; (800) CDC-1311
E-mail: ccdinfo@cdc.gov
Web: www.cdc.gov/tobacco

American Lung Association
1740 Broadway
New York, NY 10019-4274
Phone: (212) 315-8700; (800) LUNG-USA
Web: www.lungusa.org

American Cancer Society
1599 Clifton Road, NE
Atlanta, GA 30329
Phone: (404) 320-3333; (800) ACS-2345
Web: www.cancer.org/frames.html

American Heart Association
National Center
7272 Greenville Avenue
Dallas, TX 75231
Phone: (800) AHA-USA1
Web: www.americanheart.org/

University-based Program List
Eating Disorder Programs and Services (by State)

California

• Center for Eating and Weight Disorders
San Diego State University
6363 Alvarado Court Suite 103
San Diego, CA 92120
(619) 594-3254 or (619) 594-3257 fax

• Loma Linda University
School of Medicine
Loma Linda, CA 92350
(909) 824-4505

• Stanford University School of Medicine
Department of Psychiatry TD209
Stanford, CA 94305
(650) 723-5868

• University of California, Los Angeles
760 Westwood Blvd.
Los Angeles, CA 90024
outpatient (310) 825-0478
inpatient (800) 825-9989

• University of California, San Francisco
School of Medicine
Langley Porter Psychiatric Institute
401 Parnassus Ave.
San Francisco, CA 94143
(415) 476-7394

Connecticut

• Yale Center for Eating and Weight Disorders
P.O. Box 208205
New Haven, CT 06520
(203) 432-4610

District of Columbia

• George Washington University
School of Medicine and Health Sciences
2150 Pennsylvania Ave NW
Washington, DC 20037
(202) 994-1709

• Georgetown University School of Medicine
3900 Reservoir Road, NW
Washington, DC 20007
(202) 687-8609
outpatient treatment only

•Georgetown University School of Medicine
Pediatric Eating Disorder Clinic
3800 Reservoir Road, NW
Washington, DC 20007
(202) 687-5437
Program: Children under the age of 18 for
over weight and eating disorders

Florida

• University of Florida College of Medicine
Box 100215 JHMHC
Gainesville, FL 32610
(352) 392-2055

• University of Miami School of Medicine
1600 NW 10th Avenue
P.O. Box 016099
Miami, FL 33101
(305) 243-4060

• University of South Florida College of
Medicine
3515 East Fletcher Ave
Tampa, FL 33613
(813) 974-2926

Georgia

• Emory University School of Medicine
Woodruff Health Sciences Center
Administration Building
1701 Clifton Road, NE
Atlanta, GA 30322
(404) 712-5628
outpatient treatment only

• Medical College of Georgia School of
Medicine Department of Psychiatry and
Health Behavior
1120 Fifteenth Street
Augusta, GA 30912-3800
(706) 721-6716 ask for Dr. Lemon

Hawaii

• University of Hawaii
John A. Burns School of Medicine
1960 East-West Road
Honolulu, HI 96822
(808) 983-8368

Illinois

• Eating Disorders Program for the Treatment of
Anorexia, Bulimia, and Obesity
Northwestern Medical Faculty Foundation
Department of Psychiatry and Behavioral Sciences
303 East Ohio Street, Suite 550
Chicago, IL 60611
(312) 908-7850

• Rush Presbyterian St. Luke's Medical Hospital
Rush University Nutrition Clinic
1725 West Harrison, Suite 129
Chicago, IL 60612
(312) 942-3438

• Southern Illinois University School of Medicine
Memorial Medical Center
701 North First Street
P.O. Box 19230
Springfield, IL 62781
(217) 788-3670

• University of Chicago
Division of Biological Sciences
Pritzker School of Medicine
5841 South Maryland Avenue
Chicago, IL 60637
(773) 702-9277

• University of Illinois College of Medicine
Eating Disorders Clinic
P.O. Box 6998 (M/C 784)
Chicago, IL 60680
(312) 996-3070

Iowa

• University of Iowa Hospital and Clinic
John Papa John Pavillion, 2nd Floor
Iowa City, IA 52242
(319) 356-1354

Kansas

• University of Kansas School of Medicine
3901 Rainbow Boulevard
Kansas City, KS 66160-7300
(913) 588-6400 - Treatment on an individual basis.

Kentucky

• University of Kentucky College of Medicine
A.B. Chandler Medical Center
800 Rose Street (MN-150)
Lexington, KY 40536-0084
(606) 323-6021 ext. 259

• University of Louisville
School of Medicine
Health Sciences Center
Norton Psychiatric Clinic, 6th Floor
Louisville, KY 40203
(502) 629-8850

Louisiana

• Louisiana State University School of
Medicine at Shreveport
Outpatient Clinic
1820 Jordan St.
Shreveport, LA 71101
(318) 676-5175

Maryland

• Johns Hopkins School of Medicine
Eating and Weight Disorders Center
720 Rutland Avenue
Baltimore, MD 21205
(410) 955-3863

Massachusetts

• Tufts University School of Medicine
New England Medical Center
Eating Disorders Clinic
750 Washington Street
Boston, MA 02111
(617) 636-5750

• University of Massachusetts Medical School
55 Lake Avenue North
Worcester, MA 01655
(508) 856-5610

Michigan

• Michigan State University College of
Human Medicine
A-110 East Fee Hall
East Lansing, MI 48823
(517) 353-6654

Missouri

• Saint Louis University Health Sciences Center
School of Medicine
St. Louis Behavioral Medicine Institute
1129 Macklind
St. Louis, MO 63110
(314) 534-0200

• BJC Home Center
605 Old Ballas Suite 250
Creve Ceur, MO 63141
(314) 534-0200

Minnesota

• Eating Disorder Research Program
University of Minnesota
2701 University Avenue, SE, Suite 206
Minneapolis, MN 55414
(612) 626-6188

• Mayo Medical School
200 First Street, SW
Rochester, MN 55905
(507) 266-5100

Mississippi

• University of Mississippi School of Medicine
2500 North State Street
Jackson, MS 39216
(601) 984-5805

Nebraska

• Creighton University School of Medicine
Eating Disorders Clinic
45th and Dewey
Clarkson Medical Center
Omaha, NE 68178
(402) 559-5088

• University of Nebraska Medical Center
Eating Disorders Program
600 South 42nd Street
Omaha, Nebraska 68198-5600
(402) 559-5524

New Hampshire

• Dartmouth Medical School
Department of Behavioral Medicine
1 Medical Center Drive
Lebanon, NH 03756
(603) 650-7520

New Jersey

• Rutgers Eating Disorders Clinic
Rutgers University
41 Gordon Road
Piscataway, NJ 08854
(732) 445-2292

• University of Medicine and Dentistry of
New Jersey
Robert Wood Johnson Medical School
675 Hoes Lane
Piscataway, NJ 08854-5635
(732) 235-7578

New York

• Albany Medical College
Department of Medicine
Division of Clinical Nutrition and Pediatric
Gastroenterology
47 New Scotland Ave., A23
Albany, NY 12208-3479
(518) 262-5299

• Albany Medical College
47 New Scotland Avenue
Albany, NY 12208
(518) 262-5299
treats children with bulimia nervosa

• Eating Disorders Clinic
New York State Psychiatric Institute
Columbia Presbyterian Medical Center
722 W. 168th Street, Unit #98
New York, NY 10032
(212) 543-5739

• Program for Managing Eating Disorders
Gracey Memorial Hospital
420 East 76th Street
New York, NY 10024
(212) 434-5584

• Ben Rush
650 South Salina Street
Syracuse, NY 13202
(315) 476-2161

• University of Rochester School of Medicine
and Dentistry
Strong Memorial Hospital
Eating Disorder Clinic
601 Elmwood Avenue
Rochester, NY 14642
(716) 275-7886

North Carolina

• Bowman Gray School of Medicine of Wake
Forest University
Medical Center Boulevard
Winston-Salem, NC 27157
(910) 716-4635

• Duke University School of Medicine
P.O. Box 3005
Durham, NC 27710
(919) 660-7440

North Dakota

• University of North Dakota School of Medicine
120 South 8th Street Suite 1
Fargel, ND 58103
(701) 234-5111 or (800) 437-4010 ext. 4111

Ohio

• Wright State University School of Medicine
3640 Kernel Glen Highway
Dayton, OH 45435
(937) 775-3333

Oregon

• Oregon Health Sciences University School
of Medicine
3181 S.W. Sam Jackson Park Road
Portland, OR 97201-3098
(503) 494-6176

Pennsylvania

• Binge Eating Program/Eating Disorders Clinic
Western Psychiatric Institute and Clinic
3811 O'Hara Street
Pittsburgh, PA 15213
(412) 624-5420

• Jefferson Medical School of Thomas
Jefferson University
1025 Walnut Street
Philadelphia, PA 19107-5083
(215) 955-6912

• Pennsylvania State University College of
Medicine
Eating Disorders Program
500 University Drive, P.O. Box 850
Hershey, PA 17033
(717) 531-7380

• University of Pennsylvania School of Medicine
Weight and Eating Disorders Program
3600 Market Street, Suite 738
Philadelphia, PA 19104-2648
(215) 898-7314

South Carolina

• Medical University of South Carolina
College of Medicine
171 Asley Avenue
Charleston, SC 29425
(803) 792-0092

Tennessee

• The Institute for Nutrition Research
The Kim Dayani Human Performance Center
Vanderbilt University Medical Center
1500 22nd Avenue South
Nashville, TN 37232-8285
(615) 936-3952

• University of Tennessee at Memphis
College of Medicine
135 North Pauline
Memphis, TN 38163
(901) 448-2474

Texas

• Behavioral Medicine Research Center
Baylor College of Medicine
6535 Fannin Street, MS F700
Houston, TX 77030
(713) 770-3600

•Eating Disorder Program
Department of Psychiatry , Medical School
Univ. of Texas Health Science Center at San Antonio
7703 Floyd Curl Drive
San Antonio, TX 78284-7792
(210) 567-5450

•Scott and White,
2401 South 31st Street
Temple, TX 76508
(254) 724-2585

•Self Help Group
10th and Poke
Amarillo, TX 79106
(806) 354-5620

•Texas Tech University Health Sciences Center
4800 Alberta Avenue
El Paso, TX 79905
(915) 533-2471

•University of Texas Medical Branch
University of Texas Medical School at Galveston
301 University Boulevard
Galveston, TX 77555
(409) 747-5756

•University of Texas Medical School at San Antonio
Nutrition Department
7703 Floyd Curl Drive
San Antonio, TX 78284-7790
(210) 567-5450

•University of Texas Southwestern at Dallas
Southwestern Medical School
5323 Harry Hines Boulevard
Dallas, TX 75235
(214) 648-3898

Washington

• Ballard Swedish Hospital
5300 Tallman Ave, NW
Seattle, WA 98195
(206) 782-2700

West Virginia

• Marshall University School of Medicine
Department of Psychiatry
1801 Sixth Avenue
Huntington, WV 25755-9000
(304) 696-7148

Adult Weight-control Programs and Services (by State)

Alabama

• University of Alabama at Birmingham
The Kirklin Clinic
2000 6th Avenue South
Birmingham, AL 35233
(205) 934-5112

• University of South Alabama College of Medicine
Family Practice
307 University Boulevard
Mobile, AL 36688
(334) 434-3475

Arkansas

• University of Arkansas
College of Medicine, Endocrine Obesity
4301 West Markham Street
Little Rock, AR 72205
(501) 686-7911

California

• Center for Eating and Weight Disorders
San Diego State University
Joint Doctoral Program
6363 Alvarado Court
Suite 103
San Diego, CA 92120
(619) 594-3254
(619) 594-3257 (fax)

• Loma Linda University
Center for Health Promotion
Weight Management Center
Loma Linda, CA 92350
(909) 824-4959

• The Medical Center at the University of
California, San Francisco
UCSF Weight Management Programs
Box 0212/M294
San Francisco, CA 94143
(415) 476-9987

• Obesity Treatment Center
Affiliated with the University of California, Davis
Division of Clinical Nutrition
1325 Howe Avenue, Suite 102
Sacramento, CA 95825
(916) 925-0300

• Stanford University School of Medicine
300 Pasteur Drive
Stanford, CA 94305
(650) 732-2300

• The UCI Weight Management Program
University of California, Irvine, Medical Center
Route 81
101 The City Drive Orange, CA 92668
(714) 824-8770

• University of California, Los Angeles
School of Medicine, Clinical Nutrition
10833 Le Conte Avenue
Los Angeles, CA 90024
(310) 206-1987

• University of California, San Diego
Medical Center
200 West Arbor Drive
San Diego, CA 92103-8802
(619) 543-6222

• Western Institute for Health Maintenance
Physicians' Weight Reduction Center
14104 Magnolia Boulevard
Sherman Oaks, CA 91423
(818) 501-3881

Colorado

• University of Colorado School of Medicine
4200 East 9th Avenue, E151
Denver, CO 80262
(303) 372-7240

Connecticut

• Guilford Nutrition Center
Affiliate of Yale-New Haven Hospital
450 Boston Post Road
Guilford, CT
(203) 458-2875

• University of Connecticut Health Center
Nutrition Counseling Service
263 Farmington Avenue
Farmington, CT 06030
(860) 679-3245

• Yale-New Haven Hospital
Centers of Nutrition
20 York Street
New Haven, CT 06504
(203) 688-2422

District of Columbia

• George Washington University Obesity
Management Program
3 Washington Circle, NW, Suite 208
Washington, DC 20037
(202) 223-3077

Florida

• University of Florida College of Medicine
Weight Loss Clinic
Box 100215 JHMHC
Gainesville, FL 32610
(352) 395-0213

Georgia

•Emory University School of Medicine
Emory Clinic-Nutrition Services
1365 Clifton Road
Atlanta, GA 30322
(404) 778-3719

•Medical College of Georgia School of Medicine
1120 Fifteenth Street
Augusta, GA 30912
(706) 721-6716

Hawaii

• University of Hawaii John A. Burns School
of Medicine
1907 South Beretania
Honolulu, HI 96822
(808) 535-7000

Illinois

• Loyola University Medical Center
Center for Preventive and Rehabilitative Services
Nutrition Assessment Clinic
8601 West Roosevelt Road
Forest Park, IL 60130
(708) 216-9103

• Rush Presbyterian St. Luke's Medical
Center
Rush University
Nutrition Clinic
1725 West Harrison, Suite 129
Chicago, IL 60612
(312) 942-3438

• University of Chicago
Nutrition and Weight Control Clinic
5841 South Maryland Avenue
MC 4080
Chicago, IL 60637
(773) 702-1000

• University of Illinois College of Medicine
at Urbana-Champaign
1802 South Mattis Avenue
Champaign, IL 61821
Carle Weight Manager Center
(217) 373-1480

Iowa

• University of Iowa College of Medicine
200 Medicine Administration Building
Iowa City, IA 52242-1101
(319) 356-1616

Kansas

• University of Kansas School of Medicine
3901 Rainbow Boulevard
Kansas City, KS 66160-7300
(913) 588-5200

Kentucky

• University of Kentucky College of Medicine
A.B. Chandler Medical Center
800 Rose Street (MN-150)
Lexington, KY 40536-0084
HMR Program: (606) 323-6824

Louisiana

• Louisiana State University of Medicine
in New Orleans
Weight Management Center
3715 Prytania Street
New Orleans. Louisiana 70115
(504) 896-3163

• Louisiana State University School of
Medicine in Shreveport
1501 Kings Highway
Shreveport, LA 71130
(318) 675-5138

Maryland

• The Johns Hopkins Weight Management Center
(On the campus of Johns Hopkins Bayview
Medical Center)
Triad Technology Center
333 Cassell Drive
Baltimore, MD 21224
(410) 550-2330

Massachusetts

• Brigham and Women's Hospital
Cardiac Risk Reduction Center
850 Boylston Street, Suite 130
Chestnut Hill, MA 02167
(617) 278-0770

• Evans Medical Group of University Hospital
An Affiliate of Boston University School of Medicine
720 Harrison Avenue
Doctors Office Building, Suite 607
Boston, MA 02118
(617) 638-5980

Michigan

• Michigan State University College of
Human Medicine
Sparrows Hospital
300 N. Clipper St. Suite 15
Lansing, MI 48823
(517) 333-7007

- University of Michigan Medical Center
Obesity Rehabilitation Program
5570 MSRB-2, Box 0678
Ann Arbor, MI 48109-0678
(313) 936-5035

Minnesota

- Mayo Medical School Diet Clinic
200 First Street, SW
Rochester, MN 55905
(507) 284-4990

- University of Minnesota Hospital and Clinic
Nutrition Services
Box 84
Minneapolis, MN 55455
(612) 626-4876

Missouri

- Saint Louis University Health Sciences Center
St. Louis Behavioral Medicine Institute
1129 Macklind
St. Louis, MO 63110
(314) 534-0200-General Intake System

- University of Missouri - Columbia School of Medicine
MA204 Medical Sciences Building
One Hospital Drive
Columbia, MO 65203
(573) 882-3818

- Washington University School of Medicine
4570 Childrens Place
Saint Louis, MO 63101
(314) 747-4747

Nebraska

- University of Nebraska College of Medicine
600 South 42nd Street
Omaha, NE 68198
(402) 559-8700

Nevada

- Nutrition Associates Weight Management Center
University of Nevada School of Medicine
Redfield Building - 153
Reno, Nevada 89557
(702) 784-4474

New Hampshire

- Dartmouth Medical Center
1 Medical Center Drive
Lebanon, NH 03756
(603) 650-8630

New Jersey

- Univ. of Medicine and Dentistry of New Jersey
Robert Wood Johnson Medical School
675 Hoes Lane
Piscataway, NJ 08854-5635
(732) 828-3000 ext. 2751

New York

- Albany Medical Center Weight
Management Program
Albany Medical College
47 New Scotland Avenue, A-23
Albany, NY 12208
(518) 262-5299

- Cornell University Medical College
Diet and Nutrition Center
1300 York Avenue
New York, NY 10021
(212) 746-5454 X60838

- Mount Sinai School of Medicine of the City
University of New York
One Gustave L. Levy Place
Annenberg Building, Room 450
Box 1180
New York, NY 10029-6574
(212) 241-6162

- New York University School of Medicine
Department of Nutrition and Weight
Management
560 First Street
New York, NY 10016
(212) 263-7007

- The Presbyterian Hospital
Columbia-Presbyterian Medical Center
Behavioral Medicine Program
Weight Control Program
New York, NY 10032-3784
(212) 543-5739

- St. Luke's-Roosevelt Institute for Health Sciences
425 West 59th St. Suite 9D
New York, NY 10019
(212) 523-8440

- State University of New York at Stony Brook
Dietary Nutrition Office
Stony Brook Hospital
Nichols Road
Stony Brook, NY 11794
(516) 444-1440

- Weight Management Center
  Strong Memorial Hospital
  University of Rochester
  601 Elmwood Avenue, Box 693
  Rochester, NY 14642
  (716) 275-1630

North Carolina

- East Carolina University
  School of Medicine
  Department of Medicine
  Greenville, NC 27858-4354
  (919) 816-3229

- Duke University Medical Center
  Rice Diet Program
  1821 Green Street
  Durham, NC 27705
  (919) 286-2243

- The North Carolina Baptist Hospitals
  Department of Clinical Nutrition
  Medical Center Boulevard
  Winston-Salem, NC 27157
  (910) 716-7984

Ohio

- Medical College of Ohio
  Department of Family Medicine
  1015 Garden Lake Parkway
  Toledo, OH 43614
  (419) 381-5545

- Ohio State University Medical Center
  Comprehensive Weight Management Program
  495 McCampbell Hall
  1581 Dodd Drive
  Columbus, OH 43210-1296
  (614) 292-1001

- University Hospital of Cleveland
  Department of Psychiatry
  1110 Euclid Avenue
  Cleveland, OH 44106
  (216) 844-8550

- Wright State University School of Medicine
  3640 Kernel Glen Highway
  Dayton, OH 45435
  (937) 775-3333

Oklahoma

- University College of Medicine - Tulsa
  2808 South Sheridan
  Tulsa, OK 74129-1077
  (918) 582-1980

- University of Oklahoma College of Medicine
  P.O. Box 26901
  Oklahoma City, OK 73901
  (405) 271-5300

Oregon

- Providence Health System
  Health and Life Style Center
  1885 NW 185th Ave
  Aloha, OR 97006
  (503) 645-4864

Pennsylvania

- The Milton S. Hershey Medical Center The
  Pennsylvania State University
  University Weight Management Center
  University Hospital
  P.O. Box 850
  Hershey, PA 17033
  (717) 531-6390

- Thomas Jefferson University Hospital
  Department of Nutrition and Dietetics
  Outpatient Nutrition Services
  1015 Chestnut Street, Suite 110
  Philadelphia, PA 19107-4302
  (215) 955-5077

- University of Pennsylvania School of Medicine
  Weight and Eating Disorders Program
  3600 Market Street, Suite 738
  Philadelphia, PA 19104-2648
  (215) 898-7314

- University of Pittsburgh Medical Center
  Obesity/Nutrition Research Center
  WPIC-UPMC
  3811 O'Hara Street
  Pittsburgh, PA 15213-9937
  (412) 383-1431

- Binge Eating Program
  Western Pyschiatric Institute and Clinic
  3811 O'Hara St.
  Pittsburgh, PA 15213
  (412) 624-5420

Rhode Island

• Weight Management Program
Miriam Hospital
Center for Behavioral Medicine
Affiliated with Brown University School of Medicine
164 Summit Avenue
Providence, Rhode Island 02906
(401) 793-2950

South Carolina

• University of South Carolina School of Medicine
Family Practice
6 Richmond Medical Park
Columbia, SC 29203
(803) 434-6116

South Dakota

• University of South Dakota School of Medicine
University Physician's Clinic
3701 West 49th, Suite 101
Sioux Falls, SD 57106
(605) 361-6229

Tennessee

• The Institute for Nutrition Research
The Kim Dayani Human Performance Center
Vanderbilt University Medical Center
607 Medical Arts Building
Nashville, TN 37232-1320
(615) 936-3952

• Meharry Medical College School of Medicine
Center for Nutrition
1005 Dr. D.B. Todd, Jr. Boulevard
Nashville, TN 37208
(615) 327-6037

• University of Tennessee College of Medicine
800 Madison Avenue
Memphis, TN 38163
(901) 448-6781

Texas

• Texas A&M University Health Science Center
Scott and White Clinic
1600 University Drive East
College Station, TX 77840
(409) 691-3322

• University of Texas Southwestern
Medical Center at Dallas
5323 Harry Hines Boulevard
Dallas, TX 75235
(214) 648-1520

Utah

• University Hospital in Salt Lake City
Nutrition Care Service
AB190 University Hospitals
50 North Medical Drive
Salt Lake City, UT 84132
(801) 581-2155

Vermont

• University of Vermont College of Medicine
Burlington, VT 05405
(802) 656-0668

Virginia

• University of Virginia
Health Sciences Center
Department of Nutrition Services
Box 273-59
Charlottesville, VA 22908
(804) 924-2286

• Virginia Commonwealth University
Nutrition Clinic
1200 East Marshall Street
P.O. Box 980046
Richmond, VA 23298-0046
(804) 828-0970

Washington

• University of Washington School of Medicine
Seattle, WA 98195
(206) 548-4615

West Virginia

• Department of Family and Community Health
Marshall University School of Medicine
Family Practice Center
1801 6th Avenue
Huntington, WV 25703
(304) 696-7000

• West Virginia University Department of Medicine
Health Sciences Center North
Morgantown, WV 26506-9169
(304) 293-6883

Wisconsin

• University of Wisconsin-Madison Medical School
Clinical Nutrition Obesity Program
W.O. Beers Clinical Nutrition Center
1415 Linden Drive
Madison, WI 53706-1571
(608) 265-5305

University-based Program List
Weight-control Information Network Programs

- Behavioral Medicine
Stanford University School of Medicine
Department of Psychiatry TD209
Stanford, CA 94305
Tel: (415) 723-5868

- Binge Eating Program
Western Psychiatric Institute and Clinic
3811 O'Hara Street
Pittsburgh, PA 15213
Tel: (412) 624-2823

- Eating Disorders Clinic
New York State Psychiatric Institute
Columbia Presbyterian Medical Center
722 W. 168th Street
Unit #98
New York, NY 10032
Tel: (212) 960-5739/5746

- Eating Disorder Research Program
University of Minnesota
2701 University Avenue, S.E.
Suite 102
Minneapolis, MN 55414
Tel: (612) 627-4494

- Nutrition Research Clinic
Baylor College of Medicine
6535 Fannin Street
MS F700
Houston, TX 77030
Tel: (713) 798-5757

- Rutgers Eating Disorders Clinic
GSAPP, Rutgers University
Box 819
Piscataway, NJ 08854
Tel: (908) 932-2292

- Women's Recovery Center
110 N. Essex Avenue
Narberth, PA 19072
Tel: (215) 664-5858

- Yale Center For Eating and Weight Disorders
P.O. Box 11A, Yale Station
New Haven, CT 06520
Tel: (203) 432-4610

University-based Program List
Weight-control Information Network Child/Adolescent Weight-control Programs and Services (by State)

Arizona

- University of Arizona College of Medicine
Arizona Health Sciences Center
1501 North Campbell Avenue
Tucson, AZ 85724
(502) 694-5766

Arkansas

- University of Arkansas College of Medicine
Children's Hospital
Clinical Nutrition
800 Marshall St.
Little Rock, AR 72202
(501) 320-3519

California

- Center for Child and Adolescent Obesity
Department of Family and Community Medicine
University of California, San Francisco
MU3 East, Box 0
San Francisco, CA 94143-0900
(415) 476-1482 ask for Laura Mellon

- Loma Linda University
Center for Health Promotion
Child and Adolescent Weight Management
Loma Linda, CA 92350
(909) 558-8142 ask for Larry Yin

Connecticut

- Guilford Nutrition Center
Affiliate of Yale-New Haven Hospital
450 Boston Post Road
Guilford, CT
(203) 458-2875

- Yale-New Haven Hospital
Centers of Nutrition
20 York Street
New Haven, CT 06504
(203) 688-2422

District of Columbia

- Georgetown University School of Medicine
Eating Disorder Clinic
3900 Reservoir Rd., NW
Washington, DC 20007
(202) 687-5437

Florida

• University of Florida
Department of Pediatrics
Adolescent and Young Adult Program
Weight Management Program
P.O. Box 100296
Gainesville, FL 32610-0296
(352) 392-3641

• University of South Florida
College of Medicine
12901 Bruce B. Downs Blvd. * Box 66
Tampa, FL 33612-4799
(813) 272-2682

Hawaii

• University of Hawaii John A. Burns School
of Medicine
1907 South Beretania
Honolulu, HI 96822
(808) 535-7000

Illinois

• Northwestern University Medical School
Children's Memorial Hospital Nutrition Clinic
303 East Chicago Ave.
Chicago, IL 60611-3008
(773) 880-4000

• Rush Presbyterian St. Luke's Medical Center
Rush University Nutrition Clinic
1725 West Harrison, Suite 129
Chicago, IL 60612
(312) 942-3438

• Southern Illinois University School of Medicine
St. John's Wellness Program
801 North Rutledge
P.O. Box 19230
Springfield, IL 62794-9230
(217) 535-3990 or (217) 524-0654

Iowa

• University of Iowa College of Medicine
200 Medicine Administration Building
Iowa City, IA 52242-1101
(319) 356-2213

Kentucky

• University of Kentucky College of Medicine
A.B. Chandler Medical Center
Pediatric Gastroenterology
800 Rose Street (MN-150)
Lexington, KY 40536-0084
(606) 323-6021

Maryland

• The Johns Hopkins Weight Management Center
(On the campus of Johns Hopkins Bayview
Medical Center)
Triad Technology Center
333 Cassell Drive
Baltimore, MD 21224
(410) 550-2330

Massachusetts

• Harvard Medical School
25 Shattuck Street
Boston, MA 02115
(617) 355-7612 or (617) 355-6177

Michigan

• Wayne State University School of Medicine
540 East Canfield
Detroit, MI 48201
(248) 213-2872

Minnesota

• Mayo Medical School , Mayo Clinic
200 First Street, SW
Rochester, MN 55905
(507) 284-2091

Missouri

• Saint Louis University Health Sciences Center
School of Medicine
St. Louis Behavioral Medicine Institute
1129 Macklind
St. Louis, MO 63110
(314) 534-0200-General Intake System

• Washington University School of Medicine
660 South Euclid Avenue
Saint Louis, MO 63101
(314) 454-KIDS

Nebraska

• Creighton University School of Medicine
Weight Management Clinic
California at 24th Street
Omaha, NE 68178
(402) 280-4580

New Jersey

• University of Medicine and Dentistry of New Jersey
Robert Wood Johnson Medical School
675 Hoes Lane
Piscataway, NJ 08854-5635
(732) 828-3000

New Mexico

• University of New Mexico School of Medicine
Albuquerque, NM 87131
(505) 272-5551
ask for Kristin Bennett

New York

• Albany Medical College Department of Medicine
Division of Clinical Nutrition and Pediatric
Gastroenterology
47 New Scotland Avenue, A23
Albany, NY 12208-3479
(518) 262-5299

• The Childhood Weight Control Program
University at Buffalo
State University of New York
Department of Psychology
235 Park Hall
Buffalo, NY 14260-4110
(716) 645-6316
overweight ages 8-13

• Mount Sinai School of Medicine of the City
University of New York
One Gustave L. Levy Place
New York, NY 10029-6574
(212) 241-7855

• New York Medical College
Department of Endocrinology
Valhalla, NY 10595
(914) 594-4602

• State University of New York
Health Sciences Center at Brooklyn
College of Medicine
450 Clarkson Avenue, Box 97
Brooklyn, New York 11203
(718) 270-1647

• State University of New York
Health Sciences Center at Syracuse
College of Medicine
750 East Adams Street
Syracuse, NY 13210
Adolescent program: (315) 464-5831
Pediatric nutritionist: (315) 464-4220

• University of Rochester School of Medicine
601 Elmwood Avenue
Rochester, NY 14642
(716) 275-7964

North Carolina

• Duke University Medical Center
Rice Diet Program
1821 Green Street
Durham, NC 27705
(919) 286-2243

•University of North Carolina at Chapel Hill
School of Medicine
Pediatric Weight Control and Nutrition Clinic
Chapel Hill, NC 27599
(919) 966-6669
ages 12-18

Ohio

• Medical College of Ohio
Department of Family Medicine
P.O. Box 10008
Toledo, OH 43699-0008
(419) 383-5545 ask for Frank Repka

• University of Cincinnati College of Medicine
Nutrition and Weight Clinic at Children's Hospital
P.O. Box 670555
Cincinnati, OH 45267-0555
(513) 636-4681
Program: Treat children 12 and under.

Oregon

• Providence Health System
Health and Life Style Center
1885 NW 185th Ave
Aloha, OR 97006
(503) 645-4864
ages 9-12 and 13-16

Pennsylvania

• The Childhood Healthy Eating Program (CHEP)
University of Pittsburgh, School of Medicine
Western Psychiatric Institute and Clinic
3811 O'Hara St.
Pittsburgh, PA 15213
(412) 624-5420

• The Children's Hospital of Philadelphia
Division of Gastroenterology and Nutrition
34th Street and Civic Center Boulevard
Philadelphia, PA 19104-4399
(215) 590-3630

• The Milton S. Hershey Medical Center
The Pennsylvania State University
Pediatrics Department
University Hospital
P.O. Box 850
Hershey, PA 17033
(717) 531-8342

• Thomas Jefferson University Hospital
Department of Nutrition and Dietetics
Outpatient Nutrition Services
1015 Chestnut Street, Suite 110
Philadelphia, PA 19107-4302
(215) 955-5077

South Carolina

• Medical University of South Carolina
College of Medicine
171 Asley Avenue
Charleston, SC 29425
(803) 777-8141

• University of South Carolina School of
Public Health
Columbia, SC 29208
(803) 777-5001

Tennessee

• The Institute for Nutrition Research
The Kim Dayani Human Performance Center
Vanderbilt University Medical Center
607 Medical Arts Building
Nashville, TN 37232-8285
(615) 936-3952

Texas

• Baylor College of Medicine
One Baylor Plaza
Houston, TX 77030
(713) 770-3600
• Texas Tech University
Health Sciences Center
School of Medicine
3601 4th Street
Lubbock, TX 79430
(806) 743-2331

Virginia

• University of Virginia School of Medicine
Medical Center
Box 395, McKim Hall
Charleston, VA 22908
(804) 924-5321
ask for Margrett Gutgesell

Washington

•University of Washington School of
Medicine
9750 3rd Ave. NE Suite 307
Seattle, WA 98195
(206) 527-6920

West Virginia

• Department of Family and Community
Health
Marshall University School of Medicine
Family Practice Center
1801 6th Avenue
Huntington, WV 25703
(304) 696-7000

CALORIES, FAT, CARBOHYDRATE & PROTEIN GRAMS
FOOD CHART
A Brief Guide - *Adapted from USDA*

DAIRY PRODUCTS

Milk, Cheese, and Ice Cream

Fluid Milk:

	Amount	# Calories	# Fat Grams	#Carbohydrate Grams	# Protein Grams
Whole Milk...	1 cup	150	8	11	8
Skim Milk (fresh or non fat dry reconstituted)...	1 cup	86	0	12	8
Buttermilk (from skim milk)...	1 cup	98	2	12	8
Yogurt (made from partially skimmed milk)...	1 cup	137	0.44	19	14

Milk Beverages

Chocolate malted milk...	1 cup	228	9	30	9
Chocolate milk...	1 cup	918	93	18	20

Cheese:

American, cheddar-type...	1 oz	114	9	0.36	7
Cottage, not creamed...	1 cup	123	0.61	3	25
Cottage, creamed, not packed...	1 cup	217	9	6	26
Swiss, diced...	1 cup	496	36	4	38
Mozzarella...	1 cup	361	28	3	24

Eggs:

Whole, raw, fresh, large...	1	86	6	0.71	7
Fried w/1 tbsp of buttter w/o salt...	1 lg	188	17	0.72	7
Egg Beaters, 99% egg substitute...	1/2 cup	50	0.2	5	7
Hard or soft cooked "boiled"...	1	78	5	0.6	6

MEATS, BEANS, PEAS, NUTS

Beef:

Ground, extra lean, broiled, well done...	3 oz	225	13	0	24
Ground, lean, broiled well done...	3 oz	238	15	0	24
Ground, regular, broiled, well done...	3 oz	248	17	0	23
Hamburger patty...	1 patty	274	12	80	12
Corned beef, brisket...	3 oz	213	16	0.4	15
Beef and vegetable stew...	1 cup	222	5	20	23
Tenderloin, lean, broiled	3 oz	247	17	0	21

Fish and shellfish:

	Amount	# Calories	# Fat Grams	#Carbohydrate Grams	# Protein Grams
Bluefish, cooked dry heat...	3 oz	135	5	0	22
Crab, Alaskan king...	1 cup	113	0.8	0	25
Fish sticks...1 whole...	57 gr	26	3.4	7	4
Mackerel, Atlantic, cooked, dry heat, boneless...	3 oz	227	15	0	20
Mackerel, Pacific, cooked, dry heat, boneless...	1 oz	57	3	0	7
Salmon, Atlantic, wild, cooked, dry heat...	3 oz	155	7	0	22
Shrimp, boiled...	1	10	0.1	0	2
Tuna, light, canned in oil, drained solids...	3 oz	169	7	0	25
Tuna, light, canned in water, drained solids...	3 oz	99	0.68	0	22

Lamb chop:

	Amount	# Calories	# Fat Grams	#Carbohydrate Grams	# Protein Grams
Domestic, loin, lean & $\frac{1}{4}$" fat, choice, roasted...	3 oz	263	20	0	19

Meats:

	Amount	# Calories	# Fat Grams	#Carbohydrate Grams	# Protein Grams
Frankfurter, beef...5 in x $\frac{3}{4}$ in dia 10 per pound...	1	142	13	0.81	5
Italian sausage...1 whole	113 gr	361	28	3	24
Pastrami...	28 gr	99	8	0.9	5
Pepperoni Slices...	1	27	2	0.2	1
Bologna...	28 gr	70	6	0.2	4
Bratwurts...	1	226	19	2	10
Beef Jerky...	1	67	3	3	8

Pork:

	Amount	# Calories	# Fat Grams	#Carbohydrate Grams	# Protein Grams
Pork fresh center loin, bone-in, lean, broiled...	3 oz	171	7	0	25
Bacon, cured, medium slices	3	109	9	0.11	6
Liver, beef, pan fried...	3 oz	184	7	7	23

Poultry, cooked, without bone:

	Amount	# Calories	# Fat Grams	#Carbohydrate Grams	# Protein Grams
Light meat, meat only, chopped, roasted...	1 cup	242	6	0	43
Dark meat, meat only, roasted...	1 cup	287	14	0	38

Veal:

	Amount	# Calories	# Fat Grams	#Carbohydrate Grams	# Protein Grams
Leg, lean, roasted...	3 oz	127	3	0	24
Loin, lean, roasted...	3 oz	149	6	0	22

NUTS:

	Amount	# Calories	# Fat Grams	#Carbohydrate Grams	# Protein Grams
Almonds, blanched...	1 cup	850	76	27	30
Almonds, sliced, unblanched...	1 cup	560	50	19	18
Brazil nuts, dried, unblanched, shelled...	1 cup	918	93	18	20
Cashew nuts, dry roasted w/salt...	1 cup	786	64	45	21
Peanuts, all types, roasted, w/salt...	1 oz	165	14	6	7
Peanut butter, smooth style, w/salt...	2 tbs	190	16	6	8

	Amount	# Calories	# Fat Grams	#Carbohydrate Grams	# Protein Grams
Pecans, shelled...	1 cup	720	73	20	8
Walnuts, black, dried...	1 cup	759	71	15	30
Coconut:					
Fresh, shredded meat...	1 cup	283	27	13	3
Dried, shredded, not sweetened...	1 oz	187	18	7	2

VEGETABLES AND FRUITS

Vegetables:

	Amount	# Calories	# Fat Grams	#Carbohydrate Grams	# Protein Grams
Asparagus, small spear, raw...	1	3	0.02	0.54	0.27
Beans, Baked beans...	1 cup	236	1	52	12
Beans, Baked beans, with tomato sauce & pork...	1 cup	248	3	49	13
Beans, kidney...	1 cup	613	1	110	43
Beans, Lima, lrg, cooked, boiled, wo/salt...	1 cup	216	0.71	39	15
Beans, snap, green, boiled, drained, w/o salt...	1 cup	44	0.35	10	2
Beets, cooked or canned...	$^6/_{10}$cup	33	0.1	8	1
Broccoli, raw, flowerets...	1 cup	20	0.25	4	2
Brussel sprouts, boiled, drained, w/o salt...	$^1/_2$ cup	30	0.4	7	2
Cabbage, raw, shredded...	1 cup	18	0.19	4	1
Carrots, raw, grated...	1 cup	47	0.21	11	1
Cauliflower, green, cooked, no salt...	$^1/_5$ hd	29	0.28	6	3
Celery, raw, diced...	1 cup	19	0.17	4	0.9
Coleslaw...	1 cup	83	3	65	2
Corn, Sweet, baby, yellow, boiled, drained...	1 ear	8.64	0.1	2	0.27
Corn On cob, cooked...	1 ear	120	2	27	4
Corn Kernels...	$^1/_2$ cup	72	0.6	17	2
Cress, garden, raw...	1 cup	16	0.35	2	1
Cucumbers...	$5^3/_4$cps	39	0.4	8	2
Cucumbers, Dill pickles, whole 65 grams...	1	12	0.1	3	0.4
Kale, cooked, raw...	1/2 cup	7	0.7	1	0.36
Lettuce, iceberg, raw, shredded...	1/2 cup	7	0.1	1	0.56
Lettuce, cos or romaine, raw, shredded...	1 cup	4	0.06	0.66	0.45
Mushrooms, raw...	1 cup	24	0.4	4	2
Okra, raw, cut...	$^1/_2$ cup	19	0	4	1
Onions, raw, chopped...	1 cup	61	0.26	14	2
Onions, cooked, boiled, drained, wo/salt...	1 cup	92	0.4	21	3
Peas, green...	1 cup	117	0.6	21	8
Peppers, sweet, green, raw...	1 cup	63	0.28	10	1
Peppers, sweet, yellow, raw...	1 cup	14	0.11	3	0.52
Potatoes, Baked, flesh, $2^1/_3$"x $4^3/_4$", w/o salt...	1	145	0.16	34	4
Potato, Baked, skin, w/o salt...	1	115	0.06	27	2
Potatoes, Boiled, cooked in skin, 1-$^1/_2$" w/o salt...	1	118	0.14	27	3
Potato Chips...	1 chip	11	0.7	1	0.1

	Amount	# Calories	# Fat Grams	#Carbohydrate Grams	# Protein Grams
Potatoes, French fried...	76 gr	235	12	29	3
Potatoes, Hash-browns...	$^1/_2$ cup	151	9	16	2
Potatoes, Mashed...	$^1/_3$ cup	66	1	13	2
Radishes, raw, slices shredded...	1 cup	20	0.63	4	0.7
Sauerkraut, canned...	1 cup	45	0.3	10	2
Spinach, cooked, boiled, drained, w/o salt...	1 cup	41	0.47	7	5
Squash, Summer, zucchini, w skin, cooked, drained, w/o salt....	1 cup	38	0.29	8	3
Squash, Winter, baked, acorn, cooked, baked, w/o salt...	1 cup	114	0.29	30	2
Sweet potatoes, Cooked, large, baked in skin...	1	185	0.2	44	3
Sweet potatoes, Boiled or cooked, w/o skin, medium, w/o salt...	1	159	0.45	37	2
Tomatoes, Raw...	1 cup	38	0.59	9	1
Tomatoes, Cooked, boiled, medium, w/o salt...	2	66	1	14	3
Tomato juice...	$^1/_2$ cup	21	0.1	5	0.9
Tomato Ketchup...	1 tbsp	16	0	4	0.2
Turnips, cooked, drained, mashed, w/o salt...	1 cup	41	1	11	2
Turnip greens, cooked...	$^1/_2$ cup	15	0.2	3	0.8

Fruits:

	Amount	# Calories	# Fat Grams	#Carbohydrate Grams	# Protein Grams
Apples, raw, with skin...	1 cup	74	0.45	19	0.24
Apple juice...	1 cup	117	0.3	29	0.2
Applesauce Sweetened...	1 cup	194	0.5	51	0.5
Applesauce Unsweetened...	1 cup	105	0.12	28	0.4
Apricots, raw, halves...	1 cup	74	0.6	17	2
Bananas, raw, sliced...	1 cup	138	0.72	35	1
Berries, Blackberries, raw...	1 cup	75	0.56	18	1
Berries, Blueberries, raw...	1 pint	225	1	57	3
Berries, Strawberries, sliced, raw...	1 cup	46	0.56	11	0.93
Cantaloupe...	$3^1/_3$cup	187	1.5	45	5
Cherries Sour, red, raw, with pits...	1 cup	78	0.5	19	2
Cherries Sweet, raw, with pits...	1 cup	84	1	19	1.4
Dates, domestic, natural, dried, pitted chopped...	1 cup	489	0.8	131	3
Figs, dried, uncooked...	1 cup	48	0.22	12	0.58
Fruit cocktail, canned in heavy syrup...	1 cup	114	0	29	1
Grape juice...	1 cup	154	0.2	38	1
Grapefruit, raw, pink& red & white in all areas, sections w/juice...	1 cup	72	0.23	19	1
Grapefruit juice, canned, unsweetened...	1 cup	94	0.25	22	1
Honeydew melon, raw, diced...	1 cup	59	0.17	16	0.78
Olives...	1 cup	361	28	3	24
Oranges, raw, California, Valencias, 2-$^5/_8$" dia...	1	65	0.3	16	0.99
Orange juice, raw...	1 cup	112	0.5	26	2

	Amount	# Calories	#Fat Grams	#Carbohydrate Grams	# Protein Grams
Papaya, raw...	1 cup	55	0.2	14	0.43
Peaches, raw, large 2-3/4"dia...	1	67	0.14	17	1
Pears...	1 cup	98	0.7	25	0.6
Pineapple, raw, diced...	1 cup	76	0.67	19	0.6
Pineapple juice, canned, unsweetened...	1 cup	140	0.2	34	0.8
Plums, raw, fruit 2/18" dia	1	36	0.41	9	0.52
Prunes, dried, uncooked...	1	20	0.04	5.27	0.22
Prune juice...	1 cup	182	0.1	45	2
Raisins, packaged...	1 cup	495	0.76	131	5.31
Watermelon, balls...	1 cup	49	0.66	11	1

BREADS AND CEREALS

Breads/Pretzels:

Bagels, plain, 3" dia...	1	157	0.91	31	6
Bagels, oat bran, 3" dia...	1	145	0.68	30	6
Corn tortillas...	1	56	0.6	12	1
English muffin...	1	134	1	26	4
Hamburger or hotdog roll...	1	123	2.19	22	3.66
Muffin, blueberry...	1	158	4	27	3
Pita bread, white, slice...	1	165	0.72	33.5	5.5
Pizza crust...	1	720	8	128	24
Pretzels, 60 grams each...	10	229	2	47	5
Rolls, wheat, each roll 1 oz...	1	77	2	13	2
Rye bread slice...	1	83	1	15	3
Taco shell, baked...	1	98	4.75	13	1.5
Tortillas, corn, bake ready, 6" dia...	1	58	0.65	12	1.5
White bread slice...	1	120	2	22	4
Whole wheat bread slice...	1	65	1	15	2

Cereals:

Buckwheat groat, roasted, cooked...	1 cup	155	1	33	6
Grits...	1 cup	579	2	124	14
Oatmeal...	1 cup	299	5	52	13
Oatbran, Cooked...	1 cup	87	1.9	25	7
Cereal, all bran ®...	1/3 cup	71	0.5	0	25
Pancake mix...	1 cup	501	2	104	14

RICE & PASTA

Rice:

Rice, white, cooked...	1 cup	169	0.33	37	3
Rice, brown, long-grain, cooked...	1 cup	217	1.77	45	5

Soups:	Amount	# Calories	# Fat Grams	#Carbohydrate Grams	# Protein Grams
Bean with pork...	1 cup	268	4	51	13
Beef noodle...	1 cup	83	3	9	5
Chicken noodle...	1 cup	75	2	9	4
Clam broth...	1 cup	46	0.2	5	5
Cream of asparagus...	1 cup	58	2	9	4
Cream of mushroom...	1 cup	129	9	9	2
Minestrone...	1 cup	82	2	11	4
Oyster stew...	1 cup	58	4	4	2
Tomato...	1 cup	85	2	17	2
Vegetable with beef broth...	1 cup	82	2	13	3
Pasta:					
Macaroni, elbow, cooked...	1 cup	197	1	39.7	6.7
Noodles, egg, cooked...	1 cup	213	2.4	39.8	7.6
Noodles, Chinese, chow mein...	1 cup	237	13.8	26	3.8
Spaghetti, cooked, enriched w/salt...	1 cup	197	0.94	40	7

FATS, OILS, AND RELATED PRODUCTS

	Amount	# Calories	# Fat Grams	#Carbohydrate Grams	# Protein Grams
Butter, w/o salt...	1 tbsp	102	11	0.01	0.12
Canola Oil...	1 tbsp	124	14	0	0
Margarine, blend, 60% corn oil & 40% butter...	1 tbsp	110	11	0.09	0.12
Peanut oil, salad oil, cooking oil...	1 tbsp	119	13.5	0	0
Cooking fats:					
Vegetable...	1 cup	1927	218	0	0
Salad dressings:					
Blue cheese...	1 cup	1235	128	18	12
Caesar...	1 cup	1320	144	8	3
French...	1 cup	1074	102	44	1
Mayonnaise...	1 cup	1577	175	6	2
Miracle whip, lite...	1 tbsp	44	4	2	0.1
Thousand Island...	1 cup	943	89	38	2

SUGARS, SWEETS, AND RELATED PRODUCTS

Candy, Jam and Syrup:	Amount	# Calories	# Fat Grams	#Carbohydrate Grams	# Protein Grams
Caramel candy, piece...	1	31	0.6	6	0.4
Chocolate syrup...	1 cup	654	3	177	6
Cool Whip ®...	1 cup	239	19	17	0.9

	Amount	# Calories	# Fat Grams	#Carbohydrate Grams	# Protein Grams
Fudge, chocolate, 17 gram piece...	1	65	1	13	0.3
Honey...	1 cup	1031	0	279	1
Jelly...	1 tbsp	51	0	13	0.1
Jelly beans, each piece...	10	104	0.1	26.4	0
Jam...	1 tbsp	48	0	13	0.1
Peanut brittle...	28 gr	128	5	20	0.6
Sugar...	1 cup	774	0	200	0

DESSERTS

Cake:

	Amount	# Calories	# Fat Grams	#Carbohydrate Grams	# Protein Grams
Angel food cake, 596 grams...	1	1532	2	350	36
Cake Plain, without icing, 777 grams...	1	3023	139	407	40
Cake Plain, with icing...	1 cup	1812	205	0	0
Chocolate cake mix...	2³/₄cup	2214	81	378	30
Cookie crumbs...	1 cup	397	16	60	4
Fruitcake, whole...	1	10886	348	1960	109
Gingerbread mix...	2³/₄cup	2261	71	386	23
Pound cake, whole 300 grams...	1	1169	54	174	16
Sponge cake, whole 454 grams...	1	1311	12	277	24

Pudding & Ice Cream:

	Amount	# Calories	# Fat Grams	#Carbohydrate Grams	# Protein Grams
Custard ...	1 cup	308	14	31	15
Pudding...	1 cup	347	8	64	9
Figbars, whole...	1	56	1	11	0.6
Gelatin dessert, plain, 85 grams...	¹/₃ cup	42	0.2	7	4
Ice cream, plain	¹/₂ cup	134	7	16	2
Sherbert...	¹/₂ cup	134	2	29	1
Yogurt, plain, whole milk...	1 cup	151	8	11.4	8.5
Yogurt, plain, fat-free...	1 cup	137	0.4	19	14

Pies:

	Amount	# Calories	# Fat Grams	#Carbohydrate Grams	# Protein Grams
Pie crust, 160 grams, whole...	1	802	49	81	11
Apple pie filling...	2 cups	601	0.6	156	0.6
Cherry pie filling...	2 cups	684	1	174	3
Lemon pie filling...	2 cups	2067	40	412	28
Pumpkin pie filling...	2 cups	562	0.7	142	6

BEVERAGES

	Amount	# Calories	# Fat Grams	#Carbohydrate Grams	# Protein Grams
Coffee, brewed hot...	1 cup	4.7	0	1	0
Coffee, instant...	³/₄ cup	3.6	0	0.7	0.2
Cola-type...	16 fl oz	201	0	51	0

	Amount	# Calories	# Fat Grams	#Carbohydrate Grams	# Protein Grams
Ginger ale...	16 fl oz	166	0	43	0
Low-calorie type beverage...	16 fl oz	1	0	0.47	0
Tea, brewed...	1 cup	2.4	0	0.7	0

ALCOHOLIC BEVERAGES

	Amount	# Calories	# Fat Grams	#Carbohydrate Grams	# Protein Grams
Beer, 3.6% alcohol...	12 fl oz	146	0	13	1
Whiskey, gin, rum:					
100-proof...	1 fl oz	82	0	0	0
86 proof...	1 fl oz	69	0	0	0.03
Wines:					
Wine, red...	3.5 fl oz	74	0	1.75	0.21
Wine, white...	3.5 fl oz	70	0	0.82	0.1

Note: This guide is intended as a handy tool for counting calories, fat, carbohydrates, and protein grams. Some figures are averaged. You should always calculate calories and grams from food product labels. We have done our best to ensure that the figures contained in this chart are accurate, however, some errors may have inadvertently occurred.

APPENDIX E
Calorie Chart Of Common Fast Foods

Source: Minnesota Attorney General's Office, Calorie Control Council,
Web Sites of Restaurant Chains, nutritional informational sheets at restaurants.

Note: This is a partial listing of foods available at some fast food chains. These chains are to be commended for making their nutritional data available; choose food items from them carefully. We have eliminated some selections. "Meals" typically only include the main entree—condiments and side dishes are separate. Salads do not include dressings unless indicated. We have tried to provide accurate information and any errors are unintentional. We cordially invite restaurants and chains can send up updated data for our next edition.

ARBY'S® Roast Beef Sandwiches	# Calories	# Fat Grams	#Carbohydrate Grams	# Protein Grams
Arby Melt/Cheddar	368	18	36	18
Arby-Q	431	18	48	22
Beef'n Cheddar	487	28	40	25
Giant Roast Beef	555	28	43	35
Junior Roast Beef	324	14	35	17
Regular Roast Beef	388	19	33	23
Chicken Sandwiches				
Breaded Chicken Fillet	536	28	46	28
Chicken Cordon Bleu	623	33	46	38
Chicken Fingers 2 pc	290	16	20	16
Grilled Chicken Deluxe	430	20	41	23
Roast Chicken Club	546	31	37	31
Roast Chicken Deluxe	433	22	36	24
Sub Roll Sandwiches				
French Dip	475	22	40	30
Hot Ham 'n Swiss	500	23	43	30
Philly Beef n' Swiss	755	47	48	39
Turkey Sub	550	27	47	31
Light Menu				
Roast Beef Deluxe	276	10	33	18
Roast Chicken Deluxe	276	6	33	20
Garden Salad	61	0.5	12	3
Roast Chicken Salad	149	2	12	20
Side Salad	23	0.3	4	1
Fried Potatoes				
Curly Fries	300	15	38	4
French Fries	246	13	30	2
Potato Cakes	204	12	20	2
Baked Potatoes				
Plain	355	0.3	82	7

	# Calories	# Fat Grams	#Carbohydrate Grams	# Protein Grams
w Margarine and Sour Cream	578	24	85	9
Desserts				
Hot Chocolate	110	1	23	2
Chocolate Chip Cookie	125	6	16	2
Breakfast				
Bacon, 2 strips	90	7	0	5
Biscuit Plain	280	15	34	6
Cinnamon Nut Danish	360	11	60	6
Egg Portion	95	8	0.5	0.5
French Toast, 6 pc	430	21	52	10
Ham	45	1	0	7
Sausage	163	15	0	7
Table Syrup	45	3	0.5	4

BOSTON MARKET®

	# Calories	# Fat Grams	#Carbohydrate Grams	# Protein Grams
1/4 White Meat Chicken no skin/wing	160	3.50	0	31
1/4 White Meat Chicken w/skin	330	17	2	43
1/4 Dark Meat Chicken no skin	210	10	1	28
1/2 Chicken with skin	330	22	2	31
Skinless Rotisserie Turkey Breast	170	1	1	36
Ham w/cinnamon apples	350	13	35	25
Meatloaf/Chunky tomato sauce	370	18	22	30
Meatloaf/Brown Gravy	390	22	19	30
Orig, Chicken Pot Pie	750	34	78	34
Chunky Chicken Salad	390	30	3	27
Caesar Salad Entree	520	43	16	20
Caesar Salad no dressing	240	13	14	19
Chicken Soup	80	3	4	9
Chicken Tortilla Soup	220	11	19	10
Chicken Sandwich (plain)	430	3.50	61	39
Chicken Sandwich w/Cheese & sauce	760	32	71	46
Chicken Salad Sandwich	680	33	63	38
Turkey Sandwich w/Cheese & sauce	710	28	68	45
Turkey Sandwich (plain)	400	3.50	61	32
Ham Sandwich				

	# Calories	# Fat Grams	#Carbohydrate Grams	# Protein Grams
w/Cheese & sauce	760	35	71	38
Ham Sandwich (plain)	450	9	66	25
Meatloaf Sandwich w/cheese	860	33	95	46
Meatloaf (plain)	690	21	86	40
Ham/Turkey Club				
w/Cheese & sauce	890	43	79	47
Ham/Turkey Club (plain)	430	6	64	29
Steamed Vegetables	35	0.05	7	2
New Potatoes	140	3	25	3
Buttered Corn	190	4	25	3
Zucchini Marinara	80	4	10	2
Mashed Potatoes	180	8	25	3
Rice Pilaf	180	5	32	5
Creamed Spinach	300	24	13	10
Stuffing	310	12	44	6
Butternut Squash	160	6	25	2
Macaroni & Cheese	280	10	36	12
BBQ Baked Beans	333	9	53	11
Hot Cinnamon apples	250	4.5	56	0
Fruit Salad	70	0.50	17	1
Med. Pasta Salad	170	10	16	4
Cole Slaw	280	16	32	2
Tortellini Salad	380	24	29	14
Caesar Side Salad	210	17	6	8
Corn Bread	200	6	33	3
Oatmeal Raisin Cookie	320	13	48	4
Chocolate Chip Cookie	340	17	48	4
Brownie	450	27	47	6

BURGER KING®

Whopper R Sandwich w/mayo	660	40	47	29
Whopper R w/cheese & mayo	760	48	47	35
Hamburger	320	15	27	19
BK Big Fish R Sandwich	720	43	59	23
BK Broiler R				
Chicken Sandwich	530	26	45	29
Chicken Sandwich	710	43	54	26
Chicken Tenders R -4 pieces	180	11	9	11
French Fries medium salted	400	21	50	3
Onion Rings medium	380	19	46	5
Dutch Apple Pie	300	15	39	3

Breakfast Croissan'wich R	# Calories	# Fat Grams	#Carbohydrate Grams	# Protein Grams
w/Sausage, Egg, & Cheese	530	41	23	18
Croissan'wich R w/Sausage & Cheese	450	35	21	13
Biscuit	300	15	35	6
Biscuit w/Egg	380	21	37	11
Biscuit w/Sausage	490	33	36	13
Biscuit w/Sausage & Egg	620	43	37	20
Cini-Minis 4 rolls.	440	23	51	5
Hash Browns-large	410	26	42	3

CHICK-FIL-A®

	# Calories	# Fat Grams	#Carbohydrate Grams	# Protein Grams
Chick-n-Strips (R) 4 pcs	230	8	10	29
Nuggets (R) 8 pcs	290	14	12	28
Cheesecake 1 slice	270	21	7	13
Cheesecake 1 slice w/ Blueberry or Strawberry Topping	290	23	9	14
Fudge Nut Brownie	350	16	41	10
Lemon Pie 1 slice	320	16	40	7
Waffle Potato Fries(R) small	290	10	49	1
Carrot & Raisin Salad small	150	2	28	5
Chargrilled Chicken Salad	290	9	21	32
Chick-n-Strips Salad	290	9	21	32
Chicken Salad Plate	290	5	40	21
Cole Slaw	130	6	11	6
Tossed Salad	70	0	13	5
Chargrilled Chicken Club Sandwich (no dressing)	390	12	38	33
Chargrilled Chicken Deluxe Sandwich	290	3	38	28
Chargrilled Chicken Sandwich	280	3	36	27
Chicken Deluxe Sandwich	300	9	31	25
Hearty Breast of Chicken Soup	110	1	10	16

CHURCH'S CHICKEN®

	# Calories	# Fat Grams	#Carbohydrate Grams	# Protein Grams
Biscuits 2.1 oz	250	16.4	25.6	2.2
Breast 2.8 oz	200	12.4	4.3	19
Leg 2 oz	140	9.1	2.4	12.7
Tender Strip 1.1 oz	80	4	4.5	6
Thigh 2.8 oz	230	16.2	5.3	16.2

	# Calories	# Fat Grams	#Carbohydrate Grams	# Protein Grams
Wing 3.1 oz	250	16.1	7.7	18.5
Apple Pie 3.1 oz	280	12.3	40.5	2.3
French Fries 2.7 oz	210	10.5	28.5	3.3
Cole Slaw 3.0 oz	92	5.5	8.4	4.2
Cajun Rice 3.1 oz	130	7	15.6	1.3
Corn on the Cob 5.7 oz	139	3.2	23.5	4.4
Okra 2.8 oz	210	16.1	19.1	2.7

DAIRY QUEEN®

	# Calories	# Fat Grams	#Carbohydrate Grams	# Protein Grams
DQ Vanilla Soft Serve 1/2 cup	140	4.50	22	3
DQ Chocolate Soft Serve 1/2 cup	150	5	22	4
DQ Non-fat Frozen Yogurt 1/2 cup	100	0	21	3
Small Vanilla Cone	230	7	38	6
Regular Vanilla Cone	350	10	57	8
Large Vanilla Cone	410	12	65	10
Small Chocolate Sundae	290	7	51	6
Regular Chocolate Cone	360	11	56	9
Regular Yogurt Cone	280	1	59	9
Regular Misty Slush	290	0	74	0
Small Chocolate Malt	650	16	111	15
Regular Chocolate Shake	560	15	94	13
Regular Chocolate Malt	880	22	153	19
DQ Sandwich	150	5	24	3
Strawberry Shortcake	430	14	70	7
Banana Split	510	12	96	8
Chocolate Dilly Bar	210	12	20	3
Chocolate Mint Dilly Bar	190	12	20	3
Fudge Nut Bar	410	25	40	8
Buster Bar	450	28	41	10
Peanut Buster Parfait	730	31	99	16
Starkiss	80	0	21	0
DQ Caramel Nut Bar	260	13	32	5
DQ Vanilla Orange Bar	60	0	17	2
Sm. Choc. Cookie Blizzard	520	18	79	10
Small Strawberry Blizzard	400	11	66	9
Small Heath Blizzard	560	21	82	10
Sm. Choc. Chip Cookie Dough Blizzard	660	24	99	12
Sm. Reese's Peanut Butter Cup Blizzard	590	24	81	14
Sm. Strawberry Breeze	320	0.50	68	10

	# Calories	# Fat Grams	#Carbohydrate Grams	# Protein Grams
Small Heath Breeze	470	10	85	11
Strawberry-Banana DQ Treatzza Pizza (1/8)	180	6	29	30
Peanut Butter Fudge DQ Treatzza Pizza (1/8)	220	10	28	4
DQ Frozen Log Cake (1/8)	280	9	43	5

DENNY'S®

	# Calories	# Fat Grams	#Carbohydrate Grams	# Protein Grams
Biscuit & Sausage Gravy 7 oz	570	38	45	11
Biscuit Plain 3 oz	375	22	40	5
Blueberry Muffin 3 oz	309	14	42	4
Dinner Roll 1.5 oz	132	2	26	4
English Muffin 4 oz	125	1	24	5
Herb Toast 2 oz	200	11	21	4
Toast Dry 1 oz	92	1	17	3
All American Slam Breakfast (R) 15 oz	1028	57	24	48
Apple Juice 10 oz	126	0	33	0
Applesauce 3 oz	60	0	15	0
Bacon 1 oz	122	14	1	9
Banana Breakfast 4 oz	110	0	29	1
Denny's Banana-Praline Hotcakes 13 oz	951	14	206	14
Banana/Strawberries Medley 4 oz	108	1	27	1
Big Texas Chicken Fajita-Fried 21 oz	1147	85	43	56
Canadian Bacon (Scrambled) 14 oz	807	59	34	47
Cereal Breakfast 1 oz	100	0	23	2
Chicken Fried Steak & Eggs 14 oz	723	56	31	28
Cinnamon Swirl French toast 11 oz	1024	48	123	23
Egg 2 oz	134	12	1	6
Egg Beaters (TM) Egg Substitute 2 oz	71	5	1	5
Eggs Benedict 19 oz	860	56	55	36
Farmer's Omelet Breakfast (R) 18 oz	912	69	38	34
Farmer's Skillet Fried (Breakfast) 16 oz	1041	84	35	37
French Slam (R) 14 oz	1029	71	58	44
French Toast - Plain 8 oz	510	25	51	19

	# Calories	# Fat Grams	#Carbohydrate Grams	# Protein Grams
Garden Fresh Skillet (Breakfast) 18 oz	785	58	43	29
Ham 'n' Cheddar Omelet 14 oz	743	55	24	36
Hotcakes-Plain 5 oz	491	7	95	12
Meat Lovers Skillet (Breakfast)-Fried 17 oz	1344	108	34	59
Meat Lovers Skillet (Breakfast)-Scrambled 16 oz	1211	95	33	56
Oatmeal (Breakfast) 4 oz	100	2	18	5
Pork Chop & Eggs (Breakfast) 18 oz	1223	95	21	70
Potato Pancakes 14 oz	526	27	61	13
Sausage Cheddar Omelette (Breakfast)16 oz	1036	86	24	46
Scram Slam 18 oz	974	80	30	42
Veggie-Cheese Omelette 16 oz	714	53	29	31
Waffle - Plain 6 oz	304	21	23	7
Buffalo Chicken Strips 10 oz-15 oz	856	54	1	92
Chicken Quesadilla 16 oz	827	55	43	50
Chicken Strips 10 oz	720	33	56	47
Grilled Chicken Breast 4 oz	130	4	0	24
Jr. Chicken Strips 5 oz	318	12	28	24
Syrup 1.5 oz	143	0	36	0
Apple Dessert 7 oz	430	20	59	3
Apple w/Equal (R) 7 oz	370	20	43	3
Cheesecake 4 oz	470	27	48	8
Jr. Fried Fish 5 oz	465	34	25	15
Jr. Shrimp Basket 4 oz	291	16	27	10
Sr. Battered Cod 5 oz	465	34	25	15
Classic Burger 11 oz	673	40	42	37
w/Cheese 13 oz	863	53	43	47
Garden Burger 3.4 oz	160	3	22	11
Battered Cod Dinner w/Tartar Sauce 9 oz	732	47	48	30
Chicken Fried Steak w/Gravy 6 oz	327	18	16	25
Grilled Chicken 4 oz	130	4	0	24
Grilled Chopped Steak w/ Gravy 10 oz	400	26	12	30
Pork Chop dinner w/Gravy 4 oz	130	4	0	24
Porterhouse Steak 14 oz	708	54	0	56

Pot Roast	# Calories	# Fat Grams	#Carbohydrate Grams	# Protein Grams
Dinner w/Gravy 7 oz	260	11	5	39
Roast Turkey &				
Stuffing w/Gravy 12 oz	701	27	63	47
Shrimp Dinner 8 oz	558	32	49	19
Sirloin Steak Dinner 5.5 oz	271	21	0	22
Sr. Chicken Fried Steak 8 oz	341	18	29	16
Sr. Grilled Chicken				
Breast 6 oz	219	6	1	26
Sr. Liver w/Bacon &				
Onions 8 oz	322	19	20	22
Sr. Pork Chop 4 oz	193	12	0	19
Sr. Pot Roast 5 oz	149	6	6	20
Sr. Turkey & Stuffing 8 oz	596	25	61	29
Steak & Shrimp Dinner 9 oz	645	42	31	36
T-bone Steak Dinner 9 oz	645	42	31	36
Baked Potato - Plain 6 oz	186	0	43	4
French Fries - Seasoned 4 oz	261	12	35	5
Hashed Browns 4 oz	218	14	20	2
Mashed Potatoes - Plain 6 oz	105	1	21	3
Fried Chicken Salad 13 oz	506	31	30	38
Grilled Chicken				
Caesar w/Dressing 13 oz	655	47	23	37
Oriental Chicken				
Salad w/Dressing 20 oz	568	26	49	33
Side Caesar				
Salad w/Dressing 6 oz	338	25	20	8
Charleston Chicken (TM)				
and Bacon 11 oz	632	32	53	35
Chicken Melt 7 oz	520	29	43	26
Club 11 oz	718	38	62	32
Deluxe Grilled Cheese 7 oz	482	26	44	18
Fried Fish 11 oz	905	56	74	29
Grilled Chicken				
Sandwich 14 oz	434	9	56	.35
Ham & Swiss on Rye 9 oz	533	31	40	23
Jr. Grilled Cheese 4 oz	375	22	35	12
Patty Melt 8 oz	695	44	39	38
Sr. Grilled Cheese				
Deluxe 7 oz	482	26	44	18
Sr. Ham & Swiss 9 oz	497	30	34	22
Sr. Turkey 9 oz	476	26	39	23
Super Bird (R) 9 oz	620	32	48	35
Applesauce 3 oz	60	0	15	0
Broccoli 4 oz	50	2	7	3

	# Calories	# Fat Grams	#Carbohydrate Grams	# Protein Grams
Carrots 4 oz	80	3	12	1
Corn 4 oz	120	4	19	3
Cornbread Stuffing				
Plain 2 oz	182	9	20	4
Cottage Cheese 3 oz	72	3	2	9
Fresh Fruit Mix 3 oz	36	0	9	1
Green Beans 4 oz	60	4	6	1
Green Beans w/Bacon 4 oz	60	4	6	1
Green Peas 4 oz	100	2	14	5
Green Peas in				
Butter Sauce 4 oz	100	2	14	5
Grilled Mushrooms 2 oz	14	0	2	2
Onion Ring Baskets 5 oz	439	27	44	6
Rice Pilaf 3 oz	112	2	21	2
Sampler (TM) 15 oz	1120	59	104	44
Strawberries				
Frozen w/Sugar 3 oz	115	1	26	1
Vegetable Beef Soup 8 oz	79	1	11	6
Chicken Noodle 8 oz	60	2	8	2
Clam Chowder 8 oz	214	11	22	5
Cream of Broccoli 8 oz	193	12	15	4
Cream of Potato 8 oz	222	12	23	4
Split Pea 8 oz	146	6	18	8

DOMINO'S®

	# Calories	# Fat Grams	#Carbohydrate Grams	# Protein Grams
Hand Tossed Cheese (1/6)	318	9.77	44.24	13.53
Thin Crust Cheese (1/6)	255.1	10.87	28.12	11.30
Deep Dish Cheese (1/6)	463.7	19.66	54.76	18.18
Hand Tossed Gr. Peppers, Olives, Mushrooms (1/6)	334.96	11.05	45.45	13.96
Thin Crust Gr. Peppers, Olives, Mushrooms (1/6)	271.08	12.15	29.33	11.73
Deep Dish Gr, Peppers, Olives, Mushrooms,	479.68	20.94	55.97	18.61
Hand Tossed Pepperoni, Italian Sausage (1/6)	417.99	18.24	45.68	17.85
Thin Crust Pepperoni, Italian Sausage (1/6)	354.29	19.34	29.56	15.62
Deep Dish Cheese (1/4)	466.50	21.29	51.82	18.29
Thin Crust Cheese (1/4)	273.20	11.65	30.11	12.11
Breadsticks (1)	77.59	3.34	10.72	1.72
Cheesy Bread (1)	103.01	5.43	10.76	3.26
Small Garden Salad	21.75	0.26	4.20	1.25
Large Garden	39.19	0.47	7.63	2.21

GODFATHER'S PIZZA®	# Calories	# Fat Grams	#Carbohydrate Grams	# Protein Grams
Original Crust Mini 1/4	131	3	19	7
Original Crust Medium 1/8	231	5	34	13
Original Crust Large 1/10	258	6	36	15
Original Crust Jumbo 1/10	382	9	53	22
Golden Crust Medium 1/8	212	8	26	10
Golden Crust Large 1/10	242	9	28	12

HARDEE'S®

	# Calories	# Fat Grams	#Carbohydrate Grams	# Protein Grams
Rise 'N' Shine Biscuit	390	21	44	6
Jelly Biscuit	440	21	57	6
Apple Cinnamon 'N' Raisin Biscuit	200	8	30	2
Sausage Biscuit	510	31	44	14
Bacon/Egg Biscuit	570	33	45	23
Ham Biscuit	400	20	47	9
Ham/Egg/Cheese Biscuit	540	30	48	20
Country Ham Biscuit	430	22	45	15
Big Country Sausage	1000	66	62	41
Big Country Bacon	820	49	62	33
Frisco Ham Sandwich	500	25	46	24
Hot Ham 'N' Swiss Burger	490	25	39	28
Fisherman's Filet	560	27	54	26
Breast	370	15	29	29
Thigh	330	15	30	19
Baked Beans (sm 5oz)	170	1	32	8
Garden Salad	220	13	11	12
Grilled Chicken Salad	150	3	11	20
French Fries(medium)	350	15	49	5
Vanilla Shake	350	5	65	12
Chocolate Shake	370	5	67	13
Peach Shake	390	4	77	10
Cool Twist	180	2	34	4
Hot Fudge Sundae	290	6	51	7
Peach Cobbler	310	7	60	2

KENNY ROGERS®

	# Calories	# Fat Grams	#Carbohydrate Grams	# Protein Grams
1/2 Chicken w/o skin & w/o wing 7 oz	313	9.5	0.7	56
1/2 Chicken w/skin 9.1 oz	515	27.5	1.9	65
1/4 Dark Meat Chicken w/skin 4.4 oz	271	16.7	0.7	29
1/4 White Meat Chicken w/o skin & w/o wing 4.7 oz	144	2.3	0.1	31

1/4 White Meat	# Calories	# Fat Grams	#Carbohydrate Grams	# Protein Grams
Chicken w/skin 4.7 oz	244	10.7	1.2	35
Chicken Pot Pie 12 oz	708	33	77.6	25.5
Cinnamon Apples 5.3 oz	199	5.1	41	0
Corn Muffin 2 oz	175	8	24	2
Macaroni & Cheese 5.5 oz	197	5.8	24.4	6
Pasta Salad 5 oz	236	11.6	27.7	5.5
Sour Cream & Dill Pasta Salad 5 oz	233	16.3	19.6	3.5
Baked Sweet Potato 9 oz	263	0.3	62.3	4.4
Garlic Parsley Potatoes 6.5 oz	259	12	37	3
Potato Salad 7 oz	390	27.3	34	3
Real Mashed Potatoes 8 oz	295	14.4	38.9	3.6
Cole Slaw 5.1 oz	225	15.5	17.9	1.4
Chicken Caesar Salad 9.4 oz	285.4	8.7	17.6	34.3
Roasted Chicken Salad 16.9 oz	292	10.3	18.5	35.0
Side Salad 4.7 oz	23	0.3	5.2	1
Sour Cream & Dill Pasta Salad 5 oz	233	16.3	19.6	3.5
BBQ Chicken Pita 7.3 oz	401	7.2	51	32.6
Chicken Caesar Pita 9.2 oz	606	34.8	34	36.1
Roasted Chicken Pita 10.8 oz	685	35.3	41.8	47.3
Turkey Sandwich 9.2 oz	385	12	30.2	38.7
Cole Slaw 5.1 oz	225	15.5	17.9	1.4
Cornbread Stuffing 7.1 oz	326	18.6	34.1	6.9
Creamy Parmesan Spinach 5.3 oz	119	5.5	9.6	9.5
Honey Baked Beans 5 oz	148	1.2	32	6
Italian Green Beans 6.1 oz	116	8.2	10.4	2.1
Rice Pilaf 5 oz	230	4.7	43.4	3
Steamed Vegetables 4.3 oz	48	0.3	8.4	3
Sweet Corn Niblets 5 oz	112	0.7	27.5	3.4
Zucchini & Squash Santa Fe 5 oz	70	4.5	7.6	0.9
Chicken Noodle Soup 10 oz	91	1.8	11.7	7.3

KENTUCKY FRIED CHICKEN®
ORIGINAL RECIPE CHICKEN

	# Calories	# Fat Grams	#Carbohydrate Grams	# Protein Grams
Whole Wing	140	10	5	9
Breast	400	24	16	29
Drumstick	140	9	4	13

	# Calories	# Fat Grams	#Carbohydrate Grams	# Protein Grams
Thigh	250	18	6	16
EXTRA CRISPY				
Whole Wing	200	13	10	10
Breast	470	28	25	31
Drumstick	190	11	8	13
Thigh	370	25	18	19
HOT & SPICY CHICKEN				
Hot and Spicy	210	15	9	10
Breast	530	35	23	32
Drumstick	190	11	8	13
Thigh	370	27	13	18
CHICKEN STRIPS				
Chicken Strips, 3	261	16	10	20
Spicy Buffalo Strips	3	350	19	22
TENDER ROAST				
CHICKEN w/skin				
Whole Wing	121	8	1	12
Breast	251	11	2	37
Thigh	207	12	2	18
Drumstick	97	4	1	15
TENDER ROAST				
CHICKEN w/o skin				
Skin Breast	169	4.3	1	31
Thigh	106	5.5	1	13
Drumstick	67	2.4	0	11
OTHER CHICKEN ITEMS				
Hot Wings 6 pc	471	33	18	27
Original Recipe				
Chicken Sandwich	497	22.3	45.5	28.6
Value BBQ Chicken Sandwich	256	8	28	17
Chunky Chicken Pot Pie	770	42	29	69
POTATOES & SIDES				
Mashed Potatoes w/gravy	120	6	17	1
Potato Wedges	180	13	28	5
Macaroni Cheese	180	8	21	7
Corn on the Cob	150	1.5	35	5
Green Beans	45	1.5	7	1
BBQ Baked Beans	190	3	33	6
Mean Greens	70	3	11	4
BREADS				
Biscuit, 1	180	10	20	40
Cornbread, 1	228	13	25	3

LONG JOHN SILVERS®	# Calories	# Fat Grams	#Carbohydrate Grams	# Protein Grams
Long John Silver's chicken w/cajun burritos 11 oz	1440	71	165	37
Long John Silver's chicken w/ ranch 11 oz	1450	72	165	36
Fish w/Cajun 23 oz	1450	70	170	36
Fish w/Ranch 23 oz	1460	72	170	35
Fish w/ Salsa 11.5 oz	690	32	84	18
Popcorn Shrimp	720	35	86	16
Batter Dipped Chicken 2 oz 1 pc	120	6	11	8
Flavorbaked (TM) Chicken Dish 2.6 oz	110	3	1	19
Batter-Dipped Fish 1 pc	170	11	12	11
Batter-Dipped Shrimp 1 pc 0.4 oz	35	2.5	2	1
Breaded Clams 3 oz	300	17	31	11
Flavorbaked (TM) Fish 1 pc 2.3 oz	90	2.5	1	14
Fish & Chips 1 serv	710	42	66	16
French Fries 1 serv 3 oz	250	15	28	3
Flavorbaked (TM) Chicken Sandwich 5.8 oz	290	10	27	24
Flavorbaked (TM) Fish Sandwich 6 oz	320	14	28	23
Grab-n-Go Battered Chicken 4.9 oz	320	12	41	14
Grab-n-Go Battered Fish 4.6 oz	300	11	39	11
Ultimate Fish Sandwich 6.4 oz	430	21	44	18
Corn Cobbette w/Butter 3.3 oz	140	8	19	3
Corn Cobbette w/o Butter 3.1 oz	80	0.5	19	3
Popcorn Chicken Munchers (side dish) 1 serv 4 oz	380	23	20	23
Popcorn Fish Munchers (side dish) 1 serv 4 oz	300	14	29	14
Popcorn Shrimp Munchers 1 serv 4 oz	320	15	33	15
Rice (side dish) 1 serv 3 oz	140	3	26	3
Slaw 1 serv 3.4 oz	140	6	20	1
Broccoli Cheese Soup 8 oz	180	12	13	5

MCDONALDS®	# Calories	# Fat Grams	#Carbohydrate Grams	# Protein Grams
Hamburger	260	9	34	13
Cheeseburger	320	13	35	15
Quarter Pounder	420	21	37	23
Quarter Pounder w/ Cheese	530	30	38	28
Big Mac	560	31	26	45
Arch Deluxe	550	31	39	28
Grilled Chicken Deluxe	440	20	38	27
Filet-O-Fish	450	25	42	16
Fish Filet Deluxe	560	28	54	23
FRIES				
Small	210	10	26	3
Large	450	22	57	6
Chicken Nuggets				
4 pc	190	11	10	12
Hot Mustard Sauce (1 pkg)	60	3.5	7	1
Barbecue Sauce (1 pkg)	45	0	10	0
Sweet 'N Sour Sauce (1 pkg)	50	0	11	0
Honey (1 pkg)	45	0	12	0
SALADS & DRESSINGS				
Garden Salad	35	0	7	2
Grilled Chicken Salad Deluxe	120	1.5	7	21
Caesar(1 pkg)	160	14	7	2
Fat Free				
Herb Vinagrette (1 pkg.)	50	0	11	0
Ranch (1 pkg.)	230	21	10	1
DESSERTS & SHAKES				
Vanilla Reduced Fat				
Ice Cream Cone	150	4.5	23	4
Strawberry Sundae	290	7	50	7
Hot Caramel Sundae	360	10	61	7
Hot Fudge Sundae	340	12	52	8
Nuts	40	3.5	2	2
Butterfinger R McFlurry	620	22	90	16
M&M or Crunch McFlurry	630	23	90	16
Oreo R McFlurry	570	20	82	15
Baked Apple Pie	260	13	34	3
BREAKFASTS				
Egg McMuffin	290	12	27	17
Sausage McMuffin	360	23	26	13
Sausage McMuffin w/ Egg	440	28	27	19
English Muffin	140	2	25	4
Sausage Biscuit	470	31	11	35
Scrambled Eggs (2)	160	11	1	13
Hash Browns	130	8	14	1

	# Calories	# Fat Grams	#Carbohydrate Grams	# Protein Grams
Hotcakes (plain)	340	9	58	9
Hotcakes w2 pats margarine& syrup	610	18	104	9
Breakfast Burrito	320	20	23	13
Apple Danish	360	16	51	5
Cheese Danish	410	22	47	7
Cinnamon Roll	390	18	50	6

PAPA JOHN'S®
ORIGINAL CRUST
1 SLICE OF LARGE PIZZA

	# Calories	# Fat Grams	#Carbohydrate Grams	# Protein Grams
Cheese Pizza	286	9	37	14
Sausage Pizza	340	13	40	15
All meats	410	18	42	21
Garden Special	298	11	36	14
The Works	369	17	37	18

THIN CRUST
1 SLICE OF LARGE PIZZA

	# Calories	# Fat Grams	#Carbohydrate Grams	# Protein Grams
Cheese	200	11	22	9
Sausage	270	15	22	12
All Meats	333	20	23	15
Garden Special	238	12	23	9
Works	319	19	24	14

POPEYES®

	# Calories	# Fat Grams	#Carbohydrate Grams	# Protein Grams
Biscuits 8 oz	250	14.9	26.1	3.7
Mild Breast 1 serv 3.7 oz	270	15.9	9.2	23.1
Mild Leg 1.7 oz	120	7.3	4.4	10.3
Mild Thigh 3.1 oz	300	22.7	9.3	14.7
Mild Wing 1.6 oz	160	10.7	6.6	9.3
Nuggets4.2 oz	410	31.9	17.9	17.1
Spicy Breast 3.7 oz	270	15.9	9.2	23.1
Spicy Leg 1.7 oz	120	7.3	4.4	10.3
Spicy Tender 1.2 oz	110	7	6	6
Spicy Thigh 3.1 oz	300	22.7	9.3	14.7
Spicy Wing 1.6 oz	160	10.7	6.6	9.3
Apple Pie 3.1 oz	240	12.2	30.8	3.5
French Fries 3.0 oz	240	12.2	30.8	3.5
Cole Slaw 4 oz	149	11.2	13.6	0.9
Shrimp 2.8 oz	250	16.4	13.2	15.6
Cajun Rice 3.9 oz	150	5.4	17.4	10
Corn on the Cob 5.2 oz	127	2.9	21.4	4
Onion Rings 3.1 oz	310	19.3	31.1	4.9
Red Beans & Rice 5.9 oz	270	16.9	29.7	7.5

SUBWAY®

6 Inch Cold Sandwiches on White Bread (Includes Veggies, w/no Condiments)	# Calories	# Fat Grams	#Carbohydrate Grams	# Protein Grams
Veggie Delite	222	3	38	9
Turkey Breast	273	4	40	17
Cold Cut Trio	362	13	39	19
Ham	287	5	39	18
Classic Italian B.M.T	445	21	21	39
Subway club	297	5	21	40
Roast Beef	288	5	39	19
Turkey Breast & Ham	280	5	39	18
Seafood & Crab	332	10	45	19
Tuna	376	15	39	18
SALADS				
Veggie Delite	51	1	10	2
Turkey Breast	102	2	12	11
Subway Club	126	3	12	14
Cold Cut Trio	191	11	11	13
Roast Beef	117	3	11	12
Tuna	205	13	11	12
Roasted Chicken Breast	162	4	20	13
Seafood & Crab	161	8	11	13
Ham	116	3	11	12
Classic Italian BMT	274	20	11	14
Steak & Cheese	212	8	13	22
Subway Melt	195	10	12	16

TACO BELL®

	# Calories	# Fat Grams	#Carbohydrate Grams	# Protein Grams
Taco	180	10	12	9
Soft Taco	220	10	21	11
Taco Supreme	220	14	14	10
Soft Taco Supreme	260	14	23	12
Double Decker Taco	340	15	38	14
Double Decker Supreme	390	19	40	15
Grilled Steak Soft Taco	230	10	20	15
Grilled Steak Soft Supreme	290	14	24	16
Grilled Chicken Soft Taco	200	7	21	14
GORDITAS				
Supreme Beef	300	13	31	14
Supreme Chicken	300	14	28	17
Supreme Steak	310	14	27	17
Fiesta Beef	290	13	31	14
Fiesta Chicken	260	10	28	16
Fiesta Steak	270	10	28	16
Santa Fe	380	20	33	14

BURRITOS	# Calories	# Fat Grams	#Carbohydrate Grams	# Protein Grams
Bean Burrito	380	12	55	13
Burrito Supreme	440	19	51	17
7 Layer Burrito	530	23	66	16
Chili Cheese Burrito	330	13	37	14
Grilled Chicken	400	14	50	17
Big Chicken Supreme	500	20	51	27
SPECIALTIES				
Tostado	300	15	31	10
Mexican Pizza	570	35	42	21
Big Beef MexiMelt	290	15	23	16
Taco Salad, Salsa	850	52	65	30
Cheese Quesadilla	350	18	32	16
Chicken Quesadilla	410	19	33	25
FAJITA WRAPS				
Steak	470	21	50	20
Chicken	460	20	51	19
Veggie	420	19	53	10
Steak Supreme	510	25	52	21
Chicken Supreme	520	26	53	18
Veggie Supreme	510	24	53	20
SIDES				
Nachos	320	18	34	5
Big Beef Nacho Supreme	450	24	45	14
Nacho Bellgrande	770	39	84	21
Pintos and Cheese	190	9	18	9
Cinnamon Twists	140	6	19	1
Chaco Taco	310	17	37	3
BREAKFAST				
Fiesta Burrito	280	16	25	9
Country Burrito	270	14	26	8
Grande Burrito	420	22	43	13
Double Bacon, Egg Burrito	480	27	39	18
Egg Quesadilla	380	21	33	15
Hash Browns	280	18	29	2
Quesadilla, Bacon	450	27	33	19
Hash Browns	280	18	29	2
WENDY'S®				
Plain Single	360	16	31	24
Single w/ Everything	420	20	37	25
Big Bacon Classic	580	30	46	34
Jr. Hamburger	270	10	34	15
Jr. Cheeseburger	320	13	34.	17
Jr. Bacon Cheeseburger	380	19	34	20

	# Calories	# Fat Grams	#Carbohydrate Grams	# Protein Grams
Grilled Chicken Sandwich	310	8	35	27
Breaded Chicken Sandwich	440	18	44	28
Spicy Chicken Sandwich	410	15	43	28
Caesar Side Salad	100	4	8	8
Deluxe Garden Salad	110	6	9	7
Grilled Chicken Salad	200	8	9	25
Grilled Chicken Caesar Salad	260	9	17	26
Side Salad	60	3	5	4
Taco Salad	380	19	28	26
Taco Chips	210	11	24	3
Soft Breadstick	130	3	23	4
Small Fries	270	13	35	4
BAKED POTATOES				
Plain	310	0	71	7
Bacon & Cheese	530	18	78	17
Chili Cheese	630	24	83	20
CHILI				
Small	210	14	7	14
Large	310	10	32	23
CHICKEN NUGGETS				
5 piece	210	14	7	14
Barbecue Sauce	45	0	10	1
Honey Mustard	130	12	6	0
Spicy Buffalo Wing Sauce	25	1	4	0
Sweet & Sour Sauce	50	0	12	0
Chicken Caesar salad	490	18	48	34
Classic Greek	440	20	50	15
Garden Ranch Chicken	480	18	51	30
Garden Veggie	400	17	52	11
DESSERTS				
Frosty Dessert, Small	330	8	56	8

WHITE CASTLE®

	# Calories	# Fat Grams	#Carbohydrate Grams	# Protein Grams
Hamburger	135	7	11	6
Cheeseburger	160	9	11	7
Dbl. Cheeseburger	285	18	16	14
Dbl. Hamburger	235	14	16	11
Fish Sandwich	160	6	18	8
Chicken Sandwich	190	8	21	8
Breakfast Sandwich	340	25	17	14
Chicken Rings	310	21	14	16
Onion Chips	180	9	25	3
Cheese Sticks	290	17	19	15

APPENDIX F
40-30-30 Sample Meal Options & Recipes

The following pages show sample meals that can be mixed and matched to formulate a healthy eating plan that approximates the 40-30-30 recommendation. Remember that portion size is very important. We start with an example of an ancient Native American diet because it represents a "thrifty gene" meal that will not result in weight gain. Of course, in modern America, it is difficult, if not impossible, to eat in this fashion.

Ancient Native American Meal For "Thrifty Genes"

Below is a sample of a fairly typical ancient "plains" meal during times of plentiful game. Native Americans relied on a high protein, low fat, high-fiber diet. They were lean and active. On a "good day," wild game of one kind or another was available: buffalo, venison, elk, moose, rabbit, and fish. All of these meats are high protein and exceptionally low-fat. If you can utilize these meats, you could increase your daily food intake by substituting them for beef, pork, or other meats. Buffalo steak is tasty and all of the other game meats, when carefully marinated, are very palatable. Fresh fish, especially, should be consumed far more often in the American diet.

Fresh wild berries are an excellent source of carbohydrates. Many modern fruits have been selectively grown to produce high sugar varieties. When possible, choose more "natural" berries. Native Americans collected many roots, seeds, nuts (such as black walnuts), cactus berries, and highly fibrous tubers. Maize, while the beginning of modern corn, had much more fiber and was lower in sugar.

The high protein, low sugar, low fat, high fiber diet of Native Americans was a "thrifty gene" diet. This is the diet that we would like to try to approximate in our modern world — especially for the obese, people who are insulin resistant, and type 2 diabetics.

Native American (Plains) meal on a "good day"	Cals.	Protein gms.	Fat gms.	Carbo. gms.
12 oz. buffalo steak	347	69	5	0
1/2 cup wild berries	40	.5	.5	10
1 cup maize	85	4	0	16
1 cup fiberous roots, vegetables	81	2	1	16
TOTALS:	553	75.5	6.5	42
PERCENTAGE CALORIES:		57%	11%	32%

Food Plan Work Sheet
BREAKFAST PLANS

Below are three sample breakfasts that can be used to match with lunch and dinner to try to meet a daily goal of 40% protein, 30% fat, 30% carbohydrate. You can change and mix selections and increase some foods to meet your calorie goals. For example, a 4 egg omelette could be made (from egg substitute).

Because food labels are rounded off, and the actual calories from each gram of protein and carbohydrate are actually higher than 4 (4.1 and 4.2, respectively), it is very difficult to make exact calculations. In addition, different brands of products will yield different calorie totals. In this food plan, we have attempted to use "generic" brands.

A. Egg Omelet & Fruit	Cals.	Protein gms.	Fat gms.	Carbo. gms.
1 egg + 2 egg whites	101	15	5	1.3
1 oz. sharp cheddar cheese (1%)	115	7	9	0
2 slices Flavorich bread	130	4	2	24
1/2 grapefruit	40	1	0	10
2 tbs. salsa	10	0	0	3
coffee or tea	0	0	0	0
TOTALS:	396	27	16	35.3
PERCENTAGE CALORIES:		27%	37%	36%
B. Cereal & Fruit				
1 cup Fiber One®	120	4	1	23
1 cup skim milk	80	8	0	12
1/2 cantaloupe	95	2	1	22
coffee or tea	0	0	0	0
TOTALS:	295	14	2	57
PERCENTAGE CALORIES:		19%	6%	75%
C. Scrambled Egg Sandwich				
Egg substitute (2 eggs)	60	12	0	2
2 slices low-fat, low-cal toast	100	6	1	24
1 cup fresh raspberries	60	1	0	14
coffee or tea	0	0	0	0
TOTALS:	220	19	1	40
PERCENTAGE CALORIES:		31%	4%	65%

Food Plan Work Sheet: LUNCH PLANS

Various appropriate lunches are outlined below. Mix and match with breakfast and supper. We have included some acceptable fast food options. Check the "fast food" data in **Appendix E** for more options.

	Cals.	Protein gms.	Fat gms.	Carbo. gms.
A. Chef Salad				
6 oz. broiled				
chicken breast (w/o skin)	146	26	4	0
1 med. tomato	25	2	0	9
3 spring onions (chopped)	15	0	0	3
2 cups lettuce	18	0	0	4
1.5 tbs. oil & vinegar	105	0	12	0
1/8 cup Chinese noodles	24	2	0	5.5
TOTALS:	333	30	16	22
PERCENTAGE CALORIES:		34%	41%	25%
B. Sub Sandwich				
6" Subway Club				
(w/veggies, mustard)	297	41	6	23
1/2 cup fresh strawberries	24	1.5	.5	5.5
TOTALS:	321	42.5	6.5	28.5
PERCENTAGE CALORIES:		50%	17%	33%
C. Sauerkraut & Hotdogs				
3 Healthy Choice® hotdogs	210	18	7.5	7
1 cup sauerkraut (low sodium)	45	2	0	10
1.5 servings pork 'n beans	180	7.5	3	36
TOTALS:	435	27.5	10.5	53
PERCENTAGE CALORIES:		26%	23%	51%
D. Wendy's®				
Grilled Chicken Caesar salad	260	26	9	17
PERCENTAGE CALORIES:		41%	32%	27%
E. Hardee's®				
Grilled chicken salad	150	20	3	11
PERCENTAGE CALORIES:		53%	18%	29%
F. Kenny Rogers®				
Turkey sandwich	385	39	12	30
PERCENTAGE CALORIES:		41%	28%	31%

Food Plan Work Sheet: DINNER PLANS

Five separate dinner plans are detailed. These should be matched to breakfast and lunch to approximate the 40-30-30 range. For example combining breakfast A, lunch B, and supper C totals 1,222 calories (37% protein; 30% fat; 33% carbohydrates). A combination of breakfast B, lunch C, and supper E totals only 985 calories (38% protein; 16% fat; 46% carbohydrates). Since the carbohydrates in this meal combination are acceptable, the food range is satisfactory. Diet drinks, tea, and water with lemon should be used. Snacks can be carefully added, however, some snack foods are unacceptable: high fat, high sugar, starch. Most non-fat snack foods have too much sugar. An acceptable snack (depending on the meals you choose) *could* be a small bag of roasted peanuts. (140 calories with 70% fat and 15% from each of protein & carbos.) Fiber One® cereal (with skim milk) is an acceptable snack. At the end of this list we have recommended some excellent substitutions. These meats and fruits are extremely healthy and more "natural."

	Cals.	Protein gms.	Fat gms.	Carbo. gms.
A. Steak				
8 oz. sirloin (trimmed, broiled)	308	48	11	0
1 cup green beans	40	2	0	10
1 cup mushrooms	18	1	0	3
1/2 cup mashed potatoes	90	2	1	18
2 cups mixed green salad	35	2	1	8
1.5 tbs. oil/vinegar	105	0	12	0
1 cup fresh strawberries	71	1.5	0	15
TOTALS:	667	56.5	25	54
PERCENTAGE CALORIES:		34%	34%	32%
B. Cod Steak				
8 oz. cod steak (broiled)	215	41	2.6	0
2 cups mixed green salad	35	2	1	8
1.5 tbs. oil/vinegar	105	0	12	0
1 tbs baco bits®	36	4	1.5	2
3/4 cup asparagus	25	2	0	3.5
1/2 cup skim milk	40	4	0	6
1 cup raspberries	60	4	0	14
TOTALS:	516	57	17	33.5
PERCENTAGE CALORIES:		44%	30%	26%

	Cals.	Protein gms.	Fat gms.	Carbo. gms.
C. Salmon Steak				
8 oz. salmon filet (grilled)	197	34	6	0
2 cups broccoli	50	5	1	9
1 cup mushrooms	18	1	0	3
2 cups mixed green salad	35	2	1	8
1.5 tbs. oil/vinegar	105	0	12	0
1/2 cup skim milk	40	4	0	6
1 cup raspberries	60	4	0	14
TOTALS:	505	50	20	40
PERCENTAGE CALORIES:		39%	35%	31%
D. Turkey Breast				
5 oz. turkey breast (w/o skin)	197	22	9	0
1 cup asparagus	34	4.5	0	5
2 cups cabbage	36	2	0	8
2 cups onion soup	116	8	3	16
1 cup fresh peaches	37	0	0	9
TOTALS:	420	36.5	12	38
PERCENTAGE CALORIES:		36%	27%	37%
E. Chicken Breast				
5 oz. chicken breast (w/o skin)	223	40	6	0
1 cup green beans in broth	41	2	0	10
1 cup Healthy Choice® beef soup	102	9	1	16
1 cup cauliflower w/lemon juice	21	2	0	4
1/2 cup diced fresh pineapple	43	0	0	10
TOTALS:	430	53	7	40
PERCENTAGE CALORIES:		49%	14%	37%
GREAT MEAT OPTIONS				
8 oz. venison steak	409	67	13	0
8 oz. buffalo steak	225	46	3	0
8 oz. moose steak	231	50	1.7	0
8 oz. elk steak	252	52	3.3	0
GREAT FRUIT OPTIONS				
1 cup boysenberries	66	1	0	16
1 cup blackberries	75	1	.5	18
1 cup elderberries	106	1	1	26
1 cup fresh red cherries	71	1.5	1	17
1 med. orange	62	1	0	15
1 large apple	81	0	.5	21

**Recipes From the
Calorie Control Council
www.caloriecontrol.org •
by permission**

Oriental-Style Sea Scallops

1-1/2 cups broccoli flowerets
2 tablespoons sesame or vegetable oil
3 cups thinly sliced Napa cabbage or bok
choy
1 cup shitake or common mushrooms, sliced
2 teaspoons ground star anise
1/2 cup chicken broth
2 to 3 teaspoons light reduced-sodium soy
sauce
1/4 cup cold water
4 cups hot cooked rice
1 cup thinly sliced onion
1 pound sea scallops
2 cups snow peas, ends trimmed
2 cloves garlic, minced
1/4 cup rice wine vinegar
2 tablespoons cornstarch
2 to 3 tablespoons NutraSweet® Spoonful ®
Makes 6 servings

Stir fry broccoli and onion 3 to 4 minutes in oil
in wok or large skillet. Add scallops, cabbage,
snow peas, mushrooms, garlic, anise; stir-fry 2
to 3 minutes. Add chicken broth, vinegar and
soy sauce; heat to boiling. Reduce heat and
simmer, uncovered, until scallops are cooked
and vegetables are tender, about 5 minutes.
Heat to boiling. Mix cornstarch and cold water.
Stir cornstarch mixture into boiling mixture;
boil, stirring constantly, until thickened. Remove from heat; let stand 2 to 3 minutes. Stir in
NutraSweet® Spoonful®, serve over rice.
Diabetic Food Exchange: 2 lean meat, 2-1/2
starches, 1 vegetable

Raspberry Swirl Peach Soup

3 pounds peaches, peeled, seeded, sliced
1/3 to 1/2 cup NutraSweet® Spoonful®
1/4 cup NutraSweet® Spoonful®
Mint sprigs
3 cups peach nectar
1 pint fresh or frozen, thawed raspberries
Freshly grated nutmeg
Yield: Makes 6 servings

Process peaches, peach nectar and 1/3 to 1/2
cup NutraSweet® Spoonful® in blender or
food processor until smooth; refrigerate until
chilled. Process raspberries in blender or food
processor until smooth; stain and discard seeds.
Stir 1/4 cup NutraSweet® Spoonful® into raspberry puree; refrigerate until chilled. Spoon
peach mixture into bowls; swirl raspberry
mixture through soup, using 2 to 3 tablespoons
raspberry puree for each bowl. Sprinkle lightly
with nutmeg; garnish with mint. GARNISH (if
desired) 1/2 cup fruit to include mixed berries
(strawberries, raspberries and blackberries).
Per serving: 1/6 recipe
140 calories
1 g protein, 36 g carbohydrates, trace total fat
0 g saturated fat, 0 mg cholesterol
4 g fiber, 9 mg sodium
Diabetic Food Exchange: 2-1/2 fruit

Strawberry-Rhubarb Crisp

12 Ounces fresh or frozen, slightly thawed
unsweetened strawberries, halved (about 2-1/
2 cups)
2 teaspoons grated orange peel
1/4 cup + 1 tablespoon brown sugar, packed
to measure, divided
1 cup quick-cooking oats
2 tablespoons whole-wheat flour
1/4 cup + 2 tablespoons margarine, melted
12 ounces fresh or slightly thawed frozen
rhubarb, sliced (about 2-1/2 cups)
1/4 cup cornstarch
9 packets Sweet One® granulated sugar
substitute, divided
3 tablespoons chopped walnuts
1 teaspoon ground cinnamon
1/2 cup whipped cream (optional)
Yield: Makes 9 servings

Preheat oven to 350 F. Spray 8-inch square
baking dish with nonstick cooking spray; add

strawberries, rhubarb an orange peel and toss. In small bowl, combine cornstarch, 1/4 cup brown sugar and 6 packets Sweet One®; add to fruit and toss to coat. In same bowl, combine oats, walnuts, flour, cinnamon, remaining 1 tablespoon brown sugar and remaining 3 packets Sweet One®; stir in melted margarine until mixture is crumbly. Sprinkle over fruit. Bake 35 to 40 minutes or until topping is browned an rhubarb is tender. Cool before serving. Serve with whipped cream, if desired.

Per serving: 190 calories

Orange Mousse

1 tablespoon + 1-1/2 teaspoons unflavored gelatin
1/3 cup granulated sugar, divided
1/4 cup + 2 tablespoons frozen orange-juice concentrate, thawed
4 large egg whites, at room temperature
1/3 cup heavy cream, whipped
1-1/2 cups evaporated skim milk, divided
4 packets Sweet One®, divided
Juice of 1 lemon
1/4 teaspoon cream of tartar
Orange sections and mint leaves for garnish

In small saucepan, sprinkle gelatin over 3/4 cup milk; let stand 5 minutes to soften gelatin. Over low heat, cook, stirring, until gelatin dissolves completely. Stir in half the sugar; cook, stirring, until sugar dissolves; remove from heat. In a large bowl, stir together remaining milk, orange-juice concentrate, lemon juice, 2 packets Sweet One® and gelatin mixture until well blended. Refrigerate 20 minutes or until mixture mounds slightly when dropped from a spoon. In medium-size bowl with mixer at high speed, beat egg whites, remaining sugar, Sweet One® and cream of tartar until stiff peaks form. In another small bowl with mixer at high speed, beat heavy cream until soft peaks form. Fold egg white an whipped cream into gelatin mixture. Spoon to Garnish with orange sections and mint leaves, if desired.

Per serving: 120 calories (225 calories saved per serving by using this sugar substitute)

Grilled Salmon with Pineapple-Cilantro Sauce

1 medium pineapple peeled, cored, cut into 1" chunks
2 tablespoons lime juice
1/2 to 1 teaspoon minced jalapeno* pepper
1 tablespoon cornstarch
2 to 3 tablespoons NutraSweet® Spoonful® Pepper
3/4 cup unsweetened pineapple juice
2 cloves garlic, minced
2 tablespoons minced cilantro
2 tablespoons cold water
Salt
6 Salmon, halibut, haddock steaks or fillets (about 4 ounces each), grilled

Heat Pineapple, pineapple juice, lime juice, garlic and jalepeno* pepper to boiling in medium saucepan; reduce heat and simmer, uncovered, 5 minutes. Stir in cilantro; heat to boiling. Mix Cornstarch and cold water; stir into boiling mixture. Boil, stirring constantly, until thickened.Removed from heat; cool 2 to 3 minutes. Stir In NutraSweet® Spoonful®; season to taste with salt and pepper. Serve warm sauce over grilled fish. NOTE: Pineapple-Cilantro Sauce is also excellent served with pork and lamb.

Serving Size: Per serving 1/6 recipe - 3 oz. fish fillet
185 calories, 24 g protein
16 g carbohydrate, 3 g total fat
trace saturated fat, 36 mg cholesterol
1 g fiber, 159 mg sodium
Diabetic Food Exchange: 2-1/2 lean meat, 1 fruit

Grilled Loin of Pork with Tart Cherry Sauce

1 boneless pork loin roast (about 4 pounds), fat trimmed
Pepper
1/2 cup orange juice
1 clove garlic, minced
1/8 teaspoon ground allspice

3 tablespoons cornstarch
1 pound fresh or frozen cherries
Salt 1 cup dry red wine
3 tablespoons chopped shallots or onions
1/4 teaspoon minced ginger root
1/8 teaspoon pepper
1/3 cup cold water
1/4 to 1/3 cup NutraSweet® Spoonful®
Makes 12 servings

Lightly Sprinkle Roast with salt and pepper; place on rack in roasting pan. Insert meat thermometer so tip is in center of eat. Roast at 325 degrees until thermometer registers 170 degrees, about 2 hours. Heat wine orange juice, shallots, garlic, ginger root, allspice and 1/8 teaspoon pepper to boiling in medium saucepan; reduce heat to low and simmer, covered, 10 minutes. Heat to Boiling once more. Mix cornstarch and cold water; stir into boiling mixture. Boil, stirring constantly, until thickened. Stir in cherries; cook over low heat 2 to 3 minutes. Remove from heat; cool 2 to 3 minutes. Stir in NutraSweet® Spoonful®. Slice port an arrange on platter; serve with Cherry Sauce. Note: Tart Cherry Sauced is also excellent served with venison or other game.

Serving size: 1/12 recipe (approx. 4 oz. meat)
315 calories, 33 g protein
9 g carbohydrate, 16 g total fat
5 g saturated fat, 90 mg cholesterol
Diabetic Food Exchange: 4 lean meat, 1/2 fat,
1/2 fruit

Breakfast Shake

1/2 cup low-fat frozen yogurt
2 tablespoons frozen orange juice concentrate
2 packets Sweet 'N Low R
3 ice cubes
1/4 cup skim milk
1 tablespoon wheat germ
1/2 teaspoon vanilla

In a blender at medium speed, blend all the ingredients until smooth and frothy. Pour into a glass. Variation: Add 1/2 cup sliced bananas or strawberries; blend as directed.

Serving size: 1-1/2 cups
220 calories, 10 g protein
42 g carbohydrate, 1 g total fat
Diabetic Food Exchange: 1 non-fat milk
exchange, 1 starch/bead exchange, 1 fruit
exchange.

Oatmeal Cake

1 cup boiling water
1/4 cup + 2 tablespoons margarine
6 packets Sweet One® granulated sugar
substitute
1 large egg
1 cup all-purpose flour
1-1/2 teaspoons baking powder
1/4 teaspoon salt
1/4 teaspoon cream of tartar
1 cup rolled oats
1/4 cup granulated sugar
2 tablespoons molasses
1 teaspoon vanilla extract
2 teaspoons ground cinnamon
1 teaspoon baking soda
2 large egg whites, at room temperature
Oatmeal Cake Topping
2 tablespoons margarine
1-1/2 teaspoons molasses
1/4 cup walnuts, chopped
2 tablespoons evaporated skim milk
2 packets Sweet One®
2 tablespoons coconut (optional)

Preheat oven to 325 F Spray 8-inch-square baking dish with nonstick cooking spray; set aside. In large bowl, combine water, rolled oats and 1/4 cup plus 2 tablespoons margarine, egg and vanilla. In small bowl, stir together flour, cinnamon, baking powder, baking soda and salt; stir into oatmeal mixture until well blended. In a large metal bowl with electric mixer at high speed, beat egg whites and cream of tartar until stiff peaks form; fold into batter. Spoon batter into prepared pan. Bake in center of over 25 to 30 minutes or until wooden pick inserted in center comes out clean. Cool on wire rack. Preparing topping: Preheat oven to broil. In small saucepan over medium heat, cook 2 tablespoons margarine, milk, 1-1/2 teaspoons molasses and 2 packets Sweet One® 2 to 3 minutes or until bubbly and slightly thickened. Stir in Walnuts and coconut, if desired. Spread on cake. Broil 3 to 4 inches from heat source 30 seconds or until nuts begin to brown. Cool on wire rack.

Calories 190 per serving

Dessert Fruit Trifle

1 package (18.25 ounces) light yellow cake mix
1-1/3 cups water
3 egg whites
2 cups sliced strawberries
2 to 3 Tbs. NutraSweet® Spoonful®
Milk Custard (see recipe below)
1 cup raspberries
2 nectarines or peaches, sliced
1 medium banana, sliced
1 pint blueberries
Light whipped topping
Makes 12 servings

Prepare Cake Mix according to package directions, using water and egg whites; bake in a 13 x 9-inch baking pan. Cool on wire rack. Cut half the cake into 1-inch cubes (freeze or reserve remaining cake for another use). Process Strawberries in blender or food processor until smooth; stir in NutraSweet® Spoonful®. Layer 1/3 of the cake cubes in bottom of 2 quart glass serving bowl. Spoon 1/3 of the Milk Custard and strawberry puree over cake and top with 1/3 of the raspberries, nectarines, banana and blueberries. Repeat layers 2 times. Refrigerate at least 1 hour before serving. Garnish with whipped topping.

Milk Custard

Makes about 1-1/2 cups
1 cup skim milk
2 eggs
1/4 tsp. ground nutmeg
3 to 4 Tbs. NutraSweet® Spoonful®
2 Tbs. flour

Heat Milk just to boiling in a small saucepan; remove from heat. Mix eggs and flour in small bowl. Slowly stir about 1/4 cup hot milk into egg mixture into milk in saucepan. Cook over low heat stirring constantly, until thickened. Cool until warm; stir in nutmeg and NutraSweet® Spoonful®. Refrigerate until chilled.

Serving Size: 1/12 recipe
175 calories, 4 g protein
35 g carbohydrates, 3 g total fat
(1 g saturated), 36 mg cholesterol, 3 g fiber
178 mg sodium
Diabetic Food Exchange
1/2 skim milk, 1 starch, 1 fruit

Lemon Tea Loaf

1-1/4 cups cake flour
2 Tbs. lemon juice
1 tsp. baking powder
1 Tbs. grated lemon peel
1 tsp. baking soda
1/3 buttermilk
1 large egg
1/2 cup margarine, softened
2 large egg whites
1/4 cup granulated sugar at room temperature
6 packets Sweet One®
1/4 tsp. cream of tartar
granulated sugar substitute

Glaze

1 Tbs. granulated sugar 1 Tbs. water
2 packets Sweet One 2 tsp. lemon juice

In a large bowl with electric mixer at medium speed, beat margarine, 1/4 cup sugar, 6 packets Sweet One, egg, 2 Tbs. lemon juice and lemon peel until well blended. Add flour mixture alternately with buttermilk, beginning and ending with flout an beating until smooth. In large metal bowl with electric mixer at high speed, beat egg whites and cream of tartar until stiff peaks form; fold into batter. Pour batter into prepared loaf pan. Bake 35 to 45 minutes or until wooden pick inserted in center comes out clean. Cool on wire rack 10 minutes. Remove from pan; cool completely on wire rack. Meanwhile, prepare glaze: In small saucepan over medium heat, combine 1 Tbs. sugar, 2 packets Sweet One, water an 2 tsp. lemon juice; bring to a boil. Cook 2 to 3 minutes or until mixture is thick and syrupy. Brush on top of tea loaf.

Per serving (1/2 inch slice) 140 calories

Herb Vinaigrette

1/3 cup Balsamic vinegar
2 Tbs. minced onion or shallots
1 garlic clove, minced
1 tsp. Dijon-style mustard
1 tsp. each dried, crumbled: basil chervil, marjoram and thyme
1/4 tsp. each: salt and pepper
1 packet Sweet N Low®
2/3 cup reduced-sodium chicken broth
1 Tbs. olive oil
Yield: 1 cup (16 servings)

In a small bowl, stir together the vinegar, onion or shallots, garlic, herbs, salt, pepper, and Sweet 'N Low®. Cover refrigerate 24 hours. Strain the mixture, reserving the onion, garlic, and herbs. Whisk the broth and mustard into the vinegar. Whisk in the oil. For a more flavorful dressing, stir 2 teaspoons reserved onion-herb mixture back into the dressing. Refrigerate, covered, up to 1 week. Serve on salads and vegetables. Tip: The reserved onion-herb mixture from the Herb Vinaigrette can be pureed with 3/4 cup nonfat cottage cheese and served as a dip with raw vegetables. Refrigerate at least 1 hour before serving. It makes about 3/4 cup, or six 2-tablespoon servings.

Per serving: (1 tablespoon): 15 calories, 1 g protein, 2 g carbohydrate, 1 g saturated fat, 0 milligrams cholesterol, 10 mgs sodium.

Diabetic exchange: Free exchange.

Southwest Shrimp Dip

1 pound boiled shrimp, peeled and coarsely chopped
2 cups reduced fat sour cream
2 tablespoons mayonnaise (regular or reduced fat)
1 to 2 teaspoons chile powder (to taste)
1/2 teaspoon ground cumin

2 tablespoons finely chopped red Spanish onion (or other sweet salad onion)
2 tablespoons fresh lime juice
1/4 cup chopped cilantro leaves
1 teaspoon brown sugar
Salt to taste
Extra cilantro leaves for garnish

Stir together all ingredients except garnish. Cover and shill for at least 2 hours. Garnish and serve with fat free chips for dipping.

Makes about 4 cups.

Green Onion-Cheese Dip

2 cups lowfat cottage cheese
2 tablespoons mayonnaise (regular or low fat)
1/2 cup coarsely chopped green onions (crisp green tops included)
1/4 cup parsley leaves
1/2 teaspoon hot pepper sauce (or to taste)
1 tablespoon fresh lemon juice

Put all ingredients into the food processor. Pulse on and off until onions and parsley are finely chopped and cheese is smooth.cover and chill for at least one hour. Serve with fat-free chips or crisp dipping vegetables.

Makes about 2 1/2 cups.

Crunchy Vegetable Dip

2 cups reduced fat sour cream (or fat-free plain yogurt)
2 tablespoons mayonnaise (regular or reduced fat)
1/4 cup finely chopped sweet salad onion
1/4 cup finely chopped radishes
1/4 cup finely chopped cucumber (seeded)
1/4 cup finely chopped green bell pepper
2 tablespoons chopped parsley
2 teaspoon sugar
1 teaspoon salt (or to taste)
1/4 teaspoon freshly ground black pepper
1 tablespoon fresh lemon juice

Stir together all of the ingredients

Roasted Onion:

Rub a large, unpeeled yellow onion with oil. Wrap in heavy-duty foil, crimping top to close tightly, Place in a preheated 400 F oven for 1 hour to 1 1/2 hours, depending on size of onion. The will be soft when done. Cool and peel.

Roasted Garlic:

Cut the top off a large, firm head of garlic. The tops of the cloves should be exposed. Place on a square of heavy-duty foil. Drizzle some olive oil over the garlic head and sprinkle with a bit of salt. Tightly close the foil, crimping the top. Place in a preheated 400 F oven for about 30 minutes or until soft. Cool. Gentle pressure on bottom of a roasted clove of garlic should easily push it out of its skin.

Salsa Fresca

1 pint cherry tomatoes
1 teaspoon salt (or to taste)
1/2 cup chopped red Spanish onion or sweet salad onion
1/4 cup fresh lime juice
2 medium fresh jalapenos, seeded and minced
1/4 cup chopped cilantro leaves
1 teaspoon extra-virgin olive oil

Wash tomatoes. Chop in the food processor, pulsing on and off. Remove and add the salt. Fold in the remaining ingredients. Cover and allow to sit at room temperature for 30 minutes for flavors to blend. Serve with fat-free chips or reduced fat tortilla chips.

Roasted Red Pepper Dip

2 red bell peppers
1 teaspoon paprika
1/4 teaspoon cayenne pepper
1 teaspoon salt (or to taste)
1 tablespoon fresh lemon juice
1/4 cup fresh basil leaves.
1 cup reduced fat sour cream
1 tablespoon mayonnaise
Preheat oven to 400 .

Wash peppers. Place on oven rack in the pre-heated oven. Roast, turning occasionally, for 12 to 15 minutes or until skin is charred. Remove to a plastic bag and seal. Set aside until peppers are cool. Remove and peel. Cut open and remove stem, seeds and veins. Place the roasted and prepared peppers in food processor. Add the paprika, cayenne pepper, salt, lemon juice and basil. Process until mixture is pureed. Remove to a bowl. Fold in the sour cream and mayonnaise. Serve with fat-free chips or crisp dipping vegetables.

Makes about 2 cups.

Suggestions for Fresh Vegetables for Dipping:

The following fresh vegetables look and taste best when blanched in a pot of rapidly boiling, salted water and then refreshed in a very cold water. Drain well, pat dry and chill until ready to serve:

Broccoli—florets and peeled and sliced stems—blanch 1 minute
Cauliflower—florets—blanch 1 minute
Asparagus—tender ends—blanch 2 minutes
Green beans—small to medium sized, and trimmed—blanch 2 to 4 minutes (depending on size)
Snow Peas—whole, with strings removed—blanch 30 seconds
Fennel—the bulb, sliced—blanch 1 minute

The following vegetables are best raw, washed, cut into small, easy-to-strips and chilled:

Carrots , Turnips, Zucchini, Yellow Summer Squash, Celery , Jicama

Other interesting additions to the *"Crudite's Platter"*:

Belgian Endive Leaves
Radicchio Leaves
Medium sized white mushrooms, firm and crisp and acidulated with lemon juice
Artichoke Leaves, cooked until tender and chilled
Radishes—Big ones sliced or medium ones whole
Cucumbers—Preferably the European type which don't require peeling and seeding,

The following vegetables are *poor choices* for serving with dips:

Cherry tomatoes— to difficult to eat

Eggplant—not good raw and wrong texture cooked

Wild mushrooms—should never eaten raw

Onions—tend too be strong in flavor, even the sweet salad varieties and the green ones

---

Chocolate Custard

2 cups skim milk

1/4 cup unsweetened cocoa powder

3 packets Sweet One® granulated sugar substitute

1 teaspoon chocolate extract

1/4 cup granulated sugar

2 tablespoons cornstarch

2 large eggs, slightly beaten

Yield: Makes 8 servings

In a medium saucepan, whisk together skim milk, sugar, cocoa powder, cornstarch and Sweet One®. Whisking constantly, cook 6-8 minutes, until mixture boils and thickens. Remove saucepan from heat. Stir 1/4 cup milk mixture into beaten eggs, stirring constantly to avoid curdling. Pour egg mixture back into saucepan and stir in extract. Cook, stirring constantly over low heat 2-3 minutes or until custard thickens. Do not let custard come to a boil. Pour custard into individual dessert cups or a serving bowl and cover with plastic wrap. Refrigerate for at lest two hours before serving.

Per serving: 80 calories, 4 g protein, 2 g fat, 13 g carbohydrate, 55 mg cholesterol, 50 mg sodium

---

Oriental Chicken "A La Microwave"

4 tablespoons white wine, divided

1 large clove garlic, minced

1/2 teaspoon grated lemon peel

1/4 teaspoon ground ginger

4 chicken cutlets (about 1 pound)

1 teaspoon sesame seeds

Chopped green onion and fresh parsley for garnish

1 tablespoon low-sodium soy sauce

1 teaspoon honey

1 packet Sweet 'N Low® granulated sugar substitute; 1/4 teaspoon paprika

Few grains ground black pepper

1 teaspoon cornstarch

Yield: Makes 4 servings

In shallow 1-1/2 quart micro-proof dish, combine 1 tablespoon wine, soy sauce, garlic, honey, lemon peel, Sweet 'N Low, ginger and paprika. add chicken and turn to coat. Cover and refrigerate several hours. To promote even cooking, tuck under any thin ends of chicken. Spoon marinade over chicken. Sprinkle with pepper and sesame seeds. Cover tightly with wax paper. Cook on medium-high power 6 to 8 minutes or just until cooked through, turning dish if chicken appears to be cooking unevenly. Remove chicken to serving dish and keep warm. In glass measuring cup, stir together cornstarch and remaining 3 tablespoons white wine; stir into drippings in dish. Cook, uncovered, on high power 1 to 2 minutes or until sauce thickens slightly. Pour over chicken.

Per serving: 170 calories

Grilled Steak and Vegetable Salad

1-1/2 pounds beef flank steak, fat trimmed, scored

6 medium Italian plum tomatoes, cut into wedges

1 medium green pepper, sliced

1 medium sweet onion, cut into small wedges

4 ears corn, cooked, cut into 1-1/2 inch pieces

Fresh Herb Vinaigrette (recipe follows)

Yield: Makes 6 servings

Grill steak over medium-hot coals to desired degree of doneness, about 20 minutes for medium, turning steak halfway through cooking time. Slice steak, diagonally across grain, into scant 1/4-inch slices. Combine sliced meat and vegetables in shallow serving bowl. Pour dressing over and toss. Serve immediately or refrigerate several hours and serve chilled. Note: If desired, steak can be broiled rather than grilled for the same amount of time.

APPENDIX G
GLOSSARY OF TERMS

Abdominal fat: Fat (adipose tissue) that is centrally distributed between the thorax and pelvis; it induces greater health risk.

Absolute risk: The observed or calculated probability of an event in a population under study, as contrasted with the relative risk.

Addiction: Chronic, relapsing disease, characterized by compulsively seeking and using addictive agents. Neurochemical and molecular changes occuring in the brain are intimatley involved in addiction.

Aerobic exercise: Any activity that allows your body to consistently replenish oxygen to your working muscles. It is performed at a low to moderate intensity and is endurance-oriented by nature. Both fat and glycogen are burned for fuel. Type of physical activity that includes walking, jogging, running, and dancing. Aerobic training improves the efficiency of the aerobic energy-producing systems that can improve cardiorespiratory endurance.

Age-adjusted: Summary measures of rates of morbidity or mortality in a population using statistical procedures to remove the effect of age differences in populations that are being compared. Age is probably the most important and the most common variable in determining the risk of morbidity and mortality.

Allergy: An allergy is a reaction to a foreign substance in which antibodies are produced. Common side effects include runny nose, red eyes and rashes.

Amino acid: Any of a class of 20 molecules that are combined to form proteins in living things. The sequence of amino acids in a protein and hence protein function are determined by the genetic code.

Anaerobic Exercise: Any activity that utilizes oxygen at a faster rate than your body can replenish it in the exercising of muscles. By nature, this type of exercise is usually intense and short in duration. Weightlifting is an example. Glycogen is the primary source of fuel.

Anorexiant: A drug, process, or event that leads to decrease or loss of appetite.

Anthropometric measurements: Measurements of human body height, weight, and size of component parts, including skinfold measurement. Used to study and compare the relative proportions under normal and abnormal conditions.

Aneurysm: Weak or thin spot on an artery wall that has stretched or ballooned out from the wall and filled with blood, or damage to an artery leading to pooling of blood between the layers of the blood vessel walls.

Antihypertensives: Drugs that lower high blood pressure. They act by relaxing blood vessels, which makes blood flow more easily. Examples of antihypertensives include methyldopa (Aldomet) and clonidine hydrochloride (Catapres).

Atherosclerosis: Blood vessel disease characterized by deposits of lipid material on the inside of the walls of large to medium-sized arteries which make the artery walls thick, hard, brittle, and prone to breaking.

Ascorbic acid: Ascorbic acid is one of the active forms of Vitamin C.

Aspartame: Generic name for a non-caloric artificial sweetener that is sold under trade names such as NutraSweet and Equal.

Atherogenic: Causing the formation of plaque in the lining of the arteries.

Barbell: A long bar, usually measuring about six feet in length, that can accommodate weighted plates on each end. The Olympic barbell is the industry standard and weighs 45 pounds.

Basal Metabolic Rate: (BMR); the rate of metabolism (calorie utilization) under resting or basal conditions 14 to 18 hours after eating.

Behavior therapy: Behavior therapy constitutes those strategies, based on learning principles such as reinforcement, that provide tools for overcoming barriers to compliance with dietary therapy and/or increased physical activity.

Bench: An apparatus designed for performing exercises in a seated or lying fashion. Many benches are adjustable so that exercises can be performed at wide array of different angles.

Biliopancreatic diversion: Surgical procedure for weight loss that combines a modest amount of gastric restriction with intestinal malabsorption.

BMI: (Body Mass Index;) calculated by divding body weight in kilograms divided by height in meters squared (wt/ht^2). Utilized as a simple screening device to assess obesity; often referred to as the Quetelet Index. Different from lean mass or percent body fat calculations because it only considers height and weight.

Body composition: The ratio of lean body mass (structural and functional elements in cells, body water, muscle, bone, heart, liver, kidneys, etc.) to body fat (essential and storage) mass. Essential fat is necessary for normal physiological functioning (e.g., nerve conduction). The body's fat reserves are the fat that people need to try to lose.

Bodysculpting: The art of exercising to shape muscles to optimal proportions.

Bran: The fiber-rich part of grain. Bran makes up about 14.5% of the kernel weight. Bran is included in whole wheat flour and can also be purchased separately. The bran contains protein, large quantities of the three major B-vitamins (thiamin, riboflavin and niacin), trace minerals and dietary fiber.

BRL 26830A: An atypical B adrenoreceptor agonist drug that in obese rodents showed an increased metabolic rate and caused a reduction in weight by decreasing body lipid content. It is not approved as a weight loss drug by FDA.

Calorie: The measurement for energy in foods.

Carbohydrates: Nutrient that supplies 4 calories/gram. They may be simple or complex. Simple carbohydrates are called sugars, and complex carbohydrates are called starch and fiber (cellulose). An organic compound—containing carbon, hydrogen, and oxygen—that is formed by photosynthesis in plants. Carbohydrates are heat producing and are classified as monosaccharides, disaccharides, or polysaccharides. (See glycogen).

Cardiovascular disease (CVD): Any abnormal condition characterized by dysfunction of the heart and blood vessels. CVD includes atheroclerosis (especially coronary heart disease, which can lead to heart attacks), cerebrovascular disease (e.g., stroke), and hypertension (high blood pressure).

Carotid endarterectomy: surgery used to remove fatty deposits from the carotid arteries.

Central fat distribution: An index of body fat distribution. Increasing waist circumference is accompanied by increasing frequencies of overt type 2 diabetes, dyslipidemia, hypertension, coronary heart disease, stroke, and early mortality. In the body fat patterns called android type (apple shaped), fat is deposited around the waist and upper abdominal area, and appears most often in men. Abdominal body fat is thought to be associated with rapid mobilization of fatty acids compared to surface fat depots, although it remains a point of contention. If abdominal fat is indeed more active than other fat depots, it would then provide a mechanism by which we could explain (in part) the increase in blood lipid and glucose levels. The latter have been clearly associated with an increased risk for cardiovascular disease hypertension and type 2 diabetes mellitus. The gynocoid type (pear-shaped) of body fat is usually seen in women. The fat is deposited around the hips, thighs, and buttocks, and presumably is used as energy reserve during pregnancy and lactation. (Central fat is the hardest to lose, but causes fewer medical problems than fat elsewhere.)

Child Nutrition (CN) Label: A CN label states a product's contribution to the meal pattern requirements. CN labels are available for eat/meat alternates and fruit juices that contain greater than 50% real fruit juice.

Cholecystectomy: Surgical removal of the gallbladder and gallstones, if present.

Cholecystitis: Inflammation of the gallbladder, caused primarily by gallstones. Gallbladder disease occurs most often in obese women older than 40 years of age.

Cholesterol: A soft, waxy substance manufactured by the body and used in the production of hormones, bile acid, and vitamin D and present in all parts of the body, including the nervous system, muscle, skin, liver, intestines, and heart.

Blood cholesterol circulates in the bloodstream. Dietary cholesterol is found in foods of animal origin. Cholesterol is found only in animal foods, such as meat and cheese.

Circuit Training: A series of exercise machines set up in a sequence to facilitate a sequence of different exercises. The exercises are performed one after the other, each stressing a different muscle group.

Cognitive behavior therapy: A system of psychotherapy based on the premise that distorted or dysfunctional thinking, which influences a person's mood or behavior, is common to all psychosocial problems. The focus of therapy is to identify the distorted thinking and to replace it with more rational, adaptive thoughts and beliefs.

Cognitive rehearsal: A technique used in cognitive behavior therapy. In a weight loss program, for example, individuals first imagine the situation that is causing temptation (such as eating a high fat food), describe the thoughts and feelings that accompany the imagined situation, and make positive self-statements about the situation (e.g., "I am feeling good about choosing a low calorie drink rather than the high fat cheese."). Then the next step is to follow the positive self-statement with an adaptive behavior (such as walking away from the buffet line to chat with a friend). Finally, individuals are encouraged to reward themselves for doing well in a difficult situation, with either positive statements or material rewards, or both. The idea is to rehearse one's thoughts and behaviors prior to experiencing the potentially difficult situation, and to be armed with healthy adaptive responses.

Cognitive restructuring: A method of identifying and replacing fear promoting, irrational beliefs with more realistic and functional ones.

Combination food: Any single serving of food that contains two or more of the required meal components is considered a combination food.

Comorbidity: Two or more diseases or conditions existing together in an individual.

Compound Movement: An exercise that involves two or more joints (and muscle groups) in the performance of the movement. Examples include squats, bench presses and chins.

Component: A food grouped in a certain food category. Milk component, meat/meat alternate component, fruit/vegetable component and the grains/breads component are examples.

Computed tomography (CT) scans: A radiographic technique for direct visualization and quantification of fat that offers high image contrast and clear separation of fat from other soft tissues. CT can estimate total body adipose tissue volume and identify regional, subcutaneous, visceral, and other adipose tissue depots. Radiation exposure, expense, and unavailability restrict the wide spread use of CT.

Complex carbohydrates: Complex carbohydrates are long chains of sugars arranged as starch or fiber.

Confounding: Extraneous variables resulting in outcome effects that obscure or exaggerate the "true" effect of an intervention.

Contraction: The act of shortening a muscle by tightening it.

Coronary heart disease (CHD): Heart disease characterized by narrowing of blood vessels feeding the heart oxygen and nutrients. A decrease in blood supply decreases the heart's ability to function and may cause death of heart muscle (a heart attack). Cholesterol is the causing agent.

Craving: a powerful, often uncontrollable desire.

Cue avoidance: A stimulus control technique often used in weight loss programs in which individuals are asked to reduce their exposure to certain food cues by making a variety of changes in their habits. The rationale is to make it easier on oneself and reduce temptation by reducing contact with food cues. For example, coming home from work and feeling tired is a time when many people reach for the high fat foods if they are available. By not having the high fat foods within reach, one can avoid eating them.

Dexfenfluramine: A serotonin agonist drug used to treat obesity. The drug has been voluntarily withdrawn from the market.

Diabetes: A complex disorder of carbohydrate, fat, and protein metabolism that is primarily a result of relative or complete lack of insulin secretion by the beta cells of the pancreas, or, a result of defects of the insulin receptors.

Diastolic blood pressure: The minimum pressure that remains within the artery when the heart is relaxed.

Diethylproprion: An appetite suppressant prescribed in the treatment of obesity.

Disaccharide: A sugar made made up of two or more sugars. Sucrose (table sugar) is an example. It contains two simple sugars, glucose and fructose.

Dopamine: A catecholamine neurotransmitter that is found primarily in the basal ganglia of the central nervous system. Major functions include the peripheral inhibition and excitation of certain muscles; cardiac excitation; and metabolic, endocrine and central nervous system actions (pleasure).

Dual energy X-ray absortiometry (DEXA): A method used to estimate total body fat and percent of body fat. Potential disadvantages include whole body radiation and the long time required for scanning while the subject lies on a hard table.

Dyslipidemia: Disorders in the lipoprotein metabolism; classified as gypercholesterolemia, h y p e r t r i g l y c e r i d e m i a , c o m b i n e d hyperlipidemia, and low levels of high-density lipoprotein (HDL) cholesterol. All of the dyslipidemias can be primary or secondary. Both elevated levels of low-density lipoprotein (LDL) cholesterol and low levels of HDL cholesterol predispose to premature atherosclerosis.

Efficacy: Extent to which a specific intervention, procedure, regimen, or service produces a beneficial result under ideal conditions. Ideally, the determination of efficacy is based on the results of a randomized control trial.

Empty calorie food: This is a popular term describing foods that have only minimal nutrient value and many calories. Alcohol is an example. One gram of alcohol contains 7 calories.

Energy balance: Energy is the capacity of a body or a physical system for doing work. Energy balance is the state in which the total energy intake equals total energy needs.

Endorphin: A substance produced in the brain or nervous system that stops pain naturally.

Endosperm: The endosperm is the bulk of the edible starchy part of a grain. Endosperm makes up 83 percent of the kernel weight and is the source of white flour. The endosperm contains the greatest share of protein, carbohydrate and iron as well as B-vitamins.

Energy deficit: A state in which total energy intake is less than total energy need.

Enrichment: Enrichment refers to the addition of nutrients to a food. The term may specifically indicate that thiamin, riboflavin, niacin and iron were added to refined grains or bread products.

Enzymes: Enzymes are made of proteins and are catalysts for many chemical reactions in the body.

Epidemiology: Scientific discipline that studies the factors determining the causes, frequency, and distribution of diseases in a community or given population.

Ephedrine: A sympathomimetic drug that raises body heat in laboratory animals and humans. Animal studies show that it may reduce fat content and, therefore, body weight by mechanisms that probably involve increased expenditure of energy and reduced food intake.

Estrogen: The female hormone.

Extreme obesity: A body mass index ≥ 40.

Exercise: Movement of the body designed to improve its physical condition. The goals of an exercise program are to improve physical conditioning, muscle strength, flexibility, well-being, and function. Exercise can also produce fat loss.

EZ-curl bar: A specially configured barbell that has curves in the middle used to alleviate strain on the wrists.

Fat: Fat is an efficient storage form of energy.

Fenfluramine: A serotonin agonist drug used in the treatment of obesity. FDA approval has been withdrawn.

Fiber: Fiber is the non-nutrient component of foods that aids in digestion and helps prevent constipation.

Fibric Acid Derivatives: One type of cholesterol-lowering drug. It includes gemfibrozil. The fibric acids lower triglycerides and raise HDLs.

Fibrinogen: A plasma protein that is converted into fibrin by thrombin in the presence of calcium ions. Fibrin is responsible for the semisolid character of a blood clot.

Fluoxetine: An antidepressant drug (Prozac) used to promote weight loss whose action is mediated by highly specific inhibition of serotonin reuptake into presynaptic neurons. Serotonin acts in the brain to alter feeding and satiety by decreasing carbohydrate intake, resulting in weight reduction.

Food and Nutrition Service (FNS): The Food and Nutrition Service is the Federal administering agency for the Child and Adult Care Food Program. It is a division of the United States Department of Agriculture.

Fortification: Fortification refers to the addition of nutrients to a food, often not originally present, and/or added in amounts greater than might be found there naturally.

Framingham Heart Study: Study begun in 1948 to identify constitutional, environmental, and behavioral influences on the development of cardiovascular disease. Framingham data show that increased relative weight and central obesity are associated with elevated levels of risk factors (e.g., cholesterol, blood pressure, blood glucose, uric acid), increased incidence of cardiovascular disease, and increased death rates for all causes combined.

Gallstones: Constituents in the gallbladder that are not reabsorbed, including bile salts and lipid substances such as cholesterol that become highly concentrated. They can cause severe pain (obstruction and cramps) as they move into the common bile duct. Risk factors for cholesterol gallstone formation include female gender, weight gain, overweight, high energy intake, ethnic factors (Pima Indians and Scandinavians), use of certain drugs (clofibrate, estrogens, and bile acid sequestrants), and presence of gastrointestinal disease. Gallstones sometimes develop during dieting for weight reduction. There is an increased risk for gallstones and acute gallbladder disease during severe caloric restriction.

Gastric banding: Surgery to limit the amount of food the stomach can hold by closing part of it off. A band made of special material is placed around the stomach near its upper end, creating a small pouch and a narrow passage into the larger remainder of the stomach. The small outlet delays the emptying of food from the pouch and causes a feeling of fullness.

Gastric bubble/balloon: A free-floating intragastric balloon used in the treatment of obesity.

Gastric bypass: A surgical procedure that combines the creation of small stomach pouches to restrict food intake and the construction of bypasses of the duodenum and other segments of the small intestine to cause food malabsorption. Patients generally lose two thirds of their excess weight after 2 years.

Gastric exclusion: Same as gastric partitioning and Rouxen Y bypass. A small stomach pouch is created by stapling or by vertical banding to restrict food intake. A Y-shaped section of the small intestine is attached to the pouch to allow food to bypass the duodenum as well as the firstportion of the jejunum.

Gastric partitioning: See gastric exclusion.

Gastroplasty: See also jejuno-ileostomy. A surgical procedure that limits the amount of food the stomach can hold by closing off part of the stomach. Food intake is restricted by creating a small pouch at the top of the stomach where the food enters from the esophagus. The pouch initially holds about 1 ounce of food and expands to 2-3 ounces with time. The pouch's lower outlet usually has a diameter of about 1/4 inch. The small outlet delays the emptying of food from the pouch and causes a feeling of fullness.

Gene therapy: Treatment that alters genes (the basic units of heredity found in all cells in the body). Addition of a functional gene or group of genes to a cell by gene insertion to correct an hereditary disease.

Genotype: The entire genetic makeup of an individual. The fundamental constitution of an organism in terms of its hereditary factors. A group of organisms in which each has the same hereditary characteristics.

Germ: The germ is the nutrient rich inner part of a grain. It makes up about 2.5 percent of the kernel weight. The germ is the embryo or sprouting section of the seed. It is often separated from flour during milling because the fat content (10%) limits flour's shelf-life. The germ contains protein, B-vitamins and trace minerals. Germ can be purchased separately and is part of whole wheat flour.

Glucose: Glucose is a single sugar used in both plants and animals as a quick energy source. Glucose is known as blood sugar.

Glucose tolerance: The power of the normal liver to absorb and store large quantities of glucose as glycogen and the effectiveness of intestinal absorption of glucose. The glucose tolerance test is a metabolic test of carbohydrate tolerance that measures active insulin, a hepatic function based on the ability of the liver to absorb glucose. The test consists of ingesting 100 grams of glucose into a fasting stomach; blood sugar should return to normal in 2 to 2 1/2 hours after ingestion.

Hemoglobin A1c: One of the fractions of glycosylated hemoglobin A. Glycosylated hemoglobin is formed when linkages of glucose and related monosaccharides bind to hemoglobin A and its concentration represents the average blood glucose level over the previous month. HbA1C levels are used as a measure of long-term control of plasma glucose (normal, 4 to 6 percent). In controlled diabetes mellitus, the concentration of glycosylated hemoglobin A is within the normal range, but in uncontrolled cases the level may be 3 to 4 times the normal concentration. Generally, complications are substantially lower among patients with HbA1C levels of 7 percent or less than in patients with HbA1C levels of 9 percent or more.

Hemorrhagic stroke: A disorder involving bleeding within ischemic brain tissue. Hemorrhagic stroke occurs when blood vessels that are damaged or dead from lack of blood supply (infarcted), located within an area of infarcted brain tissue, rupture and transform an "ischemic" stroke into a hemorrhagic stroke. Ischemia is inadequate tissue oxygenation caused by reduced blood flow; infarction is tissue death resulting from ischemia. Bleeding irritates the brain tissues, causing swelling (cerebral edema). Blood collects into a mass (hematoma). Both swelling and hematoma will compress and displace brain tissue.

Heritability: The proportion of observed variation in a particular trait that can be attributed to inherited genetic factors in contrast to environmental ones.

High-density lipoproteins (HDL): Lipoproteins that contain a small amount of cholesterol and carry cholesterol away from body cells and tissues to the liver for excretion from the body.

Low-level HDL increases the risk of heart disease, so the higher the HDL level, the better. The HDL component normally contains 20 to 30 percent of total cholesterol, and HDL levels are inversely correlated with coronary heart disease risk.

Hirsutism: Presence of excessive body and facial hair, especially in women; may be present in normal adults as an expression of an ethnic characteristic or may develop in children or adults as the result of an endocrine disorder. *Apert's hirsutism* is caused by a virilizing disorder of adrenocortical origin. Constitutional hirsutism is mild-to-moderate hirsutism present in individuals exhibiting otherwise normal endocrine and reproductive functions; it appears to be an inheritable form of hirsutism and commonly is an expression of an ethnic characteristic. Idiopathic hirsutism is of uncertain origin in women, who may exhibit menstrual abnormalities and sterility. Some authorities believe the hirsutism reflects hypersecretion of adrenocortical androgens. Seen often in PolyCystic Ovary Syndrome.

Hypercholesterolemia (high blood cholesterol): Cholesterol is the most abundant steroid in animal tissues, especially in bile and gallstones. The relationship between the intake of cholesterol and its manufacture by the body to its utilization, sequestration, or excretion from the body is called the cholesterol balance. When cholesterol accumulates, the balance is positive; when it declines, the balance is negative. In 1993, the NHLBI National Cholesterol Education Program (NCEP) Expert Panel on Detection, Evaluation, and Treatment of High Blood Cholesterol in Adults issued an updated set of recommendations for monitoring and treatment of blood cholesterol levels. The NCEP guide-lines recommended that total cholesterol levels and subfractions of high-density lipoprotein (HDL) cholesterol be measured beginning at age 20 in all adults, with subsequent periodic screenings as needed. Even in the group of patients at lowest risk for coronary heart disease (total cholesterol <200 mg/dL and HDL >35 mg/dL), the NCEP recommended that rescreening take place at least once every 5 years or upon physical examination.

Hypertension: High blood pressure (i.e., abnormally high blood pressure tension involving systolic and/or diastolic levels). The Sixth Report of the Joint National Committee on Prevention, Detection, Evaluation, and Treatment of High Blood Pressure defines hypertension as a systolic blood pressure of 140 mm Hg or greater, a diastolic blood pressure of 90 mm Hg or greater, or taking hypertensive medication. The cause may be adrenal, benign, essential, Goldblatt's, idiopathic, malignant PATE, portal, postpartum, primary, pulmonary, renal or renovascular.

Hypertriglyceridemia: An excess of triglycerides in the blood that is an autosomal dominant disorder with the phenotype of hyperlipoproteinemia, type IV. The National Cholesterol Education Program defines a high level of triglycerides as being between 400 and 1,000 mg/dL.

Hypoglycemia: Condition where the blood sugar is lower than normal. A much more dangerous condition than high blood sugar, and should be avoided or treated rapidly.

Incidence: The rate at which a certain event occurs (i.e., the number of new cases of a specific disease occurring during a certain period).

Insulin: Insulin is a hormone secreted by the pancreas in response to rising blood glucose levels; it assists cells in drawing glucose from the blood. Insulin also promotes the storage of fat and blocks the utilization of fat as fuel. It acts on the liver to produce more of the bad cholesterol and less of the good. Insulin triggers hunger.

Insulin resistance: A partial blocking of the effect of insulin. Insulin resistance typically results in high, sustained blood insulin levels.

Ischemic stroke: A condition in which the blood supply to part of the brain is cut off. Also called "plug-type" strokes. Blocked arteries starve areas of the brain controlling sight, speech, sensation, and movement so that these functions are partially or completely lost. Ischemic stroke is the most common type of stroke, accounting for 80 percent of all strokes. Most ischemic strokes are caused by a blood clot called a thrombus, which blocks blood flow in the arteries feeding the brain, usually the carotid artery in the neck, the major vessel bringing blood to the brain. When it becomes blocked, the risk of stroke is very high.

Isometrics: Isometric exercises are exercises that cause a muscle to contract and do work while joints do not move, for example, pushing against a wall.

Jejuno-ileostomy: See gastroplasty.

J-shaped relationship: The relationship between body weight and mortality.

Ketone: breakdown product of fat that accumulates in the blood as a result of inadequate insulin or inadequate calorie intake.

Lactase: Lactase is an enzyme that splits lactose into digestible parts.

Lactose: Lactose is a disaccharide composed of glucose and galactose. Lactose is known as "milk sugar."

Lactose intolerance: Lactose intolerance is the inability to digest lactose, due to a lack of the enzyme, lactase.

Legumes: Legumes are plants of the bean and pea family that are rich in protein and fiber.

Linkage analysis: A gene hunting technique that traces patterns of heredity in large, high-risk families, in an attempt to locate a disease causing gene mutation by identifying traits that are coinherited with it.

Lipid: Lipids are the family of compounds that include triglycerides (fats and oils), phospholipids and sterols.

Lipoprotein: Protein-coated packages that carry fat and cholesterol throughout the bloodstream. There are four general classes: high-density, low-density, very low-density, and chylomicrons.

Locus/loci: A general anatomical term for a site in the body or the position of a gene on a chromosome.

Longitudinal study: Also referred to as a "cohort study" or "prospective study"; the analytic method of epidemiologic study in which subsets of a defined population can be identified who are, have been, or in the future may be exposed or not exposed, or exposed in different degrees, to a factor or factors hypothesized to influence the probability of occurrence of a given disease or other outcome. The main feature of this type of study is to observe large numbers of subjects over an extended time, with comparisons of incidence rates in groups that differ in exposure levels.

Low-calorie diet (LCD): Caloric restriction of about 800 to 1,500 calories (approximately 12 to 15 kcal/kg of body weight) per day.

Low-density lipoprotein (LDL): Lipoprotein contains most of the cholesterol in the blood. LDL carries cholesterol to the tissues of the body, including the arteries. A high level of LDL increases the risk of heart disease. LDL typically contains 60 to 70 percent of the total serum cholesterol and both are directly correlated with CHD risk.

Lower-fat diet: An eating plan in which 30 percent or less of the day's total calories are from fat.

Lymphatic system: The tissues and organs, including the bone marrow, spleen, thymus, and lymph nodes, that produce and store cells that fight infection and disease. This system also has channels that carry lymph.

Macronutrients: Nutrients in the diet that are the key sources of energy, namely protein, fat, and carbohydrates.

Magnetic resonance imaging (MRI): Magnetic resonance imaging uses radio frequency waves to provide direct visualization and quantification of fat. The sharp image contrast of MRI allows clear separation of adipose tissue from surrounding nonlipid structures. Essentially the same information provided by CT is available from MRI, including total body and regional adipose tissue, subcutaneous adipose, and estimates of various visceral adipose tissue components. The advantage of MRI is its lack of ionizing radiation and hence its presumed safety in children, younger adults, and pregnant women. The minimal present use of MRI can be attributed to the expense, limited access to instrumentation, and long scanning time.

Menopause: The cessation of menstruation in the human female, which begins at about the age of 50.

Meta-analysis: Process of using statistical methods to combine the results of different studies. A frequent application is pooling the results from a set of randomized controlled trials, none of which alone is powerful enough to demonstrate statistical significance.

Midaxillary line: An imaginary vertical line that passes midway between the anterior and posterior axillary (armpit) folds.

Milligram (mg): A unit of weight equal to one thousandth of a gram.
There are about 28,350 mg in 1 ounce. Dietary cholesterol is measured in milligrams.

Mitochondria: The energy producing organelles of the cell.

Monosaccharide: A monosaccharide is a single unit sugar; i.e., glucose as opposed to a disaccharide: sucrose (table sugar).

Monounsaturated fat: An unsaturated fat that is found primarily in plant foods, including olive and canola oils.

Muscle: Tissue that can contract, producing movement or force. There are three types of muscle: striated muscle, attached to bones; smooth muscle, found in such tissues as the stomach and blood vessels; and cardiac muscle, which forms the walls of the heart.

Muscle Definition: The absence of fat in the presence of well developed muscle.

Myocardial infarction (MI): Partial heart muscle death resulting from an interruption of the blood supply to the area; it is almost always caused by atherosclerosis of the coronary arteries, upon which coronary blood clot is usually superimposed.

Nicontinic Acid: A cholesterol lowering medicine that reduces total and LDL-cholesterol and triglyceride levels and also raises HDL-cholesterol levels. This is the same substance as Niacin or vitamin B1, but in doses that lower cholesterol, used with a doctor's supervision.

Nutrients: Nutrients are components of food that help nourish the body. They include carbohydrates, fats, proteins, vitamins, minerals, and water.

Obesity: The condition of having an abnormally high proportion of body fat. Defined as a body mass index (BMI) of greater than or equal to 30. Subjects are generally classified as obese when body fat content exceeds 30 percent in women and 25 percent in men.

Observational study: An epidemiologic study that does not involve any intervention, experimental or otherwise. Such a study may be one in which nature is allowed to take its course, with changes in one characteristic being studied in relation to changes in other characteristics. Analytical epidemiologic methods, such as case control and cohort study designs, are properly called observational epidemiology because the investigator is observing without intervention other than to record, classify, count, and statistically analyze results.

Oils: Oils are lipids that are liquid at room temperature. Oils are unsaturated fats.

Orlistat: (Xenical); a lipase inhibitor used for weight loss. Lipase is an enzyme found in the bowel that assists in lipid absorption by the body. Orlistat blocks this enzyme, reducing the amount of fat the body absorbs by about 30 percent. It is known colloquially as a "fat blocker." Because more oily fat is left in the bowel to be excreted, orlistat can cause an oily anal leakage and fecal incontinence. Orlistat may not be suitable for people with bowel conditions such as irritable bowel syndrome or Crohn's disease.

Osteoarthritis: Noninflammatory degenerative joint disease occurring chiefly in older persons, characterized by degeneration of the articular cartilage, hypertrophy of bone at the margins, and changes in the synovial membrane. It is accompanied by pain and stiffness.

Osteoporosis: Osteoporosis is known as "adult bone loss." It is a disease in which bones become porous and brittle.

Overweight: An excess of body weight but not necessarily body fat; a body mass index of 25 to 29.9 kg/m2.

Polysystic Ovary Syndrome: (PCOS) female disorder characterized by excess body hair, obesity, menstral irregularity, and infertility associated with enlarged sclerocystic ovaries.

Peripheral regions: Other regions of the body besides the abdominal region (i.e., the gluteal-femoral area).

Pharmacotherapy: A regimen of using medications to manage a disease process; in this case obesity.

Phenotype: The entire physical, biochemical, and physiological makeup of an individual as determined by his or her genes and by the environment in the broad sense.

Phentermine: An distant cousin to amphetimine used to decrease appetite and increase BMR. Administered orally as a complex with an ion-exchange resin to produce a sustained action.

Plaque: Fatty cholesterol deposits found along the inside of artery walls that lead to atherosclerosis and stenosis of the arteries.

Potassium: Vital element in the body. Potassium supplements help prevent and treat potassium deficiency in people taking diuretics.

Polysaccharide: A carbohydrate formed by covalent bonding of numerous monosaccharides; i.e., glycogen and starch.

Polyunsaturated fat: An unsaturated fat found in greatest amounts in foods derived from plants, including safflower, sunflower, corn, and soybean oils.

Postprandial plasma blood glucose: Glucose levels after eating a meal.

Prevalence: The number of events, e.g., instances of a given disease or other condition, in a given population at a designated time. When used without qualification, the term usually refers to the situation at specific point in time (point prevalence). Prevalence is a number not a rate.

Prognosis: The probable outcome or course of a disease; the chance of recovery.

Prospective study: An epidemiologic study in which a group of individuals (a cohort), all free of a particular disease and varying in their exposure to a possible risk factor, is followed over a specific amount of time to determine the incidence rates of the disease in the exposed and unexposed groups.

Protein: A class of compounds composed of linked amino acids that contain carbon, hydrogen, nitrogen, oxygen, and sometimes other atoms in specific configurations.

Randomization: Also called random allocation; Is allocation of individuals to groups, e.g., for experimental and control regimens, by chance. Within the limits of chance variation, random allocation should make the control and experimental groups similar at the start of an investigation and ensure that personal judgment and prejudices of the investigator do not influence allocation.

Randomized clinical trial (RCT): An epidemiologic experiment in which subjects in a population are randomly allocated into groups, usually called study and control groups, to receive or not to receive an experimental prevention or therapeutic product, maneuver, or intervention. The results are assessed by rigorous comparison of rates of disease, death recovery, or other appropriate outcome in the study and control groups, respectively. RCTs are generally regarded as the most scientifically rigorous method of hypothesis testing available in epidemiology.

Recessive gene: A gene that is phenotypically expressed only when homozygous.

Recommended Dietary Allowance (RDA): RDAs are the nutrient intakes suggested by the Food and Nutrition Board (FNB) of the National Academy of Sciences/National Research Council for the maintenance of health in people in the U.S.

Refractory obesity: Obesity that is resistant to treatment.

Refined grains: Refined grains have the coarse parts of the kernel removed. They are often enriched.

Relative risk: The ratio of the incidence rate of a disease among individuals exposed to a specific risk factor to the incidence rate among unexposed individuals; synonymous with risk ratio. Alternatively, the ratio of the cumulative incidence rate in the exposed to the cumulative incidence rate in the unexposed (cumulative incidence ratio). The term relative risk has also been used synonymously with odds ratio. This is because the odds ratio and relative risk approach each other if the disease is rare (<5 percent of population) and the number of subjects is large.

Risk: The probability that an event will occur. Also, a nontechnical term encompassing a variety of measures of the probability of a generally unfavorable outcome.

Risk Factor: A habit, trait, or condition in a person that is associated with an increased chance (or risk) for a disease.

Roughage: Roughage is the rough part of foods that is indigestible. It aids in digestion and preventing constipation.

Roux-en-Y bypass: See gastric exclusion; the most common gastric bypass procedure.

Saturated fat: A type of fat found in greatest amounts in foods from animals, such as fatty cuts of meat, poultry with the skin, whole-milk dairy products, lard, and in some vegetable oils, including coconut, palm kernel, and palm oils. Saturated fat raises blood cholesterol more than anything else eaten.

Secular trends: A relatively long-term trend in a community or country.

Serotonin: A monoamine vasoconstrictor, found in various animals, in bacteria, and in many plants. In humans, it is synthesized in the intestinal chro-maffin cells or in the central or peripheral neurons and is found in high concentrations in many body tissues, including the intestinal mucosa, pineal body, and central nervous system. Produced enzymatically from tryptophan by hydroxylation and decarboxylation, serotonin has many physiologic properties (e.g., inhibits gastric secretion, stimulates smooth muscle, serves as central neurotransmitter, and is a precursor of melatonin).

Serving size or portion: The portion size is described by the weight, measure or number of pieces or slices. The serving sizes specified in the meal patterns must be provided to meet the meal pattern requirements.

Sibutramine: A drug used for the management of obesity that helps reduce food intake and is indicated for weight loss and maintenance of weight loss when used in conjunction with a reduced calorie diet. It works to suppress the appetite primarily by inhibiting the reuptake of the neurotransmitters norepinephrine and serotonin. Side effects include dry mouth, headache, constipation, insomnia, and a slight increase in average blood pressure. In some patients it causes a blood pressure increase.

Sleep apnea: A serious, potentially life-threatening breathing disorder characterized by repeated cessation of breathing due to either collapse of the upper airway during sleep or absence of respiratory effort.

Social pressure: A strategy used in behavior therapy in which individuals are told that they possess the basic self-control ability to lose weight, but that coming to group meetings will strengthen their abilities. The group is asked to listen and give advice, similar to the way many self-help groups, based on social support, operate.

Starch: Starch is a plant polysaccharide composed of glucose. Starch is found in breads, potatoes, and pasta products.

Statins: One type of cholesterol-lowering drug that includes lovastatin, pravastatin, and simvastatin. These drugs lower LDL levels by limiting the amount of cholesterol the body can make.

Stress management: A set of techniques used to help an individual cope more effectively with difficult situations in order to feel better emotionally, improve behavioral skills, and often to enhance feelings of control. Stress management may include relaxation exercises, assertiveness training, cognitive restructuring, time management, and social support. It can be delivered either on a one-to-one basis or in a group format.

Strengthening exercises: Exercises that build stronger muscles, for example, exercises that require movement against a force (weight lifting or isometric exercises).

Surgical procedures: See jejuno-ileostomy, gastroplasty, gastric bypass, gastric artitioning, gastric exclusion, Roux-en-Y bypass and gastric bubble.

Symmetry: The way in which muscle groups compliment one another, creating a proportional physique.

Systolic blood pressure: The maximum pressure in the arterial system produced as the heart contracts and blood begins to flow.

Testosterone: A hormone that is responsible for promoting muscle mass. It is commonly referred to as the male hormone although both men and women produce it.

Tofu: Tofu is a curd made from soybeans, rich in protein and calcium. Tofu is used in many Asian and vegetarian dishes in place of meat.

Tolerance: a condition that occurs with repeated drug use in which higher doses of a drug are required to produce the same effect as experienced initially. Tolerance does not cause addiction, but is a component of it.

Total fat: The sum of the saturated, monounsaturated, and polyunsaturated fats present in food. All foods have a varying mix of these three types.

Total serum cholesterol: Combined measurement of a person's high-density lipoprotein (HDL) and low-density lipoprotein (LDL).

Toxic: Temporary or permanent drug effects that are detrimental to the functioning of an organ or group of organs.

Triglyceride: A lipid carried through the blood stream to tissues. Most of the body's fat tissue is in the form of triglycerides, stored for use as energy. Triglycerides are obtained from fat in foods and made from unused energy sugar.

Type I diabetes: A disease characterized by high levels of blood glucose resulting from defects in insulin secretion, insulin action, or both. Autoimmune, genetic, and environmental factors are involved in the development of type I diabetes. Formerly called Insulin dependent diabetes mellitus

Type 2 diabetes: Usually characterized by a gradual onset with minimal or no symptoms of metabolic disturbance and no requirement for exogenous insulin. The peak age of onset is rapidly declining to the early 40's. Obesity and possibly a genetic factor are usually present.

Unsaturated fat: A type of fat that is usually liquid at refrigerator temperature. Monounsaturate fat and polyunsaturated fat are two kinds of unsaturated fat. When used in place of saturated fat, monunsaturated and polyunsaturated fats help to lower blood cholesterol levels.

Validity: The degree to which the inferences drawn from study results, especially generalization extending beyond the study sample, are warranted when account is taken of the study methods, the representativeness of the study sample, and the nature of the population from which it is drawn.

Vegetable Protein Products (VPP): Vegetable protein products are food components which may be used to substitute, in part, for meat, poultry, or seafood in some cases.

Vertical banded gastroplasty: A surgical treatment for extreme obesity; an operation on the stomach that involves constructing a small pouch in the stomach that empties through a narrow opening into the distal stomach and duodenum.

Very low-calorie diet (VLCD): The VLCD of 800 (approximately 6-10 kcal/kg body weight) or fewer calories per day is conducted under physician supervision and monitoring and is restricted to severely obese persons. VCLD diets are not usually considered effective or safe over the long term.

Very low-density lipoprotein (VLDL): The lipoprotein particles that initially leave the liver, carrying cholesterol and lipid. VLDLs contain 10 to 15 percent of the total serum cholesterol along with most of the triglycerides in the fasting serum; VLDLs are precursors of LDL, and some forms of VLDL, particularly VLDL remnants, appear to be atherogenic.

Visceral fat: One of the three compartments of abdominal fat. Retroperitoneal and subcutaneous are the other two compartments.

VO 2 max: Maximal oxygen uptake is known as VO 2 max and is the maximal capacity for oxygen consumption by the body during maximal exertion; used as an indicator of cardiorespiratory fitness.

Waist circumference: To define the level at which the waist circumference is measured, a bony landmark is first located and marked. The subject stands, and the technician, positioned to the right of the subject, palpates the upper hip bone to locate the right ileum. Just above the uppermost lateral border of the right ileum, a horizontal mark is drawn and then crossed with a vertical mark on the midaxillary line. The measuring tape is then placed around the trunk, at the level of the mark on the right side, making sure that it is on a level horizontal plane on all sides. The tape is then tightened slightly without compressing the skin and underlying subcutaneous tissues. The measure is recorded in centimeters to the nearest millimeter.

Waist-hip-ratio (WHR): The ratio of a person's waist circumference to hip circumference. WHR looks at the relationship between the differences in the measurements of waist and hips. Most people store body fat in two distinct ways, often called the "apple" and "pear" shapes, either the middle (apple) or the hips (pear). For most people, carrying extra weight around the middle increases health risks more than carrying extra weight around the hips or thighs. Overall obesity, however, is still of greater risk than body fat storage locations or WHR. A WHR ≥ 1.0 is in the danger zone, with risks of heart disease and other ailments connected with being overweight. For men, a ratio of .90 or less is considered safe, and for women .80 or less.

Whole grain flours and cereals: Products made from whole grains containing the bran, germ and endosperm of the whole kernel of grain.

Yohimbine: An alkaloid that possesses adrenergic-blocking properties and is used in rteriosclerosis and angina pectoris, formerly used as a local anesthetic and mydriatic and for its purported aphrodisiac properties.

Xenical: See Orlistat.

INDEX